NATURAL PET CARE

NATURAL
PET CARE

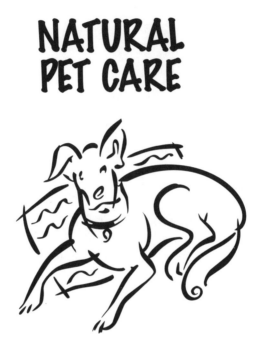

GARY NULL

SEVEN STORIES PRESS

New York/London/Sydney/Toronto

ACKNOWLEDGMENT

The author wishes to thank the following people for their help in producing this book:

Editing: Vicki Riba Koestler, Lois Zinn, Sloane Seale, Dominga Rosalita Wilson, Kim Coombs

Research: Jenny Barbosa, Matt Brown

Expert review: Dr. Robert S. Goldstein, Dr. Nancy Scanlan, Alicia McWatters

★   ★   ★

Seven Stories Press
140 Watts Street
New York, NY 10013
www.sevenstories.com

In Canada: Hushion House, 36 Northline Road, Toronto, Ontario M4B 3E2

In the U.K.: Turnaround Publisher Services Ltd., Unit 3, Olympia Trading Estate, Coburg Road, Wood Green, London N22 6TZ

In Australia: Tower Books, 9/19 Rodborough Road, Frenchs Forest NSW 2086

Library of Congress Cataloging-in-Publication Data
Null, Gary.
    Natural pet care / Gary Null.— 1st ed.
      p.   cm.
    ISBN 1-58322-074-7 (pbk.)
        1.   Pets—Health. 2. Pets—Nutrition. 3. Pets—Diseases—
        Alternative treatment. I. Title.
SF413.N86 2001
636.088'7—dc21   00-050951

9 8 7 6 5 4 3 2 1

College professors may order examination copies of Seven Stories Press titles for a free six-month trial period. To order, visit www.sevenstories.com/textbook, or fax on school letter

Book design by Cindy
Printed in the U.S.A.

TABLE OF CONTENTS

INTRODUCTION

If you're like me, you can't imagine living without pets. I have always had them. Over the course of my life, from early childhood on, I've had every kind of pet you can think of. As an adult, owning a farm in upstate New York, a ranch in Texas, and then a ranch in Florida, I've had pets ranging from buffalo to Scottish long-haired cattle, to elk, foxes, coatimundi, anteaters, ring-tailed lemurs, horses, goats, chickens, peacocks, cows, cats, dogs, and exotic fish. I've learned a great deal in these many years about how to help these animals live long and healthy lives. That knowledge is what I now want to share with you.

And I know that there are many people who are eager to put such knowledge to use. Right now, there are more pets in America than people, which means that many people have more than one pet. And many count their pets among the most beloved members of their family. These people are willing to go the extra mile for their cherished animal companions. In fact, people will frequently do things for their pets that they would not do for themselves, as I've discovered after a long career of trying to educate the public about how to prevent or reverse sickness using natural means, and discovering that despite a vast supply of resources, many folks will frequently not take beneficial measures for themselves, either because they think it's too much trouble, or even, deep down, because they think they don't deserve it. But for their pets, these same people will do the right thing. While it doesn't make any sense, on the pet side of the equation it's no mystery why people are wildly devoted to their animals.

Pets are the ones, after all, that provide us with unconditional love, joy, comfort, and an emotional vulnerability and warmth that are not easily obtained from other humans, at least not adult humans. Indeed, pets are like children in these respects, but they're like children who never grow up and go out into the world, so that they always need us to feed them, give them shelter, and give them warmth. And unlike humans, who are not always grateful for the energy that we put out, pets are filled with unlimited amounts of love for us. If you're having a rough day, if you've been around someone who may have been insensitive, unkind, or thoughtless, you can always bet that when you open the door, your pet will be glad to see you. There will be a wagging tail, the chatter of little bird voices, the rapid movement in the water of fish, a purring sound, a brush against your leg to make a connection. Suddenly you're needed, appreciated, loved for who you are, not for what you've achieved or for your income level.

There's a bond that's created with pets that is deep, meaningful, even spiritual. One of the first things that pet owners ask others with dogs or cats is, "Where do your animals sleep?" And with a lot of people it's in bed, of course. There has to be a real feeling of closeness when we allow something or someone to be with us during our most vulnerable time, our sleep. To me this illustrates the trust and love that we share with these creatures.

Most pets, with the exception of some birds and horses, have a short lifespan. The irony is that the one we care so much about we know, in all probability, will die before we do. So there's a great sense of the preciousness of the moments we spend with our animals. Staying bonded with them and having them at your side becomes doubly important. Those people who work from home know that animals are generally going to be right there with you during the day. Indeed, that friendly shadowing by an animal is one of the plusses of working at home.

A group that particularly benefits from the presence of pets is home-centered senior citizens. When you put a pet around a senior citizen you frequently see a joy and a vitality re-emerge in that person's life. Pets have unique personalities, but they all seem to say, "Pay attention to me," and they respond to your attention.

What's nice about most senior citizens is that they have a great deal of patience, and they have the time to really pay attention. They can take their time to do things with a sense of quality and care, which makes them a perfect match for pets. Even—and especially—elderly people in nursing homes can have mutually beneficial relationships with pets.

Actually, human beings have always had a symbiotic relationship with animals, even as our perceptions of them have changed over the ages. Animals were once treated as gods. The ancient Egyptians' reverence for cats is the best-known example of this; in that society, killing a cat was punishable by death. Cats certainly lost their privileged status in medieval Europe, when they became associated with witchcraft and were often killed. Not only was this a cruel practice, it harmed European civilization, which could have used cats to get rid of plague-carrying rats.

For much of history, working animals, such as horses, were essential to human survival. People didn't have horses for the joy of riding. They had horses because they needed them to take them from one place to another. What's more, a horse would plow your field. You couldn't do that job by yourself, and thus, you respected your horse. You understood that if you didn't take care of him, that horse was going to die, and so would your farm, and maybe your family. Likewise, sheep and goats performed essential services, providing wool for warmth and milk for nourishment. Dogs were workers too: Some were bred for hunting; the smaller ones were bred for going into holes after rabbits and foxes, the larger ones for hunting larger animals—bears or boars—or for protection. If you look at ancient paintings and drawings and read the literature of antiquity, you'll see that people's animals were a very important part of what they considered their possessions to be. And people knew that if they abused their animals, or were indifferent to them and they died, that could directly affect their own welfare.

It's amazing to realize that it's only in the past hundred years that we've come to look at animals less as beasts of burden or workmates and more as pets. Except for those farmers who happen to have livestock for slaughter, almost everyone else who has animals has them for the joy of their company.

Part of our changing mentality vis-à-vis animals is that today, we've come to see that we're really neither their owners nor their masters. In the legal sense, yes, we may own the cat or dog or horse. But in reality, we know that they are our companions rather than our possessions or servants. Consider, particularly, cats. You can say that you own a cat or are its master. But watch how a cat's own, totally unique attitude will determine whether you can get near it and when and how it interacts with you. You're really not its master; you have to get the signals from the cat. And it's the same with a horse. You can feed that horse, and you can pet it when it's in a stall. But let it go into the field, and then call it. See if it comes to you. If you want to ride the horse, see if it's willing to allow that or whether it becomes a major effort. I've seen people that have to chase their horse around a field for half a day! They try to get it by bribing it with carrots or apples, but it doesn't want to be ridden. It doesn't even want to be around people; it wants to be with another horse or by itself. Then again, if you've raised that horse with a lot of love, rather than with fear, anger, or indifference, it may come right over to you because it wants to be there. Animals remember how we've treated them in the past; thus, we teach them how to respond.

In turn, animals teach us many things. Humility is one: We become humble as we go about the daily rituals of pet care and cleanup. It's something like the sense of grounding you get from caring for a baby. You have to come down off your high horse and abandon your pretenses if you're going to take care of a baby or a pet, and I think this makes both pet owners and new parents relatively easy groups of people to communicate with. Having a pet can help you develop the warm side of your personality, as you surrender your own fears and ego and open up to the needs of the animal. That then allows you to be more open for human contact.

In addition, animals can help us learn patience, and balance, because an animal will always try to balance itself in its environment. We can learn focus as well, and we can learn to be more playful. Animals can teach us to be gentler in how we treat each other. And they can show us the virtues of simplicity. They do this, of course, by example, but also because it is only by simplifying our lives that many of us baby-boomer types can have room for our pets.

Now I feel it's time for us to make room for new ideas about pet care. Over the past several years I've seen that, even with the best of intentions, we in America are feeding our animals the wrong foods and engaging in other practices, such as over-vaccination, that are contributing to disease. I've found that in Europe, particularly in Italy and Germany, people frequently have pets—whether it's horses or dogs or cats or birds—that live substantially longer than those in the U.S., sometimes double the lifespan. In an effort to close that gap I've consulted the finest minds in veterinary medicine, practitioners who use a holistic, nontoxic, natural approach to optimizing animal health, preventing disease, and reversing disease—even life-challenging illness. I bring you the results of their experience here, as well as of my own. Some of what's in this book may shake up your long-held assumptions. But then that's always been one of my goals, along with a happier, healthier life for both people and their animal friends.

—Gary Null

CHAPTER 1

The Tao of Chow: Rethinking Your Pet's Food

A good diet is the key to a long and healthy life for any pet. It's vitally important for pet owners to understand that quality nutrition is as beneficial for their animal charges as it is for us humans. Sound nutrition goes a long way toward preventing diseases, and, of course, prevention is the best cure.

Most people trust that their animals will remain healthy with commercially prepared meals. They believe these foods are scientifically proven to provide complete and balanced nutrition and that one brand is all an animal will ever need to remain healthy. In reality, most of these foods lack sufficient minerals, enzymes, and vitamins for good health. In addition, they consist of unhealthy ingredients such as processed grains and harmful additives. Could this have something to do with the fact that dogs and cats in the United States are living shorter lives today than they did in the not-too-distant past? Read on and decide for yourself.

THE MANY PROBLEMS OF COMMERCIAL PET FOODS

Up until the 1940s cats and dogs ate meat and vegetable scraps with some limestone or bone meal thrown in for nutritional balance. On the farm, companion animals would mostly hunt food themselves and be fed whatever leftovers were available. After World War II, when household pets became increasingly popular and life increasingly complex, average people started to rely on industry to

NATURAL PET CARE

free them from cooking and other routine chores. At the same time, the kennel industry developed and was looking for a way to feed animals consistently and conveniently. In response to these demands, the pet food industry emerged and rapidly grew. Americans had a lot of faith in this industry's ability to simplify life, but little understanding of its motives.

In its infancy, the fast-growing pet food industry was in need of large amounts of raw ingredients. The void was filled by the human food processing industry, which had a great many wastes it wished to dispose of. At the time, organic materials were was being converted to fertilizer or farm animal feed, but very little profit was being made from these businesses. The opportunity to supply pet food makers appeared far more lucrative, and indeed it was. Today, most pet food companies are divisions of major agricultural and human food production companies (e.g., Nestle owns Alpo, Fancy Feast, Friskies, and Mighty Dog) and the industry earns billions of dollars each year.

Most commercially produced pet foods are full of cheap, inedible ingredients that are bad for your pets, and, unfortunately—though predictably—the cheaper the food, the more likely this is to be the case. Just think about it. What are the odds of spending only a few dollars on a bag full of quality protein and grain? They're not good, when you consider that the cost of purchasing such ingredients would be higher than the selling price of the typical bag. This is not to say that more expensive pet foods are better in every case. Some are, but others are just as undesirable as any bargain brand. Compare the labels of a cheap grocery store dog food and a premier pet store product, and you may see many of the same basic ingredients. These might include corn as one of the top ingredients, meat and poultry byproducts, meat meals, animal fat preserved in BHA, ethoxyquin, and various vitamins.

What you are likely to find in pet foods are the contaminated or condemned remains of "4D" animals—that means dead, dying, diseased, or disabled livestock. Foods are made from all body segments—intestines, udders, esophagi, nails, ground feathers, claws, chicken beaks, cartilage, tendons, and bones. Ingredients may also include lungs with pneumonia and even cancerous parts, as well as blood and fecal wastes. These slaughterhouse throwaways, often listed on pet food labels as byproducts, are considered unfit for human consumption. Capitalizing on the whole animal creates an additional source of income for food processors and farmers, but does little in providing healthy sustenance for companion animals, as the ingredients are toxic. Also, the nutritional consistency of protein byproducts is questionable and may vary from batch to batch.

Byproducts are primary components of moist pet food, and they're in semi-moist and dry foods as well. Dry foods also contain equally revolting material from rendering plants. Rendering is a process that melts animal carcasses in a large vat to produce meat, bone meal, and animal fats for use in the manufacture of pet food. The stew is once again composed of materials considered unfit for human consumption—roadkill, zoo animals, and euthanized companion animals, flea collars and all. Animals are cooked in high heat for up to an hour. Fat, called tallow, rises to the top, and the raw material sinks to the bottom. The raw material is then put into a spin-type dryer where it is forced through small holes and dried. This creates a product called meat meal, which is the protein component of pet food and livestock feed.

By the way, shelter companion animals are not the only candidates for rendering. Pet owners should be aware that their beloved pets, once deceased, could become another animal's food as well. To prevent this from happening an animal owner should not automatically sign authorization papers at a veterinary clinic (papers that state that a pet is no longer yours and anything can be done with it). First, an owner should find out exactly how the pet is going to be disposed of, as some animals are buried in mass grave sites, some are cremated, and others are sent to rendering plants.

High-heat cooking is supposed to make rendered foods safe, but there is no guarantee of protection. While the rendering process destroys bacteria, the processed material may come in contact with raw product—dead and diseased animals—and become recontaminated. Pet food companies should be testing for bacterial recontamination from salmonella and Escherichia coli, but they seldom do. Nor do they test for endotoxins, pathogens produced during a bacterium's growth that are released when the bacterium dies. These toxins can cause sickness and disease.[1]

Rendering destroys many germs, but it does not destroy the chemicals and heavy metals that were in livestock before their demise, such as hormones, antibiotics, and pesticides. Additionally, insecticides used in flea collars and topical ointments will remain, as will sodium pentobarbital, a barbiturate used to euthanize animals. Many poisons not only withstand the rendering process, they become more toxic. Most companies do not test for the presence of chemicals but assume the material they buy from rendering companies to be drug-free.

What makes such awful ingredients appeal to animal taste buds are added fats, and these are often produced from another sickening source—rancid restaurant grease. Restaurants collect grease in huge drums that are stored outside, where they may be exposed to extreme temperatures. Rendering companies eventually pick up the used grease, blend it with other fats, including the tallow from rendered products, and then stabilize the mix with antioxidants to prevent further spoilage before selling it to pet food companies. These fats are then sprayed onto dried kibble, extruded pellets, and other bland foods to entice animals to eat food they would normally walk away from in disgust.

Grains are used in large volume as cheap filler. Top carbohydrate ingredients are corn and wheat; the problem is that nutrients from these are not completely absorbed by dogs and cats. You might see a grain deceptively listed as if it were two products (such as ground wheat and wheat flour) since components are listed in the order of quantity, and splitting the ingredient makes it appear as if less grain and more protein is being offered. Carnivorous animals need a diet high in protein, so feeding them a mostly grain-based diet is not in their best interest; however, it does serves a purpose— that of saving money for the manufacturer. This is especially true when the parent company manufactures cereal; note that the largest producer of pet foods is Ralston-Purina.

Moldy grains are potentially deadly and a reason pet foods are sometimes recalled. Wheat, corn, cottonseed meal, peanut meal, and fish meal are particularly susceptible to mycotoxins—toxic substances produced by mold. In 1995, Nature's Recipe pulled $20 million worth of dog food from its shelves after many dogs became ill with vomitoxin, a mycotoxin that causes vomiting, diarrhea, and an inability to eat. In 1999, an even more harmful mycotoxin prompted the recall of Ol'Roy, a Wal-Mart's brand of dry dog food, but not before 25 dogs had already died.

Processing practices—heating, cooking, rendering, freezing,

dehydrating, canning, extruding, pelleting, and baking—greatly diminish the nutritive value of pet foods. For this reason pet food manufacturers add vitamins and minerals to the final product. Vitamin fortification, however, does not compensate for what has been lost in the food. Mineral deficiencies or imbalances may result from inferior food products and cause a host of ailments, notes Howard Peiper, coauthor of *Supernutrition for Animals*. Peiper explains that a lack of zinc, for instance, could cause vomiting, conjunctivitis, debility, or retarded growth, especially in cats. Another example: Calcium deficiency could result in osteoporosis, hip dysplasia, gum erosion, tooth loss, bones that break easily, and reproductive failure.

Finally, chemical additives and preservatives are added to improve appearance and shelf life. Synthetic preservatives commonly include butylated hydroxy anisole (BHA), butylated hydroxy toluene (BHT), and ethoxyquin, a synthetic antioxidant developed to keep rubber in tires from oxidizing. Although only small amounts of these substances are added to foods, animals tend to rely on a single food for their nourishment. These potentially cancer-causing toxins build up in the system and over time may take a toll on the animal's health. Also, no studies have been performed to ascertain the synergistic effects of various additives. In other words, your pet may be ingesting coloring agents, emulsifiers, flavor enhancers, and stabilizers at the same time without anyone knowing whether or not dangerous interactions could occur.

It's no wonder that today's pet foods are correlated with chronic sickness in young animals and shorter lifespans. Cancer among young animals is rampant. In the past, veterinarians sometimes saw cancer in older pets; today, they are witness to many cancer-ridden animals that are only two or three years of age. Other diseases being seen in increasing or epidemic proportions include infections, skin diseases, liver problems, irritable bowel disease, bone and joint diseases, urinary tract disorders, and thyroid problems. Some specific conditions have been directly linked to commercial food ingredients, such as ethoxyquin, which has been related to skin problems and infertility in dogs. Other diseases stem from a lack of nutrients. Heart disease and blindness, for instance, are known to result from taurine deficiency. Additionally, there may be a connection between the eating of diseased animals and mad cow disease, according to

Ann Martin, author of the book *Foods Pets Die For: Shocking Facts About Pet Food.* Martin states that over 100 cases of mad cow disease have been discovered in England, although Canada has reported only one and the U.S. none. Nevertheless, Martin says that the disease could be more widespread than believed, as it can easily be misdiagnosed as a neurological illness.[2]

Many other illnesses are not traceable to a single cause but are simply the result of a worn-out immune system that can no longer keep up with the influx of so many toxins. "There are millions of dogs and cats fed garbage every day, and nobody has ever questioned it," says Martin. This is because, for the most part, pet food companies are accountable to no one. It's an industry that grew very quickly, Martin points out, and fell through the cracks without ever being regulated.[3]

Labeling. Pet food companies do have one constraint: They must label their products for nutritional standards. But these requirements are not as stringent as one would expect. Originally, laboratory and testing facilities were set up to weed out unscrupulous pet food manufacturers. Guidelines were set by the National Research Council (NRC) of the Academy of Sciences, which required feeding trials for pet foods claiming to be balanced and complete. The group changed hands in 1992 when the American Association of Feed Control Officials (AAFCO), an organization created by the pet food industry itself, took over. At first the AAFCO adopted NRC regulations, but later they replaced feeding trials with testing through chemical analysis.

The problem with chemical analysis is that it does not address the biological value of foods. Dr. Morris, the founder of the Hills Pet Food Company, once published a chart mocking regulatory standards with an inedible list of ingredients that would pass as pet food. His concoction contained:

2 old shoes (protein)
1 quart of crankcase oil (fat)
1 bucket of coal (carbohydrates)[4]

This is an exaggeration, perhaps, but one well worth considering when planning your pet's diet.

One should also be wary of products marked USDA-inspected. While this appears to indicate that the food is good for human consumption, it actually means that the product was rejected for this purpose.

Advocating for Change. Because major pet food companies are comfortable with their profits, they are not, by and large, motivated to improve standards. To the contrary, defenders of the industry, which include rendering and veterinary associations, claim that pet food companies are conscientious suppliers of a good product. According to one member of the Pet Food Association of Canada, whose constituents include such multinationals as Ralston Purina and Heinz, "Regulations are not the answer. I believe the products are already good."[5]

One advocate for change is the Animal Protection Institute (API). As a liaison to AAFCO's Pet Food and Ingredient Definitions Committees, the API voices consumer concerns about pet foods and lobbies for federal regulation and the development of more stringent standards for ingredients. They are faced with a difficult challenge because the multibillion-dollar industry has no desire to regulate itself and makes million-dollar contributions to government agencies in order to preserve its interests.

Still, the API is an important resource for consumers who wish to know more about the pet food industry. For more information, contact the API at P.O. Box 22505, Sacramento, CA 95822, or call (916) 731-5521 and ask for the organization's pet food report. Be sure to share the literature with friends, family, and veterinarians. Another source is author Ann Martin, who can be reached via e-mail at newsage@teleport.com for information on the pet food industry and resources for consumer action. Additionally, pet food issues are discussed in the *Love of Animals* newsletters. Subscriptions can be obtained by calling (800) 211-6365 or (800) 711-2292.

Education is the first step toward action. Become involved by writing or calling pet food companies and the Pet Food Institute (whose numbers are listed in the appendix) to express concerns about commercial pet foods. And, of course, boycott undesirable products. When enough people start spending their dollars elsewhere, real change can happen.

THREE LEVELS OF HEALTHFUL PET NUTRITION

Fortunately, you can promote good health, and help reverse illness, once you start feeding your animal human-grade or *real* foods. That's how Rotweiller breeder Kim Thomson cured her animals of eye and ear infections, skin diseases, and liver problems. Thomson's own success inspired her to help others, and so she began to market her own product,[6] but of course there are a variety of other options for people seeking to improve the diet of their pets. In addition to buying healthier commercial brands, they can cook foods themselves, or feed their animal charges some combination of home-cooked and commercial foods.

Most holistic veterinarians advocate homemade meals for animals, and some animal owners have the time and interest to prepare foods themselves. But not everyone is willing or able to do this. Many people lead busy lives and, while they may love their pets, they just don't have the time or energy to follow pet recipes. Others don't like to cook or feel the extra costs are not within their budget. Dr. Robert Goldstein, a holistic veterinarian with more than 20 years of experience, and his wife, Susan J. Goldstein, an expert in animal nutrition, have responded to the widespread need for better pet nutrition with a quality dietary program that's simple for anyone to follow. Their three-level plan invites people to engage either minimally (level I), with a bit more involvement (level II), or with optimal input (level III). At level I, all an owner need do is switch to a natural brand of commercial dog or cat food, because yes, there are some good brands. A level II degree of participation has owners adding nutritious chopped vegetables to the commercial food, and level III adds healthy table scraps and other wholesome foods to levels I and II. Whatever your degree of involvement, expect to see such positive results as a shinier, more lustrous coat and an enhanced resistance to infections and chronic diseases.

Level I: Feeding Better Commercial Foods. Well-informed consumers are demanding healthier pet foods and some manufacturers are responding by creating acceptable alternatives to standard fare. Ingredients are often far superior to the average pet product. Instead of adding harsh artificial chemicals, the fats in these foods are naturally preserved with such ingredients as vitamin C (ascorbate), vitamin E (mixed tocopherols), and oils of rosemary, clove, or other spices. Rather than meat meals or byproducts, whole meats are used. You can tell what is used because the label will read "turkey" instead of "turkey meal" or "chicken" instead of "chicken byproducts." In addition, you'll find better grades of minerals and vitamins. Easily absorbed chelated minerals will replace cheap, less absorbable ones. Whole grains, the nutrients of which are easily digested and fully bioavailable, will be used. Instead of hard-to-digest corn and nutritionally useless ground wheat, the product will contain wholesome brown rice, oatmeal, and barley. These grains, which contain complex carbohydrates, are excellent sources of nutrients, soluble and insoluble fiber, and energy.

The consumer should still be cautious, however, as many foods touted as natural are not always as wholesome as they appear to be. Fats may be preserved in rosemary oil and vitamin C, for instance, while other ingredients in the product are chemically preserved. Since it is not mandatory to list all preservatives on a label, one can be easily duped. The only way to know for sure is to call or write individual pet food companies asking for a full list of the exact ingredients.   According to Dr. and Mrs. Goldstein, who have researched commercial products, the best ones, as listed in their *Love of Animals* newsletter, are:

California Natural—(800) 532-7261
Cornucopia—(800) PET-8280
Flint River Ranch—(909) 682-5048
Halo, Purely for Pets (Spot's Stew)—(813) 854-2214
Innova—(800) 532-7261
Nature's Recipe—(800) 237-3856
Nutro Natural Choice—(800) 833-5330
Old Mother Hubbard (Wellness)—(800) 225-0904
One Earth (Eight in One)—(516) 232-1200
PetGuard—(800) 874-3221
Precise—(888) 4-PRECISE
Sirius—(800) 890-7767 or (800) 395-7134
Solid Gold—(800) 364-4863
Wysong—(517) 631-0009 or www.wysong.net[7]

They also recommend Alive, an organic, three-module food plan for dogs and cats that features active enzymes and is available from

Earth Animal at (800) 622-0260. However, any of these products could be used in level I of Dr. Goldstein's program. Remember, though, that as animals have sensitive digestive tracts, new foods should be introduced gradually.

Level II: Adding Live Foods to the Base Diet. Even though better-quality dog and cat foods are a vast improvement over average fare, they are still cooked at high temperatures, a process that destroys indispensable enzymes and other valuable nutrients. Thus, level II of Dr. Goldstein's diet plan consists of adding live foods to the base diet to be sure an animal gets a full spectrum of enzymes, vitamins, and minerals.

Implementing level II is simple in that all you have to do is add some fresh, organic, chopped or grated fruits or vegetables. Be sure to keep pieces small because your dog and cat's ancestors that lived in the wild got their vegetables in a digested form out of the intestines of their herbivorous prey. Good choices are carrots, cabbage, celery, asparagus, Brussels sprouts, watercress, broccoli, and green beans. Cats are especially fond of zucchini. To make fruits and vegetables more appetizing, try mixing the chopped produce with a spoonful of organic plain yogurt and a capful of flaxseed oil before blending into the food.

Raw fruits and vegetables will boost your animal's immune system with the live enzymes needed to help digest carbohydrates, proteins, and fats, and to generate new tissue. You can also take your animal's health and healing to a higher level by juicing organic raw fruits and vegetables.

HOW JUICING HELPS. If you make fresh juices for yourself, allow your animal to share some of the marvelous benefits too. Juices are a concentrated source of splendid nutrients that requires very little work for digestion and absorption. As such, they are ideal "medicines" for the ailing dog or cat. Even serious conditions, such as cancer, arthritis, and kidney disease, may improve with the extra immune support supplied by fresh juice.

Each fruit and vegetable has healing properties. Apple contains pectin for the removal of toxins, and the fruit's alkalinity makes it a digestive aid. Carrot juice, rich in fiber, beta carotene, chelated minerals, and antioxidants, is good for the eyes and the immune system, and helpful in reducing oxidative stress in the bloodstream.

Combination juices can nourish the system even more completely. Use carrot or apple juice as a base because their sweetness pleases an animal's taste buds. Then add a little green juice for its potent healing effect. Greens are bitter, and bitters help detoxify the liver. Be careful to use only small amounts of green juices, as just a little is needed, and too much could make your animal sick. An example of a combination juice would be a sprig of parsley blended into apple or carrot juice. The apple will aid digestion while the parsley will cleanse the blood, fight viruses and bacteria, and even sweeten the breath. For special challenges, try some of the following juice combinations:[8]

Allergies, asthma	carrot, apple, kale, parsley
Arthritis, dysplasia	carrot, celery, lettuce
Constipation	carrot, lettuce, cabbage
Cancer	carrot, apple, watercress
Skin disorders, itching	carrot, apple, cucumber
Cataracts, vision	carrot, apple, endive
Epilepsy	peas, carrot, beet greens, spinach
Diabetes	carrot, Brussels sprouts, string beans
Heart problems	carrot, red pepper, asparagus
Digestive disorders	lettuce, papaya, carrot, apple
Kidney, bladder	carrot, watermelon, cranberry
Toxic liver	carrot, garlic, dandelion
Congested lungs	carrot, ginger, garlic, radish
Tooth decay	carrot, celery, spinach
Stomach upset	apple, kale, collard greens

Just a little juice can be a powerhouse of healing. For small dogs and cats start with 1 teaspoon and work up to 2 tablespoons. For medium dogs, those between 15 and 34 pounds, begin with 1 to 2 tablespoons and build up to _ cup. And for large dogs, initially give 3-4 tablespoons and work up to 1 cup.

If you are wondering how to get your pet to drink fresh juice, try waiting until mealtime and then mixing a small amount of juice in with the food. Or add a few drops to your pet's water. You could also put some juice in an eye dropper and place it in his mouth. Before long your pet may develop a liking for the juice and look forward to a little each day.

Level III: Taking it a Step Further. If your dog or cat is chronically ill, preparing meals yourself may be the fastest way to restore its well-being. This is also a great way to keep a healthy animal healthy. You may think that cooking for your pet is time consuming, but it doesn't have to be, note the Goldsteins, who suggest using healthful human-meal leftovers or making a big pot of meat and grains once a week that can be served for several days.

On level III of the Goldstein food program, healthful table scraps and other wholesome ingredients are added to commercial fare by reducing the natural base of dry food by about 25 percent and replacing it with equal amounts of protein, whole grains, and finely chopped or grated vegetables. Recommended portions are 1/4 cup per meal for a cat or small dog, _ cup per meal for a medium-sized dog, 1 cup for a large dog, and 1 to 1_ cups for a giant dog. The great thing about this plan is that it needn't be costly.

SHARE THE HEALTH—AND SAVE THE WEALTH!

Do you think you should never give your dog or cat table scraps? That's probably something you've learned from pet food companies, or from conventional veterinary medicine. But think about the kind of nutrition your animal gets from commercially produced pet foods, and then think about the kind of nutrition you want your pet to receive in order to stay healthy and happy. If you yourself are eating healthfully, there are lots of ways you can extend the benefits of your own good nutritional habits to your furry loved ones, and save money in the process.

Say you're having salad for dinner. Save some without dressing for your dog or cat, leaving out the onions and avoiding tomatoes—they're too acidic. Then grate your salad with a food processor or hand grater, and add it to your pet's regular food. You'll be reducing the amount of money you spend on pet food, and improving your pet's diet at the same time. Cats, in particular, love salad and greens.

You can do the same thing with oatmeal. If you're making yourself some for breakfast, make an extra cup, let it cool, and add it to your dog's reduced morning helping of dry food. Oats are as good for animals as they are for people. Other good grains to use are brown rice and millet. The rich roughage and fiber content from these complex carbohydrates will ensure fewer hairballs in cats. Refined grains, however, should be avoided.

Almost any fruit, except citrus, can be shared with pets. Apples make a great snack for everybody in your household, two-legged or four-. Cats are often fond of melons. And remember to save some of your baked potato (without the butter or sour cream, of course) as cats and dogs love spuds and their skins. Buy organic potatoes if you can; otherwise, scrub the skin well before cooking.

Many people shy away from feeding table scraps to their pet for fear of upsetting their delicate digestive systems. But this should not happen if you introduce the food slowly and increase leftover portions gradually. One more caveat: Raw vegetables should also be eaten as fresh as possible; after purchase, refrigerate and use them within three to five days; otherwise, they will spoil as a result of naturally occurring enzymes and bacteria.

HOMEMADE FOODS—A GREAT OPTION

The best way to feed your dog or cat is to prepare the food yourself. Obviously, in this hectic day and age, not everyone's going to be able to devote kitchen time to creating meals for their animals; many people can't even do so for their children! But to extent, however limited, that you can cook for your pet, you'll both benefit. You'll feel good about doing something life-promoting. And your animal will become healthier for the change because high-quality protein supplies the full spectrum of amino acids needed to grow and replace muscles, blood cells, and many other body tissues, while good sources of carbohydrates ensure greater energy and vitality.

If you plan on making a real dietary shift to homemade, begin the transition slowly, especially if your pet is older or used to commercial foods. Because animals have sensitive digestive systems, they sometimes have adverse reactions to changes in their customary diet, even when the transition is from poor food to excellent. So start by mixing a very small amount of the new food into the previous brand and continue to convert with the gradual addition of new food every week. If the stool is loose or your pet rejects the food it probably means that you were trying to make the switch too quickly and that you should slow down a bit.

If you are planning to prepare food on a long-term basis, you will need to supply the correct constituents—particularly amino acids, vitamins, and minerals—in the correct ratio. Before you start to make homemade foods, consult with your holistic veterinarian about a dog's, cat's, or other animal's overall nutritional needs, and to see if your animal has any special requirements. In general, a cat's diet should consist of approximately two-thirds protein and one-third grains and vegetables, while dogs can eat equal amounts of protein and a veggie/grain-or-potato mix. Puppies and kittens will need slightly more protein and geriatric animals somewhat less. Also, if your animal is ill you will need to adjust the diet accordingly. An animal with kidney disease or inflammatory bowel disease, for example, should be eating less protein, and an animal with a hyperthyroid condition would need to minimize iodine-rich foods, such as sardines, turnips, and mustard greens. You may therefore need to customize your pet's diet.

Begin as simply as possible. You might try supplementing your dog's or cat's regular diet with small amounts of lightly cooked chicken (no skin or spices) and rice. If this is agreeable to your pet, you can now add some vegetables and the correct amounts of vitamins, minerals, and fat. Raw vegetables should be put through a food processor and finely chopped or, if the animal has a weak digestive system, pureed, until his or her digestive tone has improved. Gradually expand healthy choices by alternating your base of chicken and rice with other sources of protein—beef, lamb, venison, fish, and even tofu—and complex carbohydrates—brown rice, millet, potatoes, oatmeal, and barley. Pork should be avoided because it is very rich and may cause diarrhea and digestive upsets. Also liver or kidney, unless certified organic, should not be eaten because they contain many toxins including heavy metals. Fish should be frozen, and only then thawed and served, as freezing will kill parasites. Ocean fish is preferable to freshwater fish. Egg yolks can be eaten raw, although egg whites, if you're using them, should be cooked, as they contain an enzyme that destroys the B vitamin biotin. In addition, you will want to add two of the following items: Most often you will want to give some cold-pressed olive oil, organic flaxseed oil, or brewer's yeast; occasionally, try cod liver oil, garlic, wheat germ oil, or kelp. Your cat needs between a half and a whole teaspoon, while dogs need between one and four teaspoons, depending on their size. Food should never be microwaved, and should always be served at room temperature.

Whole grains are a rich source of the fiber needed to maintain a healthy colon and intestines and ensure proper weight. To prepare, cook millet and barley for an hour and half, brown rice for about an hour, and oatmeal for only five minutes. Brown rice is high in tick- and flea-repellant vitamin B1 and can be combined with millet for animals in need of a hypoallergenic diet. Your pets may find these less appealing to their tastes than commercial food, but you can dress them up with a drizzle of flaxseed oil or a tiny amount of Parmesan cheese. They're even better when combined with protein and veggies.

Once you are sure that your pet has gotten used to a change in diet, he or she is certain to thrive on a variety of home-prepared meals. To help you get started, try some of these healthful recipes designed by the Goldsteins for their healing and rejuvenating effects: [9]

Wild Rice Trio

This is a hearty meal that is great for the skin and coat and high in energizing complex carbohydrates.

1 medium potato, cooked with skin
1 cup wild and brown rice (perhaps left over from Sunday dinner) steamed with fresh garlic
1 cup romaine lettuce, chopped
2 cups natural commercial pet food
2 flaxseed oil capsules
olive oil

Pour olive oil on a cutting board. Cut the potato while rolling it in the oil. Mix all ingredients together and serve.

For cats and small dogs (up to 25 lb)—1/2 cup
For dogs 50 lb and over—2 cups

Watercress Delight (Mock Grass)

Green foods are rejuvenating, and watercress is one of the best green foods to cleanse the intestinal tract. This meal will help fulfill your animal's wild side.

1 handful watercress
3 cups natural commercial food
1 tbsp virgin olive oil
1 tbsp Internal Powder or unprocessed brewer's yeast

Cut watercress with shearing scissors or chop into small pieces with a sharp knife. Mix all ingredients together.

For cats and small dogs (up to 25 lb)—1/2 to 1 cup
For dogs 50 lb and over—2 cups

Festival Topper

This mixture is high in minerals that sooth the stomach. It's good for weight loss and an excellent prelude to a fast and for pre- and post-surgical patients. It also has five-star taste.

1 carrot, grated
3 Brussels sprouts, chopped
2 potatoes, cut into chunks with skin
1/2 cup brown rice, cooked

Steam carrot, Brussels sprouts, and potatoes until soft. Combine the vegetables, rice, and steaming water (which is rich with minerals, especially potassium). This mixture can be stored in a glass jar or stainless steel bowl in the refrigerator for up to five days; however, always check food for freshness before serving. The last thing you want to do is serve a rancid meal.

For cats and small dogs (up to 25 lb)—1/2 cup
For dogs 50 lb and over—1-1/2 cups

Holiday Breakfast

This meal is far superior to commercially prepared foods.

1 large yam, roasted
1 cup oatmeal, cooked
1 tsp raw honey

Combine and serve.

For cats and small dogs (up to 25 lb)—1/4 to 1/2 cup
For dogs 50 lb and over—1 to 2 cups

Holiday Dinner

Delicious and nutritious. A favorite any time of the year.

2 large yams, roasted
1 egg, soft-boiled
1 tbsp grated cheese
1 tbsp virgin olive oil

Cut the yams and egg into small pieces and combine with cheese and olive oil. Serve as a topper or as the entire meal.

For cats and small dogs (up to 25 lb)—1/2 to 1 cup, as meal
For dogs 50 lb and over—2 cups

Snow Top

This makes a good pick-me-up for your pet, especially during winter months when your animal may feel stiff and achy. It's loaded with antioxidants and fiber, and the fish oil provides a rich source of omega 3 fatty acids, which act as an anti-inflammatory and promote healthy skin and coat.

1/2 cup cauliflower
1/4 cup low-fat ricotta cheese
2 tbsp feta cheese, crumbled
1 tbsp plain low-fat yogurt
1 cup natural commercial food
2 fish oil capsules

Chop the cauliflower in a food processor; mix with cheeses and yogurt. Place a mound on top of half your pet's normal amount of dry food. Cut open the two fish oil capsules, drizzle over food, and mix.

For cats and small dogs (up to 25 lb)—1/4 to 1/2 cup
For dogs 50 lb and over—1 cup

Winter Breakfast

Loaded with complex carbohydrates, this dish serves up steady energy for long walks.

1 cup oatmeal, cooked
2 potatoes, cooked
1 tbsp fish oil (about 4 capsules)
 strips Swiss cheese

Combine the oatmeal and potatoes with the fish oil and mix in strips of cheese.

For cats and small dogs (up to 25 lb)—1/4 to 1/2 cup
For dogs 50 lb and over—1 cup

Upset Tummy Topper

If your pet is prone to digestive disorders, such as gastritis, burping, hiccups, or excessive swallowing, this topper can help. Finely chopped cabbage is a great therapeutic agent when mixed with other food. It is high in silica, water, and minerals, and makes great roughage.

1-2 tbsp cabbage, chopped

Mix cabbage with natural commercial cat or dog food or serve over cooked grains. It can easily be stored in a glass container in the refrigerator. Even if it begins to ferment a little, it's okay. After all, it only becomes sauerkraut.

Caution: Too much roughage can further irritate the lining of the stomach and intestines. Until the irritation is under control, go with a bland, low-fiber diet, including white rice. When dealing with vomiting, diarrhea, and inflammatory conditions, such as inflammatory bowel disease, check with your veterinarian for dietary recommendations.

Sunday Stew

This vegetable stew contains sodium and potassium, two minerals essential for the healing of inflamed joints, stomach disorders, and inflamed skin. It's also rich in beta carotene, an essential vitamin for cancer patients.

8 medium baking potatoes
6 celery stalks
4 broccoli stalks and tops
6 carrots
3 cloves garlic, cut in half

On the stove, fill a large soup pot with 3 to 4 quarts of distilled or filtered water. Peel 1/4 inch off potatoes (the cores can be reserved for mashed potatoes). Add the peelings and remaining vegetables to the water. Simmer 1 to 2 hours, covered. Serve 1 cup at a time several times a day, or use as a topping for mixed dry and canned food. Stew will keep in refrigerator for 1 week.

For cats and small dogs (up to 25 lb)—1/2 cup, as topper
For dogs 50 lb and over—1-1/2 cups, as topper

Sweets for My Sweet

This energizing meal picks up sluggish animals that have been eating highly processed foods and are starved for key nutrients. The complex carbohydrates are easy to digest, and maintain blood sugar and energy levels for long periods. Raisins are high in iron, calcium, potassium and magnesium, which are used for the body's metabolic processes and in the creation of healthy new tissue. Apples are loaded with fiber and pectin and soothe the stomach and intestinal tract. You may substitute carrots for the apples; you'll still retain the high vitamin and mineral content. Cat people: You may be worried about giving your cat extra magnesium for fear of causing a urinary tract infection or bladder stones. But rest assured that magnesium derived from food is used and metabolized, not excreted in the urine or stored needlessly in the body.

1 large apple, cut into bite-size pieces
2 tbsp low-fat or fat-free plain yogurt, organic
1 tsp raw honey (omit this for diabetic animals)
1 tbsp wheat germ extract
1 handful sulfur-free raisins
3 cups oatmeal, cooked

Combine apple, yogurt, honey, wheat germ, and raisins. Mix thoroughly with the cooked oatmeal. Serve.

For cats and small dogs (up to 25 lb)—1/2 cup
For dogs 50 lb and over—1-1/2 cups

Yam Puree

In addition to being a treat for all pets, this is a healthful source of nutrients for an animal that has lost its teeth and cannot tolerate solid foods.

4 large sweet potatoes, cooked
2 raw egg yolks
2 tbsp low-fat plain yogurt
1 tsp bee pollen

Bake or steam the yams until soft. Leave the skins on. Blend in a food processor at low speed until smooth. Mix in the egg yolks, yogurt, and bee pollen. Serve alone or as a topping over natural base food.

For cats and small dogs (up to 25 lb)—1/2 cup, as meal
For dogs 50 lb and over—2 cups, as meal

Adoption Celebration

Animals that have just come home from a shelter or breeder should not be fed a meal immediately. Instead, try a few chunks of apple, raw carrots, or rice cakes as a welcome-home treat. The first cele-bration meal is actually a transitional one that will ward off loose stools or diarrhea, which are often caused by a change in environ-ment or diet. Wait two hours before feeding the new arrival the fol-lowing meal and feed about half the normal quantity for the first day. Adding a bit of yogurt is fine. You can feed this meal again the following morning. By the evening meal, you can mix any leftovers with the usual ration of pet food.

2 cups white rice
1 lb lean ground beef

Begin to cook the rice in 4 cups of water. After the water boils, reduce the heat, add the beef, and cover. Cook until all the water has been absorbed and the rice is soft (about 15 minutes).

For cats and small dogs (up to 25 lb)—1/4 to 1/2 cup
For dogs 50 lb and over—1 cup

Rapid Recovery/Post-Surgical

This is just like grandma's chicken soup! Carrots, parsley, and beets promote tissue repair and provide a great source of iron to help replenish the blood.

8-10 medium potatoes
2 cloves garlic
1/4 inch ginger root
4 carrots, with tops (cut into 2-inch pieces)
2 leaves kale
4 sprigs parsley
1/2 beet, quartered

In a large pot, peel potatoes about 1/4 inch (reserve cores for your family's meal). Add the rest of the ingredients. Fill to 2 inches from the top with filtered or distilled water and cook at low boil for 1 hour, covered. You can strain out the vegetables and serve the broth, or feed the whole mix if your animal has a good appetite.

Hairball Relief

The key to eliminating hairballs is supplementing your cat's diet with quality oils, raw veggies, and an occasional helping of whole grains. For extra support, add psyllium husks, rice polish, or rice bran to your cat's food.

Standard Ration natural commercial food (wet or dry)
2 tbsp psyllium, rice polish, or rice bran
2 tsp yogurt (for dry commercial food)

Put psyllium, rice polish, or rice bran into 1 cup of warm water. Let sit for 20 minutes until soft. Mix 1 to 2 tsp with morning and evening meals. If you're feeding dry food only, mix the softened fiber with 2 tsp of yogurt, then coat the dry food.

Urinary Tract Health

Animals with urinary tract disease need demineralized (distilled) water and quality minerals—junk minerals found in most commercial foods are useless, even harmful to pets with chronic urinary tract disease. Provide this meal for five to seven days during a flare-up. For animals with chronic conditions, mix this recipe with a natural commercial base food in a 50/50 ratio.

FOR CATS:

1 cup millet
3-1/4 cups steam-distilled water
2 stalks asparagus or 1 medium cucumber
1 small yellow squash
3 sprigs parsley
8 oz fresh chicken meat, boiled (no skin)
1 tsp tamari (reduced-sodium soy sauce)
1 raw egg

In a large pan, cook millet in 3 cups of distilled water for about 35 minutes or until most of the water has been absorbed and the grain has the consistency of porridge. Chop asparagus or cucumber, squash, and parsley in food processor until fine and mix with cooked millet. Add chicken, tamari, and raw egg yolk. Mix well. Makes approximately 4 to 5 days' worth of meals for average-sized cats. Store in refrigerator or freeze in serving-size portions in plastic storage bags. Feed 1/4 cup twice daily.

FOR DOGS:

Use only 6 oz. of deboned chicken and omit egg yolk. Double recipe for 50-lb dog to make enough for 5 to 5 days.

For small dogs—1/4 cup, as meal
For dogs 50 lb and over—1 cup, as meal

THE MEAT CONTROVERSY: IS RAW RIGHT?

Many animal experts would agree that an appropriate diet for any pet, from dogs to horses to reptiles, is one that is matched as closely as possible to what that animal would eat in the wild. The biggest mistake pet owners make is not respecting their animals' nature as carnivores, omnivores, or vegetarians. People may try to give their cats a vegetarian diet, for example, thinking this is healthier for the cat than eating meat products. But cats are carnivores through and through, and so their species-specific nutritional needs will best be met with a carnivorous diet. Dogs, too, have sharp, tearing teeth, jaw-crushing bones, and highly acidic digestive systems that thrive on meat.

Since carnivorous animals in the wild survive on freshly killed prey, some experts recommend raw meat, fish, and eggs for dogs and cats. But that's not an idea that is universally accepted. Our dogs and cats are domesticated, not the wolves or wild cats of ages long past that would spend a great deal of time roaming to hunt for prey and fasting when food was unavailable. While researching a book on animal health, author Ann Martin spoke to leading experts in the animal field at over 60 universities across the U.S. to discover that many were adamantly opposed to raw meat in the diet. Martin points out that while the proponents of a raw diet think this is the diet of wolves, our pet dogs have been domesticated for thousands of years, and have changed during that time.[10] She adds that animals in the wild have shorter lifespans because of raw meat diets.

On the other side of the question is Francis Pottenger, M.D., a scientist who says he accidentally discovered the value of raw meat in the feline diet while using cats to research hormones. He fed his cats what he thought at the time was the best possible diet—market-grade raw milk, cod liver oil, and cooked meat scraps. To his surprise, they became sickly, were poor surgical risks, and would give birth to weak and deformed offspring. To lower his overhead, Dr. Pottenger switched their diet to raw meat scraps, muscle organs, and bone, and within months noted a remarkable improvement in the health of his cats and their newborns.

So dramatic was the contrast that Dr. Pottenger began a formal study of raw versus cooked diets for cats between 1932 and 1942. What he discovered confirmed his hypothesis. Cats on raw foods diets were seldom sick, had a better appearance, and produced more robust offspring. By contrast, cats fed cooked foods were in poor health, lived shorter lives, and gave birth to weak and deformed kittens. After three generations on a cooked foods diet, the cats could no longer reproduce. Then, according to Pottenger, their health and reproductive ability returned with the reinstatement of a raw foods diet.

The benefit from raw meats is largely attributable to their enzyme-rich content. Advocates of raw meat diets suggest buying free-range products only and ensuring their freshness by keeping the food no longer than three days refrigerated or six months frozen. Frozen packages should be dated and small portions thawed in the refrigerator the night before serving. The meat should be kept out of the refrigerator just long enough to prepare it, and if it smells bad, it should be thrown out. Other safety precautions include discarding food left over in your dog's or cat's bowl, washing your hands in hot water after preparing the food, and cleaning the animal's food bowl, countertops, and other surfaces that come in contact with raw meat with a mild bleach solution or other disinfectant.

Those in favor of a cooked diet argue that today's meat products are polluted and could be dangerous if eaten raw. No matter how trustworthy the butcher, he is purchasing meat from a slaughterhouse, and these are notoriously underinspected. It's possible that the cut of meat you purchase has come in contact with fecal matter and is tainted with a potentially deadly dose of E. coli. Dr. Goldstein sees many animals put on a raw foods diet begin to degenerate from some disease. "This is because they're weak to begin with and they're eating contaminated food," he explains. A good compromise, Goldstein has found, is to lightly steam the outside of meat from an animal raised without hormones and antibiotics. Light cooking will destroy any surface bacteria. That way the animal will get most of the benefit of the raw food, but none of the bacterial contamination.

AVOID THE TREATS TRAP

Beware of the between-meal snack; it may be as detrimental as most commercially prepared foods. The rawhide bones sold in pet food stores, for example, can be bleached, and preserved with formaldehyde or arsenic. Recently, some of these toxic products were recalled, though they may be on the market once again. Pig's ears are likely to contain salmonella, which is probably why the bins that hold them advise consumers to wash their hands after handling. Similarly, store-bought dog biscuits and cat treats are often nutritionally void and filled with such undesirable ingredients as salt, sugar, byproducts, alcohol, MSG, and dyes. Such snacks contain empty calories that add pounds and are full of tainted ingredients.

No matter how busy you are you can always provide nutritious pick-me-ups with such snacks as chopped apples or pears, melon balls, or organically grown grapes or bananas. Brown rice cakes or Oatios can be found in health food stores, or try whole wheat matzo. Vegetable snacks can include Brussels sprouts, zucchini sticks, or whole carrots. Another favorite is homemade popcorn. (Hold the butter and salt!)

If you like to bake, you dog or cat will appreciate the following recipes:

Oatmeal Cookies[11]

3 cups oatmeal, uncooked
1 cup cold-filtered water
1 1/2 cups whole wheat flour (or rye flour)
1 tbsp parsley, chopped
2 egg yolks
2 tbsp raw honey (omit for diabetic animals)
1 cup raisins
1 tsp baking soda
2 cloves garlic, chopped (optional)

Mix all ingredients and spoon onto a greased cookie sheet. Bake for 12 to 15 minutes at 350 degrees F. Place on cooling rack and store in refrigerator for up to two months.

"Good Dog" Biscuits

1-3/4 cup whole wheat flour
1/2 cup oatmeal
1/2 cup cornmeal
1/4 cup liver powder (available at health food stores)
2 tbsp brewer's yeast powder
1/4 cup bone meal powder
3 tbsp powdered milk
2 eggs, lightly beaten
3 tbsp wheat germ oil (vegetable oil or bacon drippings may be used instead)
1/2 cup water

Preheat over to 325 degrees F. Combine flour, oatmeal, cornmeal, liver powder, brewer's yeast, bone meal, and powdered milk in a food processor or blender, or mix in a large bowl. Stir in the eggs, oil, and water, mixing thoroughly. The dough will be stiff and dry. Remove dough to a lightly floured surface or pastry cloth. Roll or pat into a rectangle 1/4 to 1/2 inch thick. Cut into bone-shaped biscuits with a small knife, or use a bone-shaped cookie cutter. Roll the leftover scraps of dough and cut into shapes until all the dough is used. Place on a lightly greased or parchment-lined baking sheet, and bake for 40 to 50 minutes until brown and dried through. Cool on a rack.

Dog Mini Cakes

2 cups whole wheat flour
1/2 cup soybean flour
1 cup skimmed milk or water
1 tbsp honey
1 tbsp canola or sunflower oil
1 tsp sea salt

Mix whole wheat flour, soybean flour, and sea salt. Then add skimmed milk or water, canola or sunflower oil, and honey. Mix and let the dough rest in a warm place for 15 minutes. Add oil and allow to sit another half hour. Flatten walnut-size portions into small cakes. Bake in a 400-degree oven for half an hour. Yield: 12 cakes.

Cat Mini Cakes

Follow directions, above, for making dog mini cakes, only roll the dough until it is 1/4 inch thick, and bake on a sheet scored into small sections, 1/4 inch square or smaller.

Kitty Treats

1 cup whole wheat flour
1/4 cup soy flour
1 teaspoon catnip
2 tbsp wheat germ
1 tbsp unsulfured molasses
1/2 cup powdered milk
1 egg
1/2 cup milk
2 tbsp vegetable oil

In a medium bowl, mix the whole wheat flour, soy flour, catnip, wheat germ, and powdered milk. Add the egg, milk, vegetable oil, and molasses, mixing well until the ingredients form a dough. Roll the dough out onto an oiled cookie sheet to about 1/4-inch thickness. Cut into small cat-bite-size pieces and spread the pieces slightly apart from each other. Bake in a 350-degree oven for about 20 minutes or until golden and firm. Remove from oven and thoroughly cool. Store in a tightly sealed container.

"HEY...WHEN DO WE EAT?"

A common mistake is giving companion animals free access to their food. This makes it easy for Fido or Puff to eat for reasons other than hunger—to alleviate boredom, for instance, or to create a feeling of emotional security. Since an animal's sense of smell is hundreds of times more sensitive than ours, smelling food all day will keep its digestive juices flowing continuously, which can lead to gluttony. "It's the same as strapping a hamburger under your chin and walking around with it 24/7," observes Phil Klein, certified Delta Society animal evaluator and owner of "Whiskers," a holistic pet care store in New York City.[12] As with humans, overweight and obese animals are more disease-prone and tend to live shorter lives.

If you are just beginning to put your animal on a feeding schedule, he or she may whine and beg at first, but be consistent and your pet will soon adjust to the change. Know that you are acting in the animal's best interests, since cats and dogs are designed to thrive as hungry predators. Make a gradual conversion with the following ideal pattern in mind: Feed kittens and puppies three times a day and adolescent and adult cats and dogs twice.

You will want to leave the food out for just half an hour. Dogs and cats will get used to eating in that half-hour period. As much as possible, refrain from offering snacks. You can give bones to chew on, toys to play with, teething items, and water, but you don't want your pet to have food all day.

NOTES

1. *What's Really in Pet Food? An API Report,* The Animal Protection Institute, Mar. 24, 2000, p. 7.

2. Gary Null interview with Ann Martin, Apr. 20, 2000.

3. Ibid.

4. Goldstein, Robert S., and Susan J. Goldstein, *Super Foods and Healing Meals for Pets,* Earth Animal, 1999, p.1.

5. Dunphy, Catherine, "Pet food or poison?" *The Toronto Star,* Aug. 31, 1998, p. A12.

6. Ibid.

7. Goldstein, Robert S., and Susan J. Goldstein, "Your Animal's Diet is the Underpinning of Health," *Love of Animals: Natural Care and Healing for Your Dogs & Cats*, 6:1, January 2000, p.3.

8. Goldstein, Robert S., and Susan J. Goldstein, "Fruit and Veggie Therapy," *Love of Animals: Natural Care and Healing for Your Dogs & Cats*, 5:7, July 1999, p.6.

9. Goldstein, Robert S., and Susan J. Goldstein, *Super Foods and Healing Meals for Pets*, Earth Animal, 1999, pp. 12-15.

10. Ibid.

11. Ibid., p.15.

12. Gary Null interview with Phil Klein, Mar. 15, 2000.

CHAPTER 2

Animals on the Move: Exercise

Animals in the wild have the benefit of full natural sunlight and moonlight, with no artificial lighting to interfere with their perception of what time of day or year it is. They also experience a full temperature range to toughen their system, life in an unpolluted, social environment, and the freedom to enjoy a full range of motion. The dog's ancestor, the wolf, is a hunter by nature, who might cover 100 miles or more every night in search of its food. Domesticated animals have come far from their natural state, and many of the conditions they must adapt to are not especially healthful for their minds or bodies. Without exercise, animals tend to feel stressed, lethargic, depressed, and bored, just as humans do. And as with humans, boredom may lead to overeating, which then leads to even lower exercise levels in a debilitating vicious cycle. So getting into an exercise routine will keep both you and your pet physically, emotionally, and mentally fit, and should therefore be a top priority right alongside a good diet and grooming.

Animals need regular exercise to help their bodies work their best. The benefits are numerous: Exercise will stimulate the muscles, increase circulation, regulate blood pressure, oxygenate tissues to get rid of toxins and build up the system, improve digestion, help the joints work better by enhancing the production of synovial fluid, and improve bone density. Bowel function will improve as well. Exercise boosts the immune system and helps to shed dead skin. It keeps insects away because bugs don't like healthy animals. Some research even shows that a small but consistent amount of exercise will aid in recuperation from injuries, such as wound healing. Plus there's the vital consideration of weight control: Exercise will keep your animal trim, and help to slim down an obese pet, an all-too-common phenomenon today. Obesity leads to circulation problems and increases the risk of heart attack and stroke.

Your usual exercise, or playing routine with your dog should be at least 15 minutes twice a day, and it can be as long as two hours, with certain breeds needing more exercise time than others. Dogs like to run, play with balls, chase sticks, play Frisbee, swim, and of course, just plain walk. But your daily walking routine with Rover needn't be thought of as a chore, or as lost time. Many people use dog walks as mental relaxation time, when they can unwind, meditate while moving, or think creatively or in a problem-solving mode. If you want to become more social, dog-walking, especially in a park, is a good way to do it, because an animal on a leash, just like a baby in a stroller, is a magnet for others of like interests. And walking a dog day after day is going to help you, as well as the animal, stay in shape.

ENOUGH WITH THE CAT NAPS!

Don't think that your cat can't get in on the walking act as well. Some cats, Siamese and Abyssinian in particular, can be trained to walk on a leash if they've become accustomed to it from the time they were young. Many cats resist any type of confinement, and will not take to being walked. It may be worth a try, however, and with time and patience you may succeed. That could open up a whole new world for you and your cat. A cat harness that wraps around the chest is best because you don't want to risk the cat getting hurt from a tug to the neck or the collar getting caught on some object. Nor do you want to risk the cat getting loose and slipping out of the collar. Note that while dogs are supposed to "heel," with cats you let the animal take the lead, as long as it's walking into safe territory, and you follow.

Indoor-only cats may look lazier than they actually are, the reason being that you don't usually see them during their peak activity times. Being nocturnal creatures, cats tend to sleep during the day and exercise in the late evening or at night by stretching, running, jumping, and playing. Cats will do a certain amount of play hunting, where they'll crouch down, creep around, and pounce on something. This play hunting is good for them. Kittens play most of the time, but older cats release their energy in short bursts of activity. You can help them to do this by encouraging them to play. There are many types of cat toys—catnip mice, toys that rattle and roll, cat bungee toys, racket socks, and cat "condos" and entertainment centers. You needn't spend lots of money for cat toys; just dangling a pencil from a string or rolling a ping pong ball might be all it takes to get your cat going.

If your cat doesn't play, it may be lonely or lethargic. One way to increase cats' vigor is to brush them daily or massage them. Cats like to play with their owners, and they just might start a play-fight if you massage them and gently move their legs. Suddenly, the cat grabs your hand and flips over. This is a form of exercise, too. If there's more than one cat, the duo will tend to get more exercise than would one cat alone. If your cat is lethargic, consider bringing a younger companion into the household. A kitten might be a little too much for an older cat, but a youthful feline, one a year or two old, could be lively enough to get an older cat (though not too old) moving.

ABOUT GETTING OUT

Don't let cold winter weather discourage you from taking a healthy dog or cat outdoors to get some exercise. Animals have natural fur coats to protect them, and the fresh air and light will do them a world of good during those dark, gray months. Everybody longs for sun, including dogs and cats and most other animals, and being inside a gloomy apartment day after day can result in seasonal affective disorder, the SAD syndrome. Just like us, our pets can get the "winter blues" if they are deprived of natural sunlight, fresh air, and exercise. That's because a sedentary, stagnant lifestyle can have a negative biochemical effect on the brain that creates boredom and a depressed immune system. Lack of sunlight can also cause vitamin and mineral deficiencies, particularly a deficiency of vitamin D, the sunshine vitamin, which is needed for good metabolism. Exercise, good air, and light will get your animal out of its rut by increasing the brain's supply of endorphins, the natural "feel good" chemicals that elevate mood. Even indoor cats can benefit if you set up a play station near a sunny, partially opened window, or on a screened porch if you have one, and if you improve the air quality of your home or apartment with a good air purifier. So be sure to let your animal move about to dispel those dark clouds and renew spirit.

Naturally you will need to practice common sense and not expose your animals to dangerous wind chill factors or ice storms for any length of time. You will also want to keep your puppies, kittens, and sick or geriatric animals indoors on bad days. But the average dog or cat should easily withstand most winter weather.

Exercising outdoors in winter and every other season has an additional important benefit—it gives animals the chance to detoxify from the effects of indoor pollution. While your home should be a haven for you and your pets, most likely it is filled with many hidden toxins that are tucked away in carpets, bedding, curtains, furniture, and household cleaners, a situation made worse by poor ventilation. Because animals are close to the ground they breathe in chemicals readily and are therefore more prone to their harmful effects than are humans. While you will want to minimize the pollutants in your household as much as possible, you can also help your pet detoxify its system and breathe more freely by letting it play outdoors.

Common sense will tell you when to cut down on or eliminate exercise if your pet is weak, geriatric, or sick with a bad heart or certain other conditions. Even if your pet has been healthy and playful for many years, there may be a time when it needs to exercise less. So look for signs that indicate a change in health. If your dog is used to two-hour walks and now, all of a sudden, is reluctant to go out, it may be communicating that something is wrong. Also, you should not expect an out-of-shape or obese animal to have the same stamina as a fit one. You will want to go slowly, starting with short walks around the block, letting the animal cool down, and building up from there. Even a short and easy exercise program will begin to improve circulation so that more oxygen and nutrients reach organs and tissues.

CHAPTER 3

Everybody Into the Tub!—Bathing and Grooming

While good nutrition keeps your pet healthy on the inside, bathing and grooming work to meet the same goal from the opposite direction. As the largest organ of elimination, the skin—sometimes referred to as the third kidney—must be washed and brushed to allow toxins to effectively work their way out. So let's look at some of the basics of bathing and grooming and all-around maintenance for your pet.

SPLISH, SPLASH...

...Get me out of this bath! Most animals don't like to be bathed, it's true. But bathing may be necessary from time to time, especially for dogs, and occasionally for outdoor cats, who may roam through dirt, grease, insect-filled grasses, and all sorts of garbage on their outdoor sojourns. A bath will be much easier for your pet—and you—if the habit is begun early in life. It will probably never become a favorite activity, but at least your animal will come to accept the unavoidable without a bark or meow of protest.

How often you bathe your animal is a matter of circumstance. The average dog, one that isn't extremely dirty, should be washed every month or two and more often during the summer. Very active dogs usually pick up more dust and dirt, and may need as many baths as one every other week. Also, some breeds get more soiled than others. Poodles, for instance, have a soft coat that picks up more dirt than many other breeds. Since cats are so adept at cleaning themselves, healthy indoor-only cats do not need to be bathed that often, if ever (although herbalist Janette Grainger, owner of PETicular, a company specializing in natural pet products, notes that you might try dipping them in distilled water once a month to prevent allergic reactions in humans). Animals with a healthy diet will secrete fewer fats and have sweeter skin than those that eat low-grade foods, which will be greasier and smellier, and need more baths. Animals with skin problems may need frequent baths. If fleas are present, as many baths as necessary should be given until the problem is eliminated.

For cats and small or medium-sized dogs, use a basin for bathing; a large tub could scare the animal into running away. A rubber mat or towel could be placed at the bottom of the basin to prevent slipping (although the rubber smell bothers some cats). Fill the basin halfway with warm water and add a little mild, nontoxic, natural shampoo made for cats or dogs. Some herbal shampoos contain natural flea-repellents. Oatmeal shampoos are also good. Other than baby shampoo, avoid human shampoos because they are designed for a person's pH, not that of an animal. Once you choose an appropriate shampoo, wash thoroughly, being careful to avoid sensitive areas, such as the eyes and ears (how to wash the eyes and ears will be discussed later). After rinsing, towel-dry thoroughly.

If your dog or cat fights you when it's time for a bath, and isn't too large, here's something you might try: Place the animal in a pillowcase, leaving its head out. Then pour water and shampoo through the pillowcase, and finish with a good water rinse. Another alternative is to use a dry shampoo. These can be sprinkled onto the coat and brushed away. For hard-to-clean spots, such as tar or grease, you can put mineral oil on the area, leave on for 24 hours, and then wash off using soap and water.

Sensitive ears and eyes should be washed gently, yet thoroughly. To remove dirty earwax, put slightly warmed olive oil into an eye-dropper and put 10 drops into the ear. By sure you are holding the earflap to prevent the animal from tossing it out. Gently massage the ear canal alongside the face, and let your animal shake out the dissolved wax and oil. Never put a cotton swab or anything smaller than your elbow into your animal's ear. And never pull out any hair. If you notice early signs of ear mites, a problem more prevalent in cats than in dogs, you will need to get rid of the parasites to prevent possible future problems, such as inflammation and hearing loss. An effective formula can be made from 10 drops of rosemary, lemon, and eucalyptus oils added to 4 ounces of warm olive oil. Follow the foregoing instructions for removing earwax. The herbal oil will kill mites that the animal will then shake out. The procedure can be repeated twice a day for four days and then daily for a week. Repeating at one- and two-week intervals will eliminate any new mites that may have hatched from eggs inside the ear after the first treatments. Eyes can be cleansed of dust and mucus with a cotton ball that has been dampened with water. Begin at the inside corner, and work your way toward the outside of the face.

Take this time to carefully scan the entire body for any unhealthy signs. Should you notice scabs, wounds, parasites, swellings, discharges, painful areas, or anything unusual, take your pet to the veterinarian for further analysis.

Eliminating Pet Odors. Most pets emit body odor from time to time. Sometimes it's from something they pick up outside while tracking through some awful-smelling matter, or it could even be the lingering aftereffect of having frightened some poor, unsuspecting skunk.

Fortunately, there are a few tried-and-true remedies for getting rid of a skunk odor. A simple approach requires only some room-temperature tomato juice and a sponge. With a damp sponge, apply the juice over the body, being careful to avoid the eyes, and allow it to set for two or three minutes before thoroughly rinsing off. If any trace of odor remains, repeat the procedure.

There is also a commercial product designed to solve this problem. Pets 'n People manufactures a product called Skunk Odor, the ingredients of which—natural citrus scent, water, and isopropyl alcohol—neutralize the strong smell. Be sure to keep Skunk Odor away from your friend's eyes.

Pets could also have a strong body odor from gum and tooth problems, a poor diet, or some underlying disease. Have your holistic vet determine the cause, and while you are working to reverse the problem, try these home remedies, too:

PARSLEY. Finely chop some fresh parsley and sprinkle it onto your pet's food. Cats and small dogs need just a teaspoon per day, while medium to large dogs should get between 2 and 4 teaspoons.

APPLE CIDER VINEGAR. Adding organic apple cider vinegar to your animal's drinking water may help to neutralize bad breath. Some animals will not drink it, though, so be sure to keep a bowl of fresh plain water nearby at all times. Cats and small dogs need a teaspoon, and medium to large dogs should get between 1-1/2 and 2 teaspoons.

To eliminate pet odors in your house or car, you might try a product called Air Sponge, which absorbs and eliminate odors; it can be ordered at (800) 622-0260.

WHAT'S GOOD ABOUT GROOMING

Brushing and combing your dog or cat's coat offers a wide range of benefits. Emotionally, it's relaxing to your pet and an opportunity for the two of you to bond. In addition, grooming is a boon to physical health, both your pet's and your own. Brushing the coat for five to ten minutes a day minimizes flying fur during the change of seasons, which, in turn, prevents or minimizes human allergies to pets. Grooming also stimulates sebaceous glands along the hair follicles to secrete oil, which gives their coats a healthy shine. Grooming every day, especially in flea season, can act as a flea repellent, since fleas are attracted to matted hair. Afterwards, spritzing the pet lightly with a dilute herbal repellent (two of the following—eucalyptus, rosemary, and sage—make a good combination formula) will keep it flea-free during a walk in the park.

There are deeper benefits to grooming, too. Brushing and massaging your cat or dog's back will improve lymphatic health and general circulation. To improve circulation, brush or rub your animal's back from head to tail several times in both directions. (Animals don't like their hair to go the wrong way, so be sure to smooth it in the right direction afterwards.) In addition, a back rub or brushing will promote health in the internal organs—the stomach, spleen, kidneys, bladder, heart, and lungs. So grooming is a really good way to help your pet stay healthy.

Professional Groomers. Just as spas for people are becoming increasingly popular, we are also seeing more doggie and kitty day spas. You may think this extra attention frivolous, but you might want to reconsider while looking at the benefits. A good spa can help your animal release anxiety and aid relaxation—pets suffer from stress, too—further detoxification, enhance beauty, relieve pain, and renew vigor. Plus the change of scenery can be a release from boredom and a chance to meet and socialize with new friends.

The key to good grooming is finding the right groomer. You will want to look for a person in line with your own ideas about what an animal needs to be physically and emotionally whole. If you are holistically oriented, you should be seeking a person who uses natural rather than chemical-laden skin products and who treats animals with sensitivity instead of harsh handling. You will also want an inviting environment, one that is clean, with a friendly staff who genuinely adore animals. How do you find such a place? Network with friends, veterinary clinics, and pet stores. Talk to like-minded pet owners. Once you're considering a place, call them up and ask for references. Then visit the facility alone to take a tour of the place and observe clients in session. Any reputable groomer will be happy to have you visit—and be sure you visit the actual room where the grooming takes place. When judging whether the facility is right for you, rely on your intuition, as well as your judgment. Often our gut reactions are the right ones.

Don't be afraid to ask your pet's prospective groomer questions. You will probably want to know:

How long have you been in the grooming business?
Where did you get your training?
What animals do you own? Have at work?
Do you have veterinary technician experience?
Do you have a first aid station or kit in the building?
    Where are the emergency exits?
What products do you use? Is the equipment stainless steel?
    Can I bring my own special products?
Will my animal come into contact with other animals
    during the visit?
What grooming techniques will be used on my pet?
Will my animal be offered water or snacks?

Do you belong to any professional organizations?
What security measures are taken to avoid theft, escape,
    or loss of animals in your care?
Where are animals not being handled kept?
    Will my dog be taken for a walk if necessary?
How will my animal be restrained while being bathed?
    While on the grooming table?
Who is the veterinarian on call?[1]

If the groomer isn't friendly and upfront, that's your signal to continue searching elsewhere.

If everything proves satisfactory, proceed to the next step and make an appointment. Before your initial visit, your animal should eat lightly, at least two hours before its scheduled time. Also, be sure your pet is wearing an up-to-date securely fastened collar with its name and your phone number. During the ride over, carry some Rescue Remedy or other essence designed to ease an emotionally distraught or carsick animal, just in case there's a problem. You might also consider bringing your own bottle of shampoo, as any new product might produce an allergic reaction, either immediately or at some later time. Be sure to stay with your animal during its first visit, making eye contact and offering words of encouragement to prevent feelings of abandonment. At the same time, notice how your pet responds to the groomer, and observe the groomer's body language as well. Your responsibility, of course, is to make sure that your animal has been socialized enough to know the rudimentary rules of good behavior. Otherwise, it is not fair to expect a groomer to handle an unruly pet, and it will be up to you to groom your pet at home while teaching it better manners.

Hopefully, all will go well, and you will have the confidence and assurance to continue making future appointments. A good groomer can become an important person in your animal's life. Once the two are comfortable together, you may leave your pet alone at the groomer's, but be sure to pick him up in a timely fashion.

Cats and Grooming. Cats learn to groom themselves as kittens when they first experience their mother's loving licks. They are fastidious about cleaning every part of their bodies, which keeps them shiny and smelling good. Self- grooming promotes tranquility and is the sign of a healthy cat, but there is one drawback to the practice: the ingestion of huge amounts of hair that can cause painful hairballs. Hairballs can create serious problems with obstructed digestion, and an extreme problem can even cause a cat's death. To prevent hairballs, brush the coat daily with a wire-bristle brush after vigorously rubbing the cat for a minute or two with your fingers. The cat will then swallow far less hair when grooming itself. If the cat already has hairballs, in addition to daily grooming, give a hairball formula, such as the simple recipe included in Chapter 1. Also, make sure your cat eats a high-fiber diet (you can mix some green vegetables into the food or grow some grass in a small container and keep it near the cat's food dish), and make sure that it gets adequate exercise. In many instances, it's also a good idea to fast your cat once a week to help cleanse, empty, and heal its intestines.

While the cat's natural inclination to groom itself is generally beneficial, there is such a thing as an over-preoccupation with self-grooming. In the same way that cleanliness is a good trait in a person but obsessive-compulsive hand-washing is an undesirable extreme, too much self-grooming is a behavioral disorder that can cause swelling and other damage to the skin. If your cat is grooming itself constantly, you will need to get to the root of the behavioral issue and at the same time repair the skin using a good herbal shampoo and conditioner.

THE LOWDOWN ON LITTERS. Something you may not have thought about is the connection between grooming and the type of cat litter used. Cats are fastidious about self-grooming and, if the cat litter contains poisonous products, the constant breathing in of dust and swallowing of particles licked from the feet and skin can irritate the bronchial tubes and intestines, setting the stage for inflammation and disease. Be especially wary of clay clumping litters and products laced with chemical deodorizers, perfumes, and antibacterial agents. They appeal to the consumer's desire for convenience and pleasant fragrance but can be harmful to the delicate tissues and organs of your cat.

Deodorizers are usually made from toxic chemicals that get into your cat's system each time it licks its pads. Keeping the litter box clean-smelling shouldn't be a problem if you change the litter regularly. If you are still bothered, try an alfalfa-based litter or add alfalfa pellets that you can purchase at a feed store. Alfalfa is a natural deodorizer.

An even more serious problem is the result of a modern marketing ploy—the clumping litter. Clay clumping litters are made from sodium bentonite, a clay that swells to 15 times its original volume and forms cement-like masses when exposed to moisture. Cats breathe these particles in and lick them off their bodies, and that has led to many a serious illness and unnecessary death. Just imagine a substance so hard and insoluble that it stops up plumbing when flushed. Now think about what it could do to the delicate plumbing of a cat, and particularly a kitten! Once inside an animal, the clay forms a hard mass and absorbs any incoming moisture, thus preventing the absorption of nutrients and causing dehydration. Early signs of a litter-induced ailment are diarrhea and eye and nasal discharges. These are the body's way to try to clean the harmful substance from the body. But if the litter is in constant use, these attempts will ultimately fail. Soon, the stool will become harder and more clay-like, and finally the hard mass inside will prevent elimination altogether. Death will follow.

The makers of such products are well aware of the risk to cats but take a buyer-beware attitude, expecting owners to keep their cats from eating the stuff. No warnings, however, are written on the package. Nor is it possible to keep an animal from ingesting the litter, as it produces a fine dust whenever the cat digs up an area to cover its waste. There is no way to prevent a cat from licking the litter from its legs and feet, unless, perhaps, its owner is there with a wet cloth after each visit to the litter box. But then the clumping litter is not so convenient after all.

There are many natural, dust-free alternatives to deadly clumping litters, such as plant-based and food-based products (see the appendix for some suggested brands). Or, if you are willing to change the box several times a day, simply lay down four thicknesses of old newspaper and add a few torn strips at the top.

Make your displeasure known to the manufacturers of these litters. Be sure to boycott dangerous litter products—encourage cat-owning friends and acquaintances to do the same—because businesses are responsive to the buying trends of the public. Also, write to the makers of clumping litters to let them know of your awareness and concern. (Their addresses are listed on the package.) If you suspect an animal in your household is suffering from the effects of a clumping litter (dogs and other pets may eat the product and get ill, too) take it to a holistic veterinarian and explain what you believe is happening. Even if your cat appears healthy, it makes a lot of sense to switch to a safer product anyway to avoid future complications.

Nailing Down Nail Trimming. To keep your dog or cat more comfortable and better protect your belongings, you will need to clip your animal's nails on a regular basis. If you're confused about how to do this, have your veterinarian demonstrate nail cutting on your next visit, or follow these instructions: First, purchase nail clippers designed for animals. These can be found at any good pet supply store. When you are ready to begin, hold your cat in your lap, and place one of her paws between your thumb and forefinger, gently squeezing until the nails emerge. *Only clip the tip of the nail,* about an eighth of an inch. Never cut the quick, which is the red line you may notice close to the paw. This contains sensitive nerves and blood vessels that will bleed if cut. Should you mistakenly cut too far, place the nail into a bar of soap, or wrap in a cold compress, to stop bleeding. There are also liquid solutions you can purchase from pet supply stores that will help. Hopefully, you will not have a mishap, but if you do, realize that the process will get easier each time.

Many animals don't like having their nails cut and will actively resist the procedure. It's best to start the process young, if possible, so that your kitten or puppy will acclimate to the program. You can also help your animal get used to having its nails cut by handling the paws several times a week and cutting only a few nails each time. Also, catch her when she is in a quiet mood. If your animal continues to resist, try giving her a few drops of Rescue Remedy or a gentle massage. And, of course, since animals pick up on our feelings so readily, make sure that you are relaxed. You might try taking a deep breath and visualizing a job well done in a few seconds' time.

Oral Hygiene: Not for Humans Only. Treating animals for gum and teeth problems? Isn't that just a new way to get yuppie pet owners to part from their money? Not at all. Animals don't get cavities, but they are highly susceptible to gum disease. In fact, 80 percent of dogs and 70 percent of cats experience the problem by the time they are just three years old. The result is the appearance of obvious local problems—loose teeth and chewing discomfort—but also less apparent conditions. Vital internal organs could be harmed because diseased gums are filled with bacteria that are easily absorbed into the bloodstream, and the constant onslaught of germs can overpower the immune system, causing inflammation throughout the body and the gradual appearance of disease. One illness that has been linked to gum disease is endocarditis, an infection of the heart chambers. Liver or kidney problems may be another outcome once these organs of detoxification become overburdened and can no longer keep up with giant work demands. Recent studies on human populations have also linked severe gum disease to a higher incidence of strokes.

As always, the best idea is prevention, which means starting an oral hygiene program when your pet is young. Even if you are starting late in the game it is often possible to take steps that will lead to the reappearance of healthy, pink gums. To begin, learn to recognize the signs of gum disease: tartar buildup, bleeding gums, inflammation that appears as redness or swelling at the gum line, foul odor, loose teeth, and difficulty eating. Your veterinarian should check the teeth and gums during a routine exam and alert you to any signs of trouble. If the problem is far along, he or she may recommend a thorough ultrasound cleaning to remove tartar and plaque and reduce the size of the periodontal pocket space between the teeth and gums (smaller pocket spaces reflect better periodontal health). While the procedure is highly effective, one drawback is the use of general anesthesia, which poses the risk of an adverse reaction, especially in older pets and animals with a weak immune system. Fortunately, there are a growing number of veterinarians and vet techs trained to perform anesthesia-free cleanings.

You know how good your own teeth and gums feel after a treatment from your dental hygienist, but you also know that they do not remain pristine unless you floss and brush at home. So too does your dog or cat require home maintenance for optimal health. That means brushing your pet's teeth three times a week. Finger brushing will work for cats and small dogs, but larger dogs will need a regular soft toothbrush. Pet stores sell natural toothpastes designed for the unique needs of dogs and cats.

Many people shy away from this essential grooming measure because it can be difficult, especially if your animal has not been made accustomed to tooth brushing from an early age. Kathy Klein, the owner of SmilePet in southern California, an anesthesia-free teeth-cleaning service, advises her clients on proper procedures. She suggests that pet owners firmly, but lovingly, place their animal in a position where it cannot escape, using a gentle voice and massage to relax them. For small to medium-size dogs, Klein suggests sitting on the floor and carefully placing the animal in an upside-down position to protect its back. The animal should then be cradled with your legs so that the back of the animal's head rests on your lap. Cats and less cooperative dogs can be wrapped in a beach towel, and larger dogs can be placed on their side. Holding the face with your left hand, the lips should be pulled out so that you can get inside the animal's mouth and brush the teeth. Don't worry if you can't see the teeth; the main goal is to push the gums back, which will stimulate them.[2]

Another important measure is to be sure your dog or cat is getting foods that do not form plaque—whole grains and fresh vegetables. At the same time, you should limit plaque-producing foods, such as brands of commercial foods that contain refined sugars and white flour. Contrary to popular opinion, biscuits and other dry foods will not effectively clean the teeth because the problem begins where chewing doesn't occur, the site where the bottom of the tooth meets the gum line. Chewing only stimulates gums sporadically in areas where pieces of food brush against them. Also, dogs and cats often swallow their food whole, without chewing.

What about that favorite canine activity, bone chewing? You might allow Fido to chew on a raw femur bone, the long bone of the leg, or a large knucklebone, one that is at least two inches long. The abrasive action of the chewing will help to remove some tartar from the teeth. Avoid steak, pork chop, rib, chicken, and fish bones, which can splinter and become a choking hazard, and dispose of the bone after it is chewed away.

In animal dental care, as in other areas, prevention and natural remedies for reversing problems are really the best ways to go, as pharmaceuticals, such as cortisone, only cover up symptoms temporarily and place an additional burden on an already overworked immune system. For an extra boost to immunity that will help keep the gums healthy, add the following supplements to your animal's diet: Ester-C (250-1000 mg mixed into regular food or with organic plain yogurt once a day), echinacea (5-12 drops in water twice a day), and coenzyme Q10 (50-125 mg added to water once a day). The amount you give will depend on the size of your animal, with cats and small dogs getting the minimum amount, medium and large dogs getting somewhat more, and giant dogs getting the maximum amount. Echinacea, which has a well-earned reputation as a natural antibiotic, should be taken for two weeks and then restarted after a two-week hiatus. Ester-C and coenzyme Q10 will strengthen the immune system year round, the latter being especially protective of the heart and gums. Check with a holistic veterinarian as you customize an immunity-strengthening plan for your pet.

For quick relief from sore gums, purchase an herbal elixir designed for this purpose, or create your own antimicrobial tea. You can brew licorice, goldenseal, or echinacea in distilled water, let the tea cool, and place in a bowl for your pet to drink. You could also apply the damp tea bag directly over the sore gums or dab some of the tea onto the inflamed area with a cotton swab. Another soothing option is aloe vera gel. Again, check with your vet about persistent problems.

NOTES

1. Goldstein, Robert S., and Susan J. Goldstein, *Love of Animals*, 4:10, October 1998, p.2.

2. Goldstein, Robert S., and Susan J. Goldstein, "Restore and Maintain the Health of Your Animal's Teeth and Gums," *Love of Animals: Natural Care and Healing for Your Dogs & Cats*, 6:4, April 2000, p.5.

CHAPTER 4

The Impetuous Pet, or
Understanding Animal Behavior

When *Men Are From Mars, Women Are From Venus* became a bestseller, that said a lot about how difficult it is for the sexes to understand one another. Because people from different sexes, races, religions, cultures, generations, and socioeconomic classes miscommunicate, problems often arise. Now imagine trying to relate to another species altogether! Living with an animal can be challenging, particularly if that animal has developed a behavioral problem.

Animals are highly sensitive and emotional creatures that, like children, often express unhappy feelings by "acting out." They may soil the house, destroy things, or become aggressive, compulsive, or overly "talkative," and it can try our patience. Indeed, a behavior problem is the number-one reason animals are euthanized. But such a drastic measure is unfortunate and unnecessary, once you realize that there are many ways to prevent problems from developing and change the patterns of already troubled animals. First, it helps to understand how emotional and behavioral problems arise.

WHAT CAUSES PROBLEMS IN THE FIRST PLACE?

An animal's troubles may begin early in life, as when a puppy or kitten is weaned too early or becomes the recipient of abuse, abandonment, or other trauma. The stress of a dysfunctional household, poor nutrition, vaccinations, medications, or illness can also take their toll on an animal's emotional health at any point in life. A situation of chronic conflict can ensue if a person chooses the wrong pet for his or her lifestyle or personality. Moreover, some animals are purposely raised to be fierce and aggressive. Another big, and sad, source of problems is breeding practices.

Over-Breeding. The fact that the pretty puppies that enliven pet stores usually come from horrid places is a "deep, dark secret," in the words of Valerie Angeli, public information manager of New York's ASPCA. These dogs are born in "puppy mills," so named because animals are there for one purpose only—to be bred for profit.

Because greed is at the core of this practice, the animals live in hideous conditions. Females are constantly made pregnant, as their sole purpose is to produce litters to stock pet stores. They are kept in very small cages and are surrounded by dead animals, animals infested with fleas and parasites, and sickly animals that are miserable and antisocial because they spend most of their time locked up without human contact. They may be exposed to the elements or receive inadequate ventilation. Food and water are usually kept to a minimum, with just enough provided to keep them alive. "These animals are bred for profit," says Angeli, "not health or temperament."

An unsuspecting person who adopts a puppy from a pet store may be in for a shock. For one thing, these animals often inherit physical weaknesses. One such Dalmatian lost all its teeth within the first two years of life from congenital gum disease that was traced to a mom at a puppy mill that had the same experience. Another problem is that their early traumatic experiences cause emotional and behavioral problems. They are generally weaned way too early. Animals taken from their mothers too soon and thrown into the world are not yet ready. They feel terribly vulnerable, and, in their attempt to cope, they may become frightened. As a defense, they can become overly aggressive.

Legislation is under way to put an end to these nightmarish conditions, but in the meantime, you can do your part by not purchasing puppies from pet stores. Buying these animals only encourages the continuation of puppy mills. There is an exception—pet stores that showcase homeless animals from shelters. Indeed, with millions of unwanted shelter animals, you can easily adopt a wonderful pet and save a life. If you are looking for a special breed, contact a rescue group that specializes in that particular type of animal. You will be able to purchase a wonderful friend at the fraction of the cost of going to a breeder. But if you do decide to adopt from a breeder, be sure the person is responsible. A good breeder will not over-breed and will only breed a certain dog when there is a request or a waiting list for that breed. Moreover, that person will consider the temperament of the animal as well as the look, and will take into account the personality of the pet and prospective owner when making a match.

The Stressed Pet. Ongoing stress, a common complaint in our society, affects animals as much as people. Of course, stress in an animal will not be precipitated by a downward turn of the stock market or not being accepted by the right country club. But it can be a result of inadequate nutrition, improper hygiene, overuse of vaccinations, pollution, and too many drugs. Animals can also pick up the negative energy transmitted in a dysfunctional household. Animals thrive on love and attention, and suffer in an atmosphere of disharmony, abuse, or neglect. A person can choose to leave an unhappy home, but for an animal such a place could become a permanent prison. Emotional problems may then develop.

As is the case with humans, the physical and the emotional are inextricably connected in animals. So you'll find chronically stressed pets with digestive upsets, vomiting problems, skin conditions, or inflammatory bowel disease. What happens is that long-term stress wears down the immune system and, thus, becomes a contributing factor in disease. Veterinarian Lester Morris has noted the relationship between the family dynamic and the animal many times throughout his career: "Often dogs are brought to me sick and very emotional. I'll place them in the hospital for a few days, and they will clear up spontaneously without medication. Then they will go back home, and their problem will return. We try to explain this to the owners. If they correct their household situations, it can help the animal a great deal."

Lifestyle and Personality Mismatches. You've just taken the kids to see *101 Dalmatians,* and now they're begging you to for a spotted dog of their own. "Aren't they cute?" they cry. "Look at the spots!"

Giving in to their pleas, you soon discover that this black and white dog is not well suited to children. Dalmatians are beautiful but high-strung animals that, originally bred to race alongside coaches to guard against robbery, need to be run often. These animals are extremely athletic and have boundless energy. They are also fierce watchdogs that are suspicious of strangers. Sometimes, then, our pets are not the problem at all; we just choose animals that are the wrong fit for our lifestyle or personality.

We should note that sometimes the reputed traits of a breed are not really innate, but are a result of training. This is the case for pit bulls. Members of this breed have a notorious reputation for being dangerous when, in actuality, they can make great, friendly pets. The problem is that reprehensible people train pit bulls to fight because their endurance levels are high. Macho teens, in particular, treat these dogs roughly to turn them into super killing machines. To that end they do hideous things—injecting the animals with steroids, running them on treadmills, weighing them down with heavy chains to strengthen their neck muscles, and hanging them on tires suspended from trees to strengthen their jaws. Most abhorrent, live animals are given to these animals for food. They learn to tear live animals to shreds and become bloodthirsty (a reason to be careful about who you give your puppies and kittens to!) Anyone aware of this or any other cruel activity should, without hesitation, contact a humane society. Pit bulls, then, can be made to live up to their reputation as the dog everyone fears, but so could other animals treated that badly. Pit bulls have a strong desire to please, and advocates for this breed say that they can just as readily be made into friendly, affectionate, and fun-loving family pets.

Be sure to get the animal that's right for your lifestyle. Don't choose a Dalmatian or Great Dane to guard a small apartment. Lack of room will frustrate the animal. Consider a silky-haired Pomeranian instead. These dogs can offer you excellent protection and not mind the limited space. Take your personality into account, too. If you love cats and have a laid-back nature, the common American shorthair is probably just right for you. You can find a variety of these beautiful cats—tabbies, calicos, tortoiseshells, or pure-colored—at any neighborhood shelter. These cats have an even temperament, attach themselves easily to loving owners, and stay close enough to their human companions to be good company without begging for constant attention. But if you're seeking lots of affection and devotion, consider a Siamese. These complex, sensitive animals have undying love for their owners and enjoy nothing more than draping themselves around their person's neck.

While animals of a particular breed are not carbon copies of one another, they do have general behavior traits that may or may not be well suited to your own. Read up on the personalities of different breeds or talk to experts about the animal type before bringing a pet into your home and your life. Taking care of an animal is a responsibility that should also be fun for you and the animal—that is, after all, one of the points of having a pet!—so you want to match your temperaments as carefully as possible.

Punishment. According to veterinarian William G. Winter, author of *The Holistic Veterinary Handbook: Safe, Effective Treatment Plans for the Companion Animal Practitioner*, animal owners who resort to harsh punishment when their animal fails to respond as expected can cause psychological and physical harm. Such punishment creates trauma that, according to Chinese medical theory, can result in energy blockages, the first stage of physical disease. In domesticated animals, Winter explains, these blockages often appear in the neck, causing it to hang shamefully rather than appear long and graceful, as it should.[1]

An owner who does not understand how to communicate with a pet may, out of frustration and anger, resort to screaming. This is particularly detrimental to a puppy or kitten that, in the first year of life, is still developing its nervous system. Plus an animal's hearing is much more sensitive than our own, so screaming at the animal can cause physical pain. What's more, yelling at a pet can actually intensify behavior problems, rather than correct them. If you scold a dominant dog, for example, it is going to respond by becoming more aggressive, while a timid dog will only become more fearful. Pet owners need to learn to show dominance through body language, not screaming.

Most behavior changes can be accomplished through positive reinforcement. Often, it's a matter of understanding what the animal requires. Your cat is not maliciously trying to destroy your carpet and furniture. It just has an innate need to scratch; it *is* a cat, after all. Rather than yelling, an owner should provide the kind of scratching post cats respond to—sisal or carpet wrapped around a log with the jute backing exposed. Applying a little catnip can make the accessory more attractive. You can discourage your cat from scratching the wrong items by placing double-edged tape over the area—they dislike getting their paws stuck—or aluminum foil. But, most important, give your pet praise each time it scratches its post.

If all your positive reinforcement fails to work, some discipline may be in order, but it should be reasonable and related to the animal's action so that it starts to make the connection. In *Conversations With Animals: Cherished Messages and Memories as Told by an Animal Communicator*, author Lydia Hiby tells of one technique she used with a rebellious cat—kitty jail. When her Russian Blue, Thomas, refused to stop bullying the other family cats, Hiby issued a warning to "stop, or else." The next time he engaged in his unruly behavior, she covered him with a plastic milk crate turned upside-down and placed him in the middle of the room just long enough for all the cats to see. This, Hiby feels, caused Thomas great embarrassment, and after two repeat offenses and short prison sentences, Thomas was reformed. Hiby advises anyone using this method to warn the animal ahead of time, keep the jail time short, only use a plastic, see-through, milk-type crate, and place the jail in a central location so that the animal is embarrassed, not isolated or terrified.[2]

Additional Factors. Animals may develop behavior problems for a number of other reasons. Separation anxiety is a common underlying cause of abnormal and destructive behavior in companion animals that might result in excessive barking or meowing, inappropriate urination and defecation, destruction of household goods, and digging. Other bad-behavior triggers: Fido may be responding to a new addition to the family, either person or animal. He may be punished too severely during housebreaking. Also, vaccines and other medicines can have psychological side effects. Then, too, an animal may be responding to some trauma in its past. If you suspect this is true of your animal, have the cat or dog medically checked to be sure that nothing is wrong. An animal that has been abused in the past may exhibit such behaviors as keeping the ears down, not eating properly, not enjoying food, tail-chasing, paw-licking, not wanting to be petted, and shaking. Animals—and not just elephants!—have great memories, and may need a lot of love to overcome adversity.

UNDERSTANDING DOGS: GOING BEYOND TRAINING

Traditional methods of obedience training only address the problem on one level—your dominance over your dog. Conventional dog training is based on conditioning, using the old Pavlovian model. But this approach to training a dog is backwards, asserts dog teacher Alan Finn, owner of Designing Dogs in Old Forge, Pennsylvania. Finn deals with many dogs exhibiting behavioral problems, such as biting, tail-chasing, and other compulsive behaviors. To properly understand how to teach our dogs, he believes we need to rethink and undo most of what we ourselves have learned about how to handle dogs.

"Teaching" is the key word here. It is far better to teach and communicate with a dog, Finn feels, than to simply condition it through bribery with food or fear-inducing yelling. Above all else, dogs need to be in tune with their owners. As a dog owner, you need to understand your dog so that your dog can understand you. There's no need to yell at a dog to discipline it. In fact, yelling, especially at a puppy, can induce negative behaviors. A dog's hearing is much more sensitive than ours, and Finn would urge us to imagine how a dog hears and experiences being yelled at. Puppies' nervous systems take a year to develop fully; if they are yelled at throughout that time, a dominant puppy will turn more aggressive, and a submissive puppy will become more fearful.

One of the most important tools an owner has is his or her voice. When speaking to your animal it is important to keep your voice low, and draw your vowels out. An example: "Ni-i-i-ice dog." Using a low, calm tone with drawn-out vowels relaxes the animal. One of the reasons this works is that you can feel your own body relaxing as you speak. You're not holding any tension or stress in your muscles, and you do not have a defensive body posture (muscles tensed, teeth clenched, head held high). Animals exhibit this same posture of conflict that releases when they are relaxed.

Dogs can think, states Finn, and they can understand much more than we humans generally realize. They can count, and they also interpret human body language. This is another way that dog owners inadvertently create behavior problems. When a dog jumps, often the first reaction of the dog's trainer is to push the dog away and say, "Down!" But to a dog, the motion of pushing it away means "jump." So being pushed away and told "down" is actually a mixed message to a dog.

Usually, the owner needs to take a good look at his or her own behavior and make some changes before being able to effectively teach and communicate with a dog. Don't yell at your dog, and don't try to condition it. Nor should you repeat commands, because dogs can count. If you say, "sit-sit-sit," the dog will become conditioned to sit on the third repetition. Finn recommends mixing up commands and changing routines, as opposed to keeping your approach static. This keeps the dog engaged, focused on you, and thinking. Use appropriate body language. Don't hold a leash tightly, and frequently change directions when walking with your dog so that it will have to focus on you and your actions.

And you *can* teach old dogs new tricks. Your dog loves you and is always ready to try again—so be positive, and don't be afraid to start over if you have negative patterns in place. September Morn, who teaches basic obedience and canine good citizenship at Dogs Love School in Bellingham, Washington, knows this for a fact. Ms. Morn helps animal shelter dogs relearn trust and openness. Animals that have been hurt become guarded and tense around humans, but they can learn to associate touch with good feelings and relaxation. She notes that "…any dog that you get second-hand is going to have second-hand behaviors. They're going to have habit patterns learned from the last people who had them. You're going to need to change those so the dog can fit into your household and your style of living." Remember that dogs want, more than anything else, to please their owners. Successfully communicating so that your dog can do what you want will make it, and you, very happy.

THE INS AND OUTS OF HOUSEBREAKING

While most kittens readily take to their litter boxes, housebreaking a puppy takes time and patience. Dogs do not automatically know to bark when they need to go out, nor do they innately understand that some places are off limits. Dogs need to be housebroken and their owners need to learn the right way to train their pets.

Dog owners can easily become frustrated and angry when their carpet or bed is soiled. Inexperienced and impatient people who yell at their pups and put their nose in an accident only confuse their animals and incite fear and trauma. Housebreaking a pup needn't be painful and traumatic. In fact, it can and should be an important part of building a trusting relationship. The art of housebreaking in a loving fashion is explained by experienced professional dog trainer September Morn, who teaches her clients how to effectively train animals in a gentle fashion. Communication with the animal is the key to success. These are her suggestions:

Keep a Log. It's helpful to keep a record of when your dog needs to go to the bathroom. The best way is to keep a log of when your puppy eats and how long afterwards it needs to "go potty." If your puppy has an accident in the house, record that time, too. Keeping a log will help you establish your dog's natural intake and output rhythms. Generally, puppies eliminate four times a day: after waking, after a pause in play or following playtime, after eating, and after drinking. Older dogs will also need to go relieve themselves after these events, but with a greater lag time.

It's important to be observant, Morn stresses. You will need to recognize behaviors that indicate the need to go to the bathroom: sniffing the floor, turning in circles, running back and forth. Puppies may appear to look for something when there's nothing to find. What they're actually seeking is a place to empty themselves. Sometimes they move quickly, spinning, or appearing anxious. Puppies will give you a very short time to figure out what they're saying, so you will need to act on their signs immediately. As soon as you notice a signal, say something like, "Do you need to go outside?" so they see that you are paying attention to them. Pick up your puppy and carry the animal outside or onto its paper. Dogs that are a little older can be put on a leash before being taken for a walk. Older dogs, except ones with poor bladder or bowel control, will give you more of a warning. Animals on medication might give you a shorter cue, as the effect of the drug might make it difficult for them to control their urges.

Teach Your Dog to Communicate its Needs. New dog owners may become frustrated because their dogs don't bark to say, "I need to go to the bathroom." Dogs have to learn how to give their owners that message. Morn suggests hanging a string of sleigh bells from the doorknob. Normally, dogs learn to associate doorknobs with going out. They may stare at the doorknob and realize that someone needs to turn it to make the door open. Bells are a great device because they add an auditory dimension to a visual cue. Each time the door opens, the animal hears a ring. In a short time, they will chain those events—the doorknob, the bell, and going out to potty. Some dogs will even begin to ring the bells themselves as a way of asking to be taken out.

It is possible, however, for a slick dog to send a false alarm. Some dogs will ring the bells just to go out and play in the sunshine. This might be alright if you don't mind letting your dog frolic in a fenced-in yard. But if the animal is in the house-training process you want the bells to signal only the need to potty. To minimize the desire to play, do not play with your pet when you take it outside to do its business. Stay out for five minutes only; that should be plenty of time for the animal to eliminate if it has to go. An exception is the puppy so excited by the outside world that it forgets its purpose. To minimize the chance of an accident, be sure to watch the pup once you return indoors. If the animal starts to give "potty signs" again—sniffing, or running back and forth, for example—say something like "You need to go potty" and go out again. This is why it is very important to stay with your dog when taking the animal to its outdoor "bathroom," especially during training times. You want to be sure the animal actually does take care of business in the appropriate place.

Indoor Potty Training. Some people who live in apartments, are away for many hours, or travel a great deal find it convenient to have their dogs eliminate on paper or litter inside the house. This option is most viable for small dogs, if they are trained while they are very young so they don't have to unlearn being housebroken. Other people begin to train their dog indoors as a first step before going outside. In this instance it's best to place papers as close to the door as possible so that the dog will learn to move in an outdoor direction.

Keep a dog's elimination area far from its food, water, and bedding so that it doesn't accidentally soil its eating or sleeping quarters. Also, if your living space is large, close off certain sections.

Puppies sometimes mistake a little-used area of the house—a guest room or sewing room, for example—for their bathroom space. So limit access during this learning phase. Otherwise, knowing what to do in such a big space might be more responsibility than a young puppy can handle.

Stay Focused. When you go outside with your puppy for the purpose of doing its business you need to help your pet understand why it is there. The best way to accomplish your goal is to stay calm and focused yourself and to help your animal do the same. Don't go for a walk first. Only visit the area you want your animal to use. You want your dog calm to the point of boredom, as opposed to being excited by the many sights, sounds, and scents that a walk provides, because an excited animal would rather engage in the world than tend to its needs. Then, once inside and settled, it suddenly remembers its needs and has an accident. So just take your dog to the elimination area and calmly wait. Generating excitement also might close off the puppy's sphincter muscle to the bladder and bowel, thus preventing elimination. If your dog is old enough, use a leash so that the animal is not tempted to wander away. After your pet becomes used to the routine, a leash might not be needed.

Some puppies will try to engage you in play instead of attending to their business. When this happens, Morn suggests doing the "boring" walk. What that means is you calmly stand there, perhaps taking a quarter turn away, shifting from foot to foot, or occasionally taking a step back. You become boring to the pup, which then loses interest in playing with you. Soon the animal realizes that the only excitement is the inner feeling of eliminating.

At the same time, use a verbal cue that your puppy will learn to associate with going to the bathroom. "Go potty," "do business," or any short phrase that you use only at this time will do. Again, you want to avoid excitement, so use a flat voice. It might take a little time for your puppy to associate your words with bathroom time, but it will eventually catch on. Afterwards, praise your pet in a subtle (still boring) voice, saying words to the effect of "good do business" or "good potty." Any excitement might prevent any remaining urine or excrement from being released until later.

Avoid rewarding Rover with food. Its value is too high for potty training. Food is so stimulating to animals that their desire to attain it might override everything else. A puppy might only half finish, or squat, do nothing, and run back to its owner, as if to say, "Give me my cookie." You would be, in effect, setting the animal up to have an accident indoors.

You should also avoid bending over and petting your dog during the training process, as the dog might mistake this for play. (Bowing is a way of saying, "Let's play.") Touching your pet at this time sends the wrong message, and that could confuse your puppy. Just stand there and repeat the phrase "good potty" or "potty more" a few times. After awhile your dog will learn that " potty" means what you do first and "potty more" means completing anything you didn't finish.

Accept that Accidents Will Happen. Don't expect your dog to respond perfectly, especially at the beginning. Accidents sometimes occur and should never be met with punishment. Some people will rub their dog's nose in the place where they had the accident as a way of scolding their pup. This doesn't make any sense to the dog and, in fact, sends a contradictory message because you're trying to teach the dog to be clean yet getting the animal dirty. The animal can't possibly make the connection and might find the lesson extremely traumatic. The pup may in fact begin to think, "They don't want me to go to the bathroom," and start holding it until the owner is gone and then hiding its deposits behind furniture. Thus, the problem worsens instead of gets better. Plus it's bad for the relationship between the person and animal. Further, physical damage could result if the puppy is treated too roughly. In truth, the accident may be your fault for not getting your pet outside quickly enough. Use each accident as an opportunity to educate yourself on what to do better next time.

When an accident occurs, clean up the area with a paper towel while saying to your friend, "This is bad potty," or "We don't potty here." Never say "Bad, bad, bad!" and never show anger. Just use an instructional tone of voice. You will want to take your animal's deposit to the proper place. On your way out the door, ring the string of bells to help your dog associate going to the bathroom with going outside. Or, if you're training on papers indoors, take it there. Drop the stool to the ground or rub the area with the urine-soaked paper (take the actual towel away). Say words to the effect of "good potty outside" in your boring praise voice. The puppy will be watching and learning from you, and seeing that you are pleased with the outdoor location.

Sometimes puppies have accidents for psychological reasons. There are dogs that are followers and dogs that are leaders. A dog that is a follower by nature may have an accident because he or she relates to you, a big towering person, as the "top dog." The dog may get so excited while greeting you that the animal wiggles all over and loses control of the bladder or bowels. Don't punish the dog, because it is only trying to express its love for you and truly means well. You appear all-powerful to the animal, and punishment makes you appear more awesome still.

The best method for dealing with this behavior is to open the door and let the dog greet you outside. That way the animal might piddle on the porch rather than on your floor. Getting the dog into the yard is even better. You could say, "Come outside; let's potty," and if your puppy eliminates on cue he or she feels worthy of praise for doing something good instead of ashamed for doing something forbidden. Another strategy is to keep a toy by the door—a stuffed toy or ball perhaps. Redirect your pet's attention by throwing the toy for the dog to retrieve. A handful of treats will also do because a dog won't feel submissive to a toy or a treat. Hopefully, your dog's excitement will subside, leaving you enough time to attach a leash to your pup and walk it to the potty area.

Creating an instructional, but loving, atmosphere is all-important. Your animal will get the message, not tense up, and know it is pleasing to you. Animals that are punished during the house-training process become afraid of eliminating in front of their owners because they begin to believe that their owners do not want to see them go. All you want to teach is that there is a right place and a wrong place. There's no need to bring negativity into the experience. Quietly telling a sensitive puppy that it's in the wrong place to potty is punishment enough. What you want to be communicating is, "We don't want to see it there, but we'd love to see it here."

The Crate Den. Puppies tend to have more accidents at night because they like to wander around the house, and all that exercise creates a need for more frequent elimination. An effective way to prevent this from happening is to let your puppy sleep in a plastic travel kennel, also known as a crate den. Dogs, unlike most cats, who hate being trapped, find this space cozy and calming. If they're quiet and relaxed in their cage at night, and not moving about, they'll be more likely to be able to wait until the next day.

By the way, you may be wondering whether you could have someone else train your puppy for you. The answer is that, sure, you could, but then you'd be missing out on an important bonding experience. Housebreaking occurs during the time you are forming your initial relationship with your companion animal. Turning the responsibility over to a trainer or some other person will probably result in your dog developing a relationship with that person instead of you.

Elimination Problems. Say you're doing all the right things, and your dog does not seem to get it. He or she is still eliminating at the wrong times in the wrong places. Is your dog being spiteful? Is this the time to become angry and resort to punishment? Absolutely not. Dogs want to please their owners and are not spiteful by nature. Your dog just may have a physical problem. In fact, 25 percent of all long-standing house-training problems are physically based. So the first thing you need to do is take your animal to a veterinarian for a thorough workup that includes fecal tests for parasites, a urine test, and a blood test.

One of the more common problems that prevent proper elimination is cystitis, also known as urinary tract infection. When a dog's urinary tract becomes inflamed, an animal will often try to hold in its urine as long as possible to prevent pain. In addition, the animal might experience loss of control over its sphincter muscle, which causes the dog to leak urine or drip a lot. Your pet might also associate his or her usual place of urination with pain and seek a more comfortable place inside. The owner's soft bed or sofa might become the animal's place of choice. Urinating there will be just as painful, of course, but the animal is hoping this more cushiony place will help him or her to feel better.

Cats commonly experience cystitis too, and behave in a similar fashion, avoiding their litter boxes and relieving themselves on the furniture or floor instead. In fact, veterinarians are generally more aware of the problem in cats than in dogs, so it's important to remind your dog's doctor to check for cystitis.

With dogs, as with other animals, you need to make sure that fresh drinking water is available at all times. Lack of water can lead to dehydration, a dangerous condition that can lead to cystitis. Symptoms of dehydration are panting and the skin being very tight against the body. By the time a dog, particularly a puppy, becomes dehydrated, the situation is already critical, and you need to get to your vet right away.

Parasites can cause other elimination problems. They irritate the stomach and intestines and cause loose stools.

Other physical problems to check for are endocrine diseases. A full blood panel will screen for thyroid, kidney, and adrenal disorders. Any of these hormonal problems can interfere with house training and the ability to properly eliminate. Spayed females sometimes develop estrogen-deficiency incontinence. Some people think that the dog is getting too old and that it should be destroyed, but an estrogen deficiency can be medically treated.

DOG BEHAVIOR PROBLEMS

Many dog behavior problems are a result of isolation, and the often-ignored reality is that dogs should not be left alone for long periods of time. The animal might go into a frenzy, chewing on anything and everything, breaking into containers, and possibly hurting itself. Dogs left alone in a yard or house often develop the habit of incessant barking. Dogs that are accustomed to living with people get used to the sound of voices and movements, while those left alone often develop antisocial behaviors. They may become fearful and run from people or, alternatively, they can become overly protective and aggressive. Dogs, like humans, need people around them to learn, to grow, and to be happy. In fact, I feel that many dog owners should actually have become cat owners, because these people are simply away from the house too much for dogs, as opposed to cats, which can remain happily alone for longer periods. But note: Cats need love and contact too. Don't adopt a cat if you are going to treat it like a piece of furniture and ignore it. And if you are going away for any length of time, taking a vacation or going on a business trip perhaps, be sure that you have a qualified person look after your cat or dog.

It is also cruel to leave a dog alone for many hours because the animal may need to relieve itself. Unless the dog is trained to use papers or litter in the house, it may suffer needlessly or lose control of its bladder. This is especially true for puppies, which need to be walked several times a day. Holding in water can also lead to the development of cystitis.

The Taming of the Chew. Up until they are approximately a year-and-a-half, dogs are generally going through a stage when they want to chew on things, especially at night. And puppies will chew on almost anything, so it's important to keep your valuable possessions out of sight, especially items that can cause choking or other dangers. Some items, such as electrical wires, can't be put away, so you have to find ways of preventing your pup from getting hurt.

If you can't corral your pet into a small, safe area, try letting the dog sleep in a travel kennel, the same crate den that helps prevent housebreaking accidents. The plastic type is best because it filters out light and noise and promotes a relaxing sleep. If all you have is a wire cage, cover three sides with a tablecloth or towel. Use this until your animal gets past the chewing stage. You will be promoting safety and comfort.

Then try a twofold approach, using commercially prepared bitter-tasting substances that will discourage chewing on the one hand, and toys that your puppy can freely chew on the other. Put the bitter gel on objects your dog likes to chew but shouldn't, such as the corner of the steps, and plants. (Be sure to buy the right stuff, as different products are designed for different types of objects.) At the same time, make the "do chew" toys available throughout the house, placing two or three in each room. This way you will be teaching your pet not to chew on items you value or that pose dangers, and at the same time you'll have something to offer as soon as Fido feels the need to chew.

This combination method of chew-taming works far better than scolding. All your pet has to do is taste a pair of horrible-tasting shoelaces once or twice and he's going to learn that shoes are no good. (Note: If you don't want Fido to chew on your good dress shoes, you shouldn't let him have any shoes, including toy shoes or old beat-up shoes, to chew on. Dogs can't make those kinds of distinctions, and you'll only confuse him.) If your pet chooses the wrong object to chew on you can show mild disapproval—"No, don't chew on that." Then you follow with something positive—

"Here's your puppy toy"—which keeps your relationship constructive and upbeat.

That Doggone Digging. Sometimes dogs dig holes in the backyard to search for rodents, or as a response to sounds they hear underground, or just for exercise. Some breeds, such as terriers, instinctively dig holes, and these dogs should be given a small sandbox area where they can have the freedom to dig. If a dog is digging holes all over your yard, and you want to discourage it, try the following: Place some dog poop a few inches under the hole made in the wrong place and cover the top with dirt. That way, when the dog starts digging there again it will smell the excrement, which will deter it. At the same time, place little treasures, such as dog biscuits, in the right holes, the ones in the dog's sandbox area. Encourage your pet to dig there with words such as, "Here, dig good holes." If your dog persists in negative behavior, hit the ground a bit to show your great displeasure. Always follow with a positive response, taking your animal back to the desired area and saying in your most inviting tone, "Come, let's dig a good hole." Creating the contrast usually works.

UNDERSTANDING CATS: FELINES JUST WANNA HAVE FUN

Cats sometimes behave in ways that puzzle and upset their owners. These are some common behaviors demonstrated by felines and some thoughts about what these actions mean and what, if anything, you should do about them:

Litter Avoidance. Are you purchasing the very best litter on the market, only to find that your cat is still avoiding the litter box, either some of the time or altogether? Litter avoidance is a common problem, notes Paulette Cooper, author of *277 Secrets Your Cat Wants You to Know*, and there could be several reasons for this behavior. If you own more than one cat—many people own two or more—you should consider having a separate litter box for each one. Cats are very clean animals that want their own toilet space. Also, if you live in a multilevel dwelling, keep a litter box on each floor to make a rest stop more convenient. You also want to be certain that your cat doesn't feel trapped in its box. Cats are skittish and always on the lookout for an escape route. Some cats will refuse to use hooded boxes because they cannot see enough of their surroundings in case the sudden need arises to escape. The box should be placed in an area that allows for an easy escape, too, close to a door, perhaps.

Presenting Dead Animals. To express your love for your cat you feed and care for it, pet and play with it—and what does it do in return? Your animal might just lay a dead bird or mouse at the foot of your door. Lots of people get upset with this behavior, but really you shouldn't. Your cat means well and is really only trying to give you a present. What your cat is saying, in effect, is, "You're my mom [or dad]." So it's a true compliment, really. By the way, when a cat kneads you with a back-and-forth motion of its paws, it's also letting you know that it thinks you are the mother or father.

Boredom and Depression. Cats can get into ruts, especially when they are indoors day after day, the lighting's not so good, the air is not so pure, and there's nothing much to do. They can't read the newspapers, after all. So they primarily sleep and center their waking hours around their caregiver. A bored cat might overeat, but obesity just complicates things by adding the risk of new health challenges. Following are some suggestions to keep your cat happy.

GET FLUFFY A FRIEND. Many cats can learn to love company, especially when their owner is away much of the time and too busy, when home, to give them the quality time they crave. Hence, two or more animals can find solace in each other. Every time they open their eyes there's someone there to lick and snuggle with and sniff and feel bonded to.

There's a right way and a wrong way to introduce a new animal into a household. Your natural inclination might be to fawn over your precious new pet, but this is not a good idea if Kitty Number One is around. Always give the older animal more attention, deferring your affections and loyalty to the other animal, so that the older one doesn't feel threatened or jealous. And it will, if you don't play your cards right. In effect, you have to be somewhat indifferent emotionally to the new arrival so that the older animal does not feel abandoned, or get anxious that there's something new that's going to take its place in your heart. Let the older animal create the bond with the new animal.

So when you bring a new cat into your house you might consider leaving it in the carrier for a short time and not paying it any special attention. Your old cat will walk by, smell the newcomer, and start to become familiar with it. The next step would be to let it out into a different room with a gate in between the two animals. Now they can see as well as sniff each other. Watch their behavior. Watch as their tails wag, as they rub up against the barrier. See if the ears and hair are up or down, showing signs of passive or aggressive behavior. Pretty soon your first cat will feel like the new cat belongs to it, and they should get along fine.

DO LITTLE THINGS TO KEEP YOUR CAT HAPPY. Little things mean a lot, especially to a cat. For instance, cats enjoy watching people and movement, so you might try placing a perch by Fluffy's favorite window so she can comfortably watch the world go by. If you have a terrace or garden, plant something that attracts butterflies and bees. Eyeing the flying insects will keep your cat happily engaged. If your cat goes outside, don't mow the grass too low. Cats enjoy hiding and pouncing, and also eating grass. Another cat-pleaser: Get down to your pet's level when playing with it. We look very large to our companion animals, and cats (as well as dogs) are happiest when we engage with them eye to eye.

CATNIP! OF COURSE! Cats love catnip. The herb releases nervous tension and stress; it causes an initial feeling of excitement and wild play, followed by calm drowsiness. Buy some in a pet store or grow it yourself, being sure to offer the fresh, green stuff, not catnip that is old and yellow or brown. You will want to give your cat approximately one heaping teaspoon weekly. Entice your cats to play by stuffing it in soft toys. And while you're at it, make a good, strong cup of catnip tea for yourself. It can cure insomnia and cramps and is excellent for the digestion and nerves. Don't leave your catnip out where your cats can (and will) steal it. Store catnip in a sealed container in the refrigerator.

WHAT IF YOUR ANIMAL IS TROUBLED?

If you are trying to help a behaviorally or emotionally troubled pet, there is plenty you can do on your own and with the help of an experienced professional. Here is some advice to consider:

Work with a Caring Holistic Professional. Veterinarian William Konrad Kruesi helps troubled animals by making the visit to his office as pleasant as possible for them. "We try to set an example. That means our appointments are long, and we take time so that the patient is not stressed. Some pets have great memories, and they've been hurt at a veterinary hospital. We don't want that. So, if we know it's a behavior case we schedule an appropriate amount of time so that no one is uptight. I mean, I'm scared of dogs that bite, too." During the initial contact, Dr. Kruesi makes sure to conference with owners about their animal's needs since they're the ones ultimately responsibility for helping the animal overcome its behavior challenge. This is different from the conventional veterinary approach, where, by and large, there is more concern with a rapid turnover rate than with the time needed to educate the owner.

One thing Dr. Kruesi discusses is the value of whole foods nutrition for good mental health. Often he advises a dietary change that involves taking the animal off commercial junk foods—foods with a lot of salt, byproducts, and rendered fats—and adding more green vegetables to the dog bowl. "I've never met an aggressive vegetarian," Kruesi notes.

In addition, lab work is done to determine the animal's unique biochemistry. "You can't separate the mind from the body," Kruesi says, stressing that medical reasons, not psychosocial factors, often cause behavior changes. A lab test will determine specifics of nutritional therapy that can make a difference. Perhaps vitamins, minerals, fatty acids, a homeopathic remedy, or a western or Chinese herb will be indicated. Often more "stress nutrients" are needed—B vitamins, magnesium, choline, and inositol.

Next on the agenda is an exploration into the animal's environment and lifestyle. Dr. Kruesi will determine whether the client is living in a new house or an old one, if there are other dogs and cats, and, if so, how many. When did the symptoms start? What time of day do they worsen? Does the animal sleep well? Are there fumes or noises or lights being turned on in the middle of the night that might cause a disturbance? Lastly, the doctor will discuss ways to cope with challenging situations. The animal might need to exercise more. Or some sort of behavior modification program could be used. "There's no magic bullet that I've seen," says Kruesi, who explains that working individually with each pet is what's required.

Consider Homeopathy. Marcie Fallek is a veterinarian who believes in the power of energy medicine to transform misbehaving animals. She cites the case of the overly aggressive dog that was brought to her after it had flunked its police dog test due to too strong a killer instinct. So hostile was the animal that "They had to chain this dog behind a door to keep it from killing anybody." After a few homeopathic treatments, Fallek reports, the animal was much more calm.

If you choose to treat your animal homeopathically, a physician will try to determine the cause of the problem. This could be a lengthy trial and error process, but once the cause and the correct formula are determined, the animal usually improves.

Related to homeopathy is the use of flower essences, which some practitioners assert is a simple way to establish balance in an animal's "personality." Sharon Callahan is an animal communicator who specializes in flower essences, the formulas for which she creates herself. Callahan explains that the essences are made by floating specific flowers on the surface of a bowl of spring water that is left in the sun for three hours. The idea is that, during this time, the vibrational imprint of the flower is transferred to the water, which is then saved and used for the therapeutic products. To purchase ready-to-use flower essences, try your health food store.

In her practice, Callahan initially treats all her animal clients for fear, even if they've been handled with love since infancy. She believes that animals are highly sensitive creatures that can sense the brutal treatment of animals over the centuries. This collective fear must be addressed so animals can live comfortably in the present, Callahan believes. She chooses a remedy called Return to Joy for this purpose.

Use Music Therapy. Fine music has a positive effect on an animal's emotional health, a concept proven by first-place high school science fair winner Dayna Barnett. With the help of her veterinarian father, Barnett was able to show that healthy kenneled dogs exposed to classical music experienced less stress than their counterparts in music-free environments. The study assessed variations in behavior, as well as heart and respiratory rates. The researchers also sent urine samples to a lab for measurements of cortisol, a hormone released in large quantities from the adrenal gland when anxiety is high.

Lab results showed significantly lower levels of cortisol in the experimental group of animals compared to the controls. Clinical observations confirmed these findings: The experimental group did not pant or pace as much. Also, their heart and respiratory rates were slower. These are all indications of the calming effect of classical music. So the next time you need to leave your animal alone for a while, call on Mozart or Vivaldi to "baby-sit" for a portion (but less than several hours) of that time. It's also a good idea to play fine music when your cat, dog, horse, bird, ferret, or other animal is suffering emotionally because of a debilitating disease. It may help the healing process.

TRY TELLINGTON TOUCH

Animals, just like people, have emotional needs. They require daily attention to help them feel a sense of belonging. Otherwise, they may begin to exhibit signs of depression or loneliness. This is especially true for the animal that spends long periods at home alone waiting for its person to return from work. And when the caretaker does get home, there is no guarantee that much time will be spent together. These days life is complicated, and it's easy to get wrapped up in whatever else is demanding our immediate attention—dinner, children, bills, etc. With so much on our minds, we just might ignore the animal sitting quietly in the corner waiting for his or her turn with us.

One of the most attractive features of Tellington Touch, also known as TTouch, is that it can create quality bonding in a short time. Even novices are able to apply its techniques successfully after just a few lessons. A person can spend just a few minutes a day communicating with an animal at a very deep level. (This is not to say, of course, that you should spend only a few minutes a day relating to your pet!)

One of the most appealing aspects of Tellington Touch therapy is that it is mutually beneficial to both recipient and practitioner. Often it is the animal's owner that gives the treatment, and both individuals receive the benefit. The idea behind this modality is that it fosters communication on a cellular level, and when you touch another being at such a basic and intimate level, both of you are affected. You establish a new connection and level of trust with each other.

Doing TTouch on a regular basis will help develop a relationship of trust and cooperation between a human and an animal that can help the animal get through stressful times. Consider a trip to the veterinarian. It is not uncommon for animals to resist these visits ahead of time. Some pets seem to have a psychic knowledge that something undesirable will be happening, and they begin to react even before they are placed in their carrier. Others experience a full-blown panic attack at first sniff of the office, which is only made worse by the scents and sounds of other frightened pets. Then, the examination itself, perhaps consisting of an unknown person poking in untoward places, adds to the anxiety. Such stresses can be alleviated with the regular use of TTouch. Learn to work on the animal's body, particularly special points located around the ear and mouth, and notice the difference at your next veterinary visit. Your pet will probably be more calm and focused.

TTouch is a remarkable therapy that has a wide variety of benefits for an animal's emotional and physical well-being. To learn more about its history and other uses, see Chapter 5.

Get Help From Behavior Specialists. If you are still in need of a course in "Animal Psychology 101" contact a behavior specialist (several holistic animal behavior experts are listed in the appendix) or go to the ASPCA's website, *www.aspca.org*. This site has many suggestions for free or low-cost help. Whether your needs are as simple as needing to know that you should keep your dog in the yard to prevent it from getting lost, or as complex as getting your cat to stop soiling the house, you're sure to find help. There are also TTouch specialists, animal communicators, and flower remedies to try. Your animal's behavior might also warrant a trip to your holistic veterinarian to rule out any physical problems that may be contributing to strange behavior.

Don't give up on your pet! An animal in your charge is your responsibility and you owe your friend the best care possible. Once you learn the proper way to work with your pet, you might just find that resolving behavioral and emotional issues is much easier than you anticipated. Often a little—forgive the pun—horse sense is all that is needed to help humans and animals lead a more harmonious existence. Some problems, of course, will take considerable time and effort to resolve—as example would be helping to undo the effects of severe early life traumas—but with love and persistence, this too is not only possible, but also extremely rewarding for both of you. If you are unwilling or unable to work with your pet's problems and you feel that you must give your pet up, always do so in a humane fashion. There is no need to shorten the life of a healthy, adoptable animal. See, Chapter 9 to read about the options.

NOTES

1. Winter, William G., *The Holistic Veterinary Handbook: Safe, Effective Treatment Plans for the Companion Animal Practitioner*, Galde Press, Lakeville, MN, 1997, p. xvii.

2. Hiby, Lydia, with Bonnie S. Weintraub, *Conversations with Animals: Cherished Messages and Memories as Told by an Animal Communicator*, NewSage Press, Troutdale, OR, 1998, p. 70.

CHAPTER 5

Holistic Vets and Their Tools

A growing number of veterinarians are adding holistic protocols to their conventional repertoire, with the idea that they want to go beyond a mechanistic, quick-fix approach to symptoms and get at the root causes of problems. Dr. Cynthia Lankenau, of Colden, New York, is a veterinarian who became certified in acupuncture, homeopathy, and chiropractic care after years of traditional training. She explains, "Orthodox medicine [was] too limited. Animals weren't getting better.... These other techniques were what I'd been looking for... a way to really cure an animal, to stimulate a deeper healing versus just hiding symptoms." Dr. Lankenau expresses what progressive-thinking veterinarians are beginning to understand, the fact that many diseases are simply not cured by conventional Western medications. This is especially true of chronic diseases, such as arthritis, immune-deficiency diseases, hip dysplasia, and cancer. An acute problem, on the other hand, such as an infection or injury, may indeed respond well to conventional Western medicine, but as pet owners know, many animal problems are not acute, but of the long-term variety. Here, the holistic practitioner's perspective of looking at the whole animal—and not just at discrete symptoms—is a welcome and helpful one.

Actually, most holistic practitioners do not advocate the abandonment of Western therapies, but rather less reliance on one mode of treatment and a greater integration of different systems—what is known as complementary medicine. Surgery may be necessary to remove a fast-growing tumor, for instance, because it buys time, but the operation alone is not a cure. Follow-up with holistic protocols that support immune function is essential. "Complementary medicine looks at what's happening in the body as a whole," says veterinarian Martin Goldstein of South Salem, New York, author of the best-selling *The Nature of Animal Healing: The Path to Your Pet's Health, Happiness, and Longevity.* "It actually looks at the purpose of the condition—like why did the animal develop a cough?—and then works to augment the healing mechanism from within and allow the body to work itself through the symptom. It's like an out-of-tune car with black smoke coming out of the tailpipe. You don't just let a mechanic work on the tailpipe; you have someone tune up the engine."

Animals can benefit remarkably from holistic care, especially when treatments are begun early. It's far easier to reverse a problem that's caught in the beginning stages (or, better yet, to prevent an illness altogether) than to wait until the animal is exhibiting full-blown symptoms. Unfortunately, many pet owners wait until it is almost too late. Most people are looking for a quick fix; they'll use antibiotics for an infection or cortisone for a skin ailment, so that the problem disappears quickly. Only after every other option has been exhausted do they seek holistic care. But at that point their animal has lost a lot of energy, making recovery far more difficult. So beginning treatment of a problem as early as possible is important. Also, pet owners must realize that holistic treatment is a process that takes time. Animals (and people) don't get sick overnight, and one can't expect them to recover immediately either.

Let's look at some of the modalities holistic vets use in treating their animal patients. Keep in mind that each practitioner has her or his own unique mix of favored approaches, so not everyone is going to use, for example, Bach flower remedies. That's one of the reasons why, as soon as you adopt an animal, you should talk to a prospective vet to see if you, that person, and Fido, are going to be a good fit. That said, the first approach we're going to examine—dietary supplementation—is one that *is* used by anyone who's truly holistic.

BEYOND THE FOOD BOWL: DIETARY SUPPLEMENTATION

A prime tenet of holistic medical care, in the case of both animals and people, is that good nutrition is vital to good health. As we discussed on Chapter 1, when an animal relies on the commonly sold commercially prepared foods, it's sure to be deficient or imbalanced in vital enzymes, minerals, and vitamins. Animals fed high-end-of-the-spectrum foods will fare better, but for optimum health, they need extra support too. That's because even the best organic foods are grown in soils that have lost their nutrient strength due to decades of soil depletion. So if you think that all you have to do is feed your animal vitamin/mineral-rich vegetables, think again, advises Howard Peiper, coauthor of *Supernutrition for Animals*, who says it's becoming more and more difficult to get quality foods. Starved for trace minerals, Peiper states, plants will pick up toxic pesticides, fertilizers, and "bad" minerals. An example is aluminum, a toxic material that can cause animals to suffer from a lack of coordination and have memory problems. Birds that eat aluminum will lay eggs with fragile shells. To safeguard your pet's health, then, supplementation with protective vitamins and minerals becomes imperative.

Lisa Newman, a doctor of naturopathy, and the author of several books in the *Natural Pet Care* series (Crossing Press), is one expert who definitely believes in the virtues of supplementation. For dogs and cats, Dr. Newman recommends a balanced multiple vitamin/mineral supplement. Vital vitamins are vitamin A, beta carotene, and the B complex; and the important minerals include calcium, phosphorous, magnesium, potassium, zinc, iodine, and copper. The vitamin A should ideally come from a fish oil source because the body can utilize this most quickly. Make sure that the B vitamin supplement you select contains B complex rather than just one or two isolated B vitamins, like B2 or B12. This is because multiple B vitamins work together to help support the nervous system and tissue regeneration. Calcium is extremely important for bone formation, muscle contraction, blood clotting, and bone strength. Magnesium works with calcium and phosphorus to develop bones. It helps the metabolism, nerves, and energy production at a cellular level. Potassium helps create electrolytes and works hand-in-hand with sodium. (Be sure to check that your multiple-nutrient supplement does contain potassium; many supplements don't contain any at all, and pets need this mineral for heart health.) Copper and zinc work together, with zinc assisting the body in using vitamin A. Zinc also maintains the skin and coat and is needed for the activity of over 100 different enzymes. Newman stresses that getting the right combination of vitamins and minerals is key to the body getting what it needs from each separate nutrient. Dosages will vary with an animal's species, breed, size, age, and condition; therefore, seek professional advice before settling on dosages. To get a general idea of what an animal might need, here is a list of Newman's recommendations for an average 25-pound dog:

> Vitamin A—5000 IU (international units)
> Beta carotene—2500 IU
> B-complex—25 mg (milligrams)
> Calcium—25 mg
> Phosphorous—10 mg
> Magnesium—3 mg
> Potassium—5 mg
> Zinc—7 1/2 mg
> Iodine—50-75 mcg (micrograms)
> Copper—1/8-1/4 mg

Other desirable ingredients in a supplement—ones that are sometimes harder to find—include choline, inositol, biotin, flavonoids (which support vitamin C assimilation), selenium, and chromium. The best idea is to get a good, basic supplement that is recommended by your holistic veterinarian, and adjust as recommended.

If your pet has allergies or arthritis, you will want to increase the amount of vitamin C it is receiving. In fact, says Newman, if you want to start with just one vitamin, make it vitamin C, in whatever dosage your animal can tolerate without developing diarrhea. If your pet has seizures, you will need to increase the B complex. Newman stresses that if you address an animal's specific needs in this way, you won't be overdosing it with unnecessary vitamins. Also, by addressing a specific symptom with a specific nutrient, you're helping to refine your diagnosis; that is, if the nutrient in question doesn't correct the problem, that gives you more information about your pet's real health needs. "The holistic animal-care lifestyle is to give the animal the nutritional foundation to make the changes it needs to make, and then work with more specific supplements to get that information from the pet," Newman explains.

You can purchase vitamin/mineral supplements as powders, liquid extracts, tablets, or capsules. Liquid extracts and powders are the easiest to administer, as they can be mixed into food. Check to see that there are no harmful fillers made from yeast, molasses, salt, sugar, or cellulose. Good fillers—those that are nutritional in themselves—include alfalfa, watercress, parsley, rice, and lecithin. Chlorophyll is desirable also. Make certain, too, that there are no preservatives in the supplement. For a guaranteed analysis of the contents, contact the manufacturer.

Again, be sure to determine—with your holistic vet's help—what your animal needs to stay in balance. Balance is a key concept because you don't want too much or too little of a nutrient, since either extreme can cause harm. While an insufficiency of a vitamin or mineral can cause dire health consequences, the other side of the coin is that excessive amounts of certain nutrients can contribute to a deficiency in others. This is what happened to the wild moose population, including the former star of the once popular *Northern Exposure* television series. Because the moose would graze on pastures that were treated with lime (to counteract the effects of acid rain), it ingested excessive amounts of the trace mineral molybdenum. As a result, the moose developed a copper deficiency, which caused a painful and early demise. Too much vitamin C could do the same thing; overdoing that nutrient could decrease absorption of copper and contribute to a copper deficiency. And note that drugs can also deplete minerals.

If for any reason your pet is not getting enough vitamins or minerals, its body will start operating as if it is depleted—storing whatever calcium, magnesium, or phosphorous, for example, it is receiving in its diet, rather than utilizing it as needed. Stored minerals may turn into stones—creating more health problems. Kidney stones, and even kidney disease, may reverse when you put your animal on a good mineral supplement.

Be Mindful of Minerals. It's a good idea to consider the form a mineral comes in, because that affects its bioavailability. There are three types of minerals you should know about:

COLLOIDAL minerals are too large to be completely absorbed at the cellular level. Only about 65 percent of these minerals will be used.

CHELATED minerals are smaller and therefore more fully absorbed by the body. Between 70 and 75 percent of chelated minerals are absorbed at the cellular level.

CRYSTALLOID minerals are the smallest form. Between 99 and 100 percent are fully absorbed by the system.

Crystalloid solutions are rich in electrolytes that provide vital electrical energy needed to carry out all the body's functions. While supplements can also be purchased in pill, capsule, or powder form, liquid crystalloid solutions generally yield the best results. Author Howard Peiper tells of his own success story with a crystalloid solution: "When my Brittany spaniel was about six she had a grand mal seizure that came out of nowhere. She started convulsing, and we held her down so she wouldn't hurt herself. When she came out of it I filled a turkey baster with the trace mineral electrolyte liquid in concentrated form and put a little on her tongue. She lapped it up and then lapped up the whole syringe, which might have been a tablespoon of liquid. Then she quieted down and went to sleep. We took her to the vet the next day, and they told us we saved her life because the electrolytes helped with her heart."[1]

Skin and coat problems can be a symptom of mineral depletion. Most animals' coats will improve after a four-to-six-week period of improved diet and supplementation. If the coat doesn't improve after about eight weeks, the animal may need more biotin, and a biotin boost for another four weeks will probably improve the condition. Then you can return to a maintenance level. If that doesn't work, the solution might be to look at what's wrong with the supplement you're using. Does it contain poor-quality fillers?

In addition to vitamins and minerals, you may also wish to supplement your animal's diet with digestive enzymes. Enzymes are essential to good health, but they're missing in cooked and packaged foods. That's because enzymes are destroyed when temperatures rise above 118 degrees. When not enough enzymes are eaten the body begins to rely on enzyme reserves that are stored in the pancreas. After awhile, though, the pancreas becomes depleted and loses its ability to make enzymes. That's when degenerative diseases set in. Fortunately, digestive enzymes can be taken to reverse the effects of many diseases. Two good sources are the products Vetzyme and Prozyme.

LIVE ENZYME THERAPY

Some holistic animal care experts are very strong advocates of enzymes as important health requisites. One of them is Susan Goldstein, editor of *For the Love of Animals* newsletter. "Enzymes are life force," Goldstein says, explaining that she realized this unexpectedly when she began giving carrot juice to her arthritic dog and saw him respond quickly, whereas conventional treatments had not been working.

Goldstein emphasizes that enzymes are bioactive ingredients in naturally occurring foods, and likens them to "spark plugs for the body." They are molecules that facilitate the chemical reactions that keep the body running smoothly. All living creatures need enzymes for healthy functioning, and a problem of modern life is that cooking food depletes it of enzymes. Domesticated animals are particularly at risk for enzyme depletion because they generally eat heavily processed and overcooked pet foods. Companion animals that eat strictly out of the bag or can are going to lack sufficient enzymes. Conversely, re-introducing enzymes into an animal's diet will re-energize that animal quickly and dramatically.

As facilitators, enzymes help the body do things it needs to do to stay healthy and function properly. Some enzymes aid digestion, some are metabolic facilitators—they help make sure nutrients are properly transported and utilized, and some are antioxidant enzymes, meaning they help the body fight against damaging free radicals.

Without enzymes, an animal can't properly digest and use its food. Older animals are particularly at risk since the pancreas is less able to pump out digestive enzymes to make up for any deficiency. When digestive enzymes are missing, metabolic and antioxidant enzymes, as well as minerals, are used to support the digestive process. This can be problematic. With antioxidant enzymes diverted, free radicals are given free reign, and you are putting your animal's immune system at risk.

An enzyme-live diet may produce seeming miracles. An arthritic dog, or a dog with hip dysplasia may recover fully because now the animal is able to make use of all the food nutrients its body is receiving. Obesity, a common problem in companion animals today, is not always the result of eating too much food; it can also be caused by eating the wrong kinds of food—that is, not enough raw, enzyme-rich food. Certified raw milk, for instance, contains a lot of butterfat, but it's also high in digestive enzymes that help to fully utilize the fat. Thus, an animal drinking the product is likely to stay at the proper weight.

You needn't add much raw food to your animal's diet. A small amount of grated or blended fruits or vegetables added to your animal's regular food will give it a good enzyme boost. And if you juice, you'll be doing even more to provide life-promoting enzymes to your pet.

Juicing: A Great Source of Enzymes—and More. Juicing is one of the most effective forms of live enzyme therapy. In animals, as in humans, juices can be effective against such chronic, bothersome ailments as allergies and urinary tract problems. They can help restore harmony to an animal plagued by arthritis or even cancer, as well as to the pet that's been over-subjected to vaccines or drugs. They will also help your pet control weight, maintain dental health, and have a healthy, shiny coat. A freshly made juice mixture incorporating a small amount of a green vegetable juice is very good for stopping parasites, boosting the immune system, and promoting healthier skin in both cats and dogs. In short, giving your animal juice can be beneficial on many, many fronts, not only because of the enzymes readily available in juice but because of its healing phytochemicals (plant chemicals) as well.

A mixture of asparagus, carrot, kale, parsley, and apple juices is good for allergies. For arthritis, celery, carrot, apple, and parsley is a helpful combination. Any juice recipe should have a base of apple and carrot for flavoring. The other ingredients can be modified, depending on what you're treating your animal for. Once you have blended an appropriate juice, you can simply mix it with the animal's water supply, or add it to your pet's regular food.

Start out with very small doses, especially of potent green juices, to give your animal's body time to adjust to this change in diet, especially if the animal is only used to commercial pet food and tap water. Remember, also, that juicing organic produce is always preferable, and that when this is not an option, removing the peel will eliminate most toxic residues.

Placing your pet on a once-a-week juice fast will help cleanse its body and give the digestive tract a helpful rest. Don't do a juice fast on a young animal or an elderly one, but for pets in their prime, you can skip a meal for 12 hours and give them juices instead. To help speed up a pet's metabolism, add small amounts of organic apple cider vinegar to its drinking water.

If your pet's main food source is processed pet foods, no matter how high-end the food is, it's essential that you add live enzymes, in the form of juice, or blended or chopped fresh fruits and vegetables, to that the animal's daily food regimen. If your pet is not initially receptive to juices, fresh fruits, or vegetables, try mixing the juice or live food into something the animal likes, such as Rice Dream ice cream. Or you could fill a dropper with juice and put it down the animal's throat. There are also powdered enzymes available, such as Vetzyme or Prozyme. "Never, ever just put down a bowl of food without adding some life force to it," advises Susan Goldstein. Remember that your animal needs fresh food every day, just as you do."[2]

HERBAL THERAPY

Herbs are nature's gift to us for healing, and they can help our animal friends too. The important thing to remember when giving herbs to animals is to work with a qualified professional who understands their benefits and limitations. Your veterinarian should be knowledgeable about the following aspects of herbal therapy:

SAFETY. We tend to think of herbs as natural, and therefore safe, but some herbs, like medicines, can be harmful if taken improperly. For example, pennyroyal is an excellent insect repellent when small quantities are applied to the coat, but very little should be used to avoid toxic effects. The herbs your veterinarian recommends should be individualized to your animal's needs and you should receive clear instructions on how to give them.

QUALITY. Some brands of an herb may be cheaper than others, but they may also be of an inferior quality and therefore a waste of your money. Often it is better to spend a little more for a better brand. Your holistic vet should be ordering products from a reputable company, one that sells standardized herbals to physicians only.

EFFICACY. Some herbs lose their effectiveness if they're taken for too long a time. Echinacea, for instance, is best given for a few days only, and then, once the body has rested, it can be given again if necessary. Also, some medicinal herbs, such as goldenseal, may create an imbalance of certain nutrients when taken for too long a time.

The herbs your veterinarian recommends will be individualized to your animal's needs. They could include pau d'arco for a compromised immune system. This South American herb strengthens the body's disease-fighting mechanisms and is a useful adjunct to other therapies in the treatment of cancer, auto-immune diseases, and chronic infections. Bilberry, eyebright, gingko, and goldenseal could help to correct eye problems by improving circulation to the area. To aid in the removal of parasites, wormwood may be the herbal remedy of choice.

The easiest and best way to give herbs to an animal is to add a few drops of the liquid tincture to your animal's food or water.

HOMEOPATHY

Homeopathy, developed by German physician Samuel Hahnemann (1755-1843), is based on the belief that there are basic vibrational patterns of disease, known as miasms, that start in the energy field surrounding an organism. Miasms can be inherited or acquired, and can remain dormant until some stressful circumstance sets them off. At such a time, the organism will react to the energy imbalance, or disease, by attempting to restore balance. In the process, symptoms will develop. The homeopath, then, doesn't think of symptoms as illness, but rather as the body's reaction to an imbalance that can be used to determine a treatment for restoring balance, and, ultimately, health. It's this premise that prompted homeopathic physician James T. Kent to advise, more than 100 years ago, "Do not say that the patient is sick because he has a white swelling, but that the white swelling is there because the patient is sick."

GARY NULL

90

In the homeopath's view, allopathic medicine's goal of suppressing symptoms only drives the symptoms deeper or shifts the problem somewhere else. In time, another, more serious illness is likely to appear, or the same disease may return, but with a stronger vengeance. Often the new problem manifests as a chronic disease. For example, irritable bowel syndrome, when treated with cortisone and antibiotics, might return several years later in the form of colon cancer. So instead of this suppressive, one-thing-at-a-time approach to treating illness, holistic medicine in general—and homeopathy as part of that paradigm—takes a curative approach based on the principle of treating a whole, living organism.

Homeopathy is a form of "energetic medicine," explains Dr. Charles Loops, a homeopathic veterinarian with over 20 years of experience. The therapy works on the principle that "like cures like." In other words, any substance that can produce a symptom in a healthy human or animal can also cure it when that substance is given in a subtler form. "The principle of homeopathy is to match the characteristics of the substance to the characteristics of an imbalance or an illness in an individual person or animal," explains Dr. Loops. The right homeopathic remedy will create a "resonance" that will positively interact with the resonance of the patient's body. This will correct the underlying imbalance, and correcting that imbalance will bring the person or animal back to normalcy.

Before prescribing any homeopathic remedy, a classically trained homeopathic veterinarian will conduct a thorough intake exam with an owner, either in person or over the phone. Age, weight, and breed of the animal are of course some of the basic information required by the practitioner. Then the owner describes in detail the symptoms his or her pet is showing. For example, if it's an ear infection, what does the discharge looks like from the ear, and what is the character of the discharge? Is it sticky? Is it yellow? Is it mucous? But basic information and presenting symptoms are only the beginning of this exam, which can take up to half an hour to complete. The practitioner will go on to ask questions about the animal's emotional state, its temperament, level of sociability, habits, fears (such as of thunderstorms or fireworks—extremely common in dogs), sleep patterns, and other characteristics. Then a thorough history is required. Are there any previous medical problems that may point to a chronic condition? What sort of diet is the animal on? How much does it like to drink? What is its vaccination history? Does it prefer warm or cool temperatures, indoors or out-doors? And there's even more—the vet will want to know about the household where the pet lives: Are there other animals? Children? Is it an apartment? A house? With a yard? And what's going on with the humans in the household? Is there an inordinate amount of stress in the home? In short, the practitioner looks at the total symp-tomatology of the patient, as well as the animal's life history, to understand a pattern of illness that begins when the animal is a puppy or kitten and continues into adulthood. Ideally, all of this information is obtained with the animal present in order to get a fuller assessment of character plus a complete physical exam before any recommendations are made, although some practitioners say that obtaining information via phone is satisfactory.

Once the veterinarian gets a complete picture of the physical and psychological makeup of the animal, a remedy is chosen. If arthritis is the presenting symptom, the homeopath may choose among Aconite, Bryonia, Belladonna, Cimicifugia, Rhus tox, or Pulsatilla. For a bladder irritation, the choices might include Belladonna once more, or Cantharis, Shaphasgria, Thuja, Aconite, or Apis. A nervous condition might respond to Ignatia, Gelsemium, or Chamomilla. Again, the right remedy depends on the total pic-ture of the animal, for what appears to be one disease may actually be somewhat different in different animals.

Homeopathic remedies are optimally effective when they're part of a total health program. They should be supported by a good diet for the animal and supplemented with minerals and vitamins. And don't overload your pet with calories when it needs maximum ener-gy for healing. The body working to digest extra calories can deplete energy from the essential task. Feed your pet only what it needs.

Homeopathy can be supported with conventional medical diag-nostic practices. In many cases, such as suspected liver, kidney, or metabolic dysfunctions, you can help your homeopathic veterinari-an by having lab work done on your animal ahead of time to help formulate a thorough and correct diagnosis. The opposite is also true: Homeopathic medicine can be used to support conventional medicines. For example, holistic veterinarians often recommend the remedy Thuja occidentalis after a vaccination to detoxify the system and thus eliminate adverse side effects.

Homeopathy is generally considered a safe system of medicine, but it should be prescribed by a trained professional when your pet is faced with chronic conditions, such as allergies or intestinal problems. Even with the proper remedy, a slight reaction could occur. Sometimes these reactions are useful; they prompt the self-healing process to begin. In many situations, side effects known as "aggravations" can actually support the healing process. For example, if your pet sleeps more, or has mild diarrhea following a treatment, this may aid in its recovery. You should note that if you buy an over-the-counter prescription to administer for a chronic disease, you run the risk of choosing the wrong remedy, one that is either inappropriate or helpful for treating only part of the symptoms. Also, lay people tend to rely on homeopathic remedies for too long. In a sensitive animal, this can cause "provings," the appearance of symptoms from a condition you are trying to treat. If, for example, you are administering the remedy Rhus tox for poison ivy, and you give it repeatedly, you might eventually elicit symptoms of poison ivy. Additionally, repeating the remedy too frequently can overstimulate the body. Homeopathy should be given short-term, just long enough to elicit a reaction so that the body can heal itself. If you're repeating a remedy over and over, you can eventually exhaust the vital force, the energy needed for self-healing. For the treatment of any chronic condition, then, seek a qualified homeopathic veterinarian who has received training and certification from a reputable organization. If you are looking for homeopathic help for your pet, get a recommendation from someone you trust, or contact one of the organizations listed in the appendix.

For acute conditions, as opposed to chronic ones, administering your own store-bought medications is simpler. Often, one homeopathic remedy is indicated for an acute condition, and you will have far greater success achieving the results you want. An emergency treatment you give may even be lifesaving. Just be sure to follow up with a visit to an animal hospital or veterinarian. Following is a look at some homeopathic remedies and the scenarios in which they might be used. Note that the key to administering doses of these is to have the remedy come into contact with the animal's gum, but not with the owner's hands. Usually, you can get a powder into the animal's mouth, and on its gums, by pouring a crushed pellet onto a small, folded index card and then onto the animal's gums. Or a liquid form of the remedy can be dropped onto the gums via eyedropper or syringe. If an animal is unusually aggressive or noncooperative, mixing the remedy in with food is a last-gasp measure. The animal will still get benefits, but the effect will not be optimal.

Arnica. Keep this homeopathic remedy in your first-aid kit because one of Arnica's most important uses is relief from trauma. This medicine can help an animal recover from shock if, for example, it has been hit by a car. It will help to stop hemorrhaging, restore circulation, and prevent further shock. Veterinarian Michael Dym of Mt. Laurel, New Jersey, praises the efficacy of this medicine: "I've treated some animals that were almost dead. In the vast majority of cases, [I'll] see the animal's gums pink up in a matter of seconds, even before I have a chance to put in an IV line. I'll put the animal back in a cage and I'll go look at it when I have a break between appointments. The animal will be sitting up and wagging its tail, ready to go home sometimes. It works that fast." Arnica also helps reduce swellings and bruises quickly, and can help an animal get over the fear of being touched after the shock of an injury. After administering Arnica for a serious injury, you should, of course, consult your holistic veterinarian right away.

Hypericum. Homeopathic hypericum (better known as St. Johnswort) is referred to as the Arnica of the nerves. In can relieve suffering from injuries involving neurological tissue, be it the tail, the digits, or the spine. If your animal gets its tail caught in a door or tears a toenail, an extremely painful injury, use Hypericum to dramatically reduce pain in a short period. Hypericum is also used for puncture wounds and lacerations, especially if the wound is painful and sensitive to touch.

Arsenicum. If your animal ate bad food and is showing signs of food poisoning, such as vomiting and diarrhea, Arsenicum album may be an excellent remedy.

Belladonna. This one is helpful in the summertime to relieve conditions of overheating, such as heatstroke or sunburn. Some people forget that extreme temperatures are just as harmful for animals as they are for people—in some cases even more so. Dogs, for example, may get overheated in temperatures that are comfortable for humans. An overheated animal can show such symptoms as vomiting, panting, and seizures. Of course, you want to prevent this from happening in the first place, but should your animal get heatstroke, reach for the belladonna.

Calendula. For a wound or laceration, the topical remedy of choice is Calendula, because of its antiseptic and healing properties. Placed on the injured area every few hours, the gel helps the wound close quickly and heal well.

BACH FLOWER REMEDIES

Restoring harmony between body and soul is the goal of flower essence therapy, a system of healing developed by Dr. Edward Bach (1886-1936) nearly a century ago in his native England. Bach professed that unless the underlying reasons for a disease were addressed, any treatment of physical symptoms alone could only be temporary. In other words, Bach, like Hahnemann before him, believed that the cause of the disease, rather than its effects, should be treated. His idea was that flower essence therapy could correct negative emotional or character traits, and that that in turn would help by promoting recovery from a corresponding physical illness, or by preventing the illness from manifesting at all.

Today, proponents of flower therapy assert that it works not only for humans but for our sensitive animal friends as well, and that it has proven itself to be especially effective for behavioral and psychological conditions, such as anxiety, depression, or aggression. The nervousness accompanying a trip to the vet and the fright brought on by a loud thunderstorm are examples of sudden emotional states that proponents say can be alleviated by this modality. Flower remedies, they say, can also help an animal during times of grief, when a beloved owner or animal friend in the household has died, easing the pet through this transitional time.

Bach's therapy involves preparations made from 38 different flowers from wild plants and trees. Each particular Bach flower remedy has certain characteristics that are given for specific emotional problems; Bach stated that these 38 essences embrace all the fundamental negative emotional conditions that can be treated. A few drops can be placed in the animal's drinking water, or the remedy can be diluted with spring or distilled water, placed in a spray bottle, and misted onto the animal. The diluted essence can also be massaged into acupuncture points.

Although Bach considered his system complete, since his time, companies have developed their own lines of remedies. In the 1970s the California Flower Essences were developed, for example, and in the 1980s the Australian Bush Flower Essences were created drawing upon the traditional knowledge of Australian Aborigines. Still, though, Bach's flower essences are the most well known and the easiest to obtain. Here therefore, is a look at the different Bach flower remedies, and at how practitioners of this modality say they should be used. Some important notes: While flower remedies may sometimes be all that your pet needs, it's important to consult your holistic veterinarian if any symptom persists for more than a few days, as emotional problems can be precipitated by physical causes, such as tumors or central nervous system disorders. Also, see a veterinarian after treating an animal for any emergency. In these instances, think of flower remedies as an adjunct to your animal's health protocol. Finally, for "problem" or unhappy pets, experts in animal behavior can sometimes do wonders; call your vet's office for recommendations.

Rescue Remedy. This emergency formula is the most famous of the Bach flower remedies. It's composed of five flower essences—Impatiens, Clematis, Rock Rose, Cherry Plum, and Star of Bethlehem—and is said to calm an animal in any fear-provoking situation. Promoted as a safe alternative to tranquilizers, Rescue Remedy can be used after an accident, convulsions, or anesthesia, or any time there is a shock to the system. If an animal is hit by a car, Rescue Remedy should be given immediately and continued during emergency-room treatment to reduce shock and stress. It can be administered orally, placed on the temples, or mixed with water and sprayed onto a terror-stricken animal to promote calm.

Agrimony. This one is for animals that hide their suffering. Proponents say that if you suspect your animal is in pain—perhaps through glimpsing a pained look in the eyes, an ill-at-ease appearance, a physical symptom, such as a skin irritation or digestive ailment, or inappropriate behavior, such as urination or defecation in the wrong place, the flower essence Agrimony may restore inner peace.

Aspen. This remedy is said to quiet fear if the source of apprehension is unknown. These edgy animals are sometimes born with an anxious character. Aspen may help with house-training in animals that are afraid to leave the house.

Beech. This flower essence may restore tolerance and flexibility to touchy animals easily annoyed at changes in routine or environment. These arrogant animals do not like other animals near them. Their rigid natures can lead to arthritic disorders and allergies.

Centaury. The insecure animal that constantly follows its owner may be helped by this remedy. These overly submissive animals are low in the pecking order and easily taken advantage of by other animals in the household. They tire easily, have a low resistance to infection, and remain weak after an illness. Centaury is reputed to restore assertiveness and resistance.

Cerato. This one is said to help immature animals that display a lack of confidence and initiative. If your animal is overly dependent, and always looking to you for approval before taking any action, Cerato might be the remedy of choice.

Cherry Plum. This remedy is given to animals that are nervous or fearful to the point of hysteria. They may demonstrate extreme fight-or-flight behaviors such as attacking people, hurting themselves, or desperately seeking to escape even if that means breaking through a window. Such animals could also be reacting to food additives, so pay close attention to the ingredients in the animal's diet.

Chestnut Bud. Animals that repeatedly make the same mistakes are said to be helped by Chestnut Bud. You might try this one if your cat frequently urinates outside of its litter box or if your dog continually makes the same mistakes during house-training.

Chicory. Some animals are desperate for constant attention; they may bark incessantly or even vomit to keep their owners from leaving. These are animals that experience severe separation anxiety in their owner's absence, or they may be clinging moms that refuse to wean their young. Bach flower advocates recommend Chicory to eliminate such attention-seeking behaviors and to restore your companion animal's normal sense of loving and caring.

Clematis. For animals that need to focus, Clematis is given. These animals appear spacey or bored, uninterested, or lazy. This one is also used if an animal has experienced a shock and its body feels cold to the touch. Clematis restores concentration and may revitalize elderly animals with memory problems.

Crab Apple. This remedy is used to restore dignity to an animal that has been suffering from diarrhea, incontinence, or kidney disease. It may assist a diabetic animal with weight loss and aid in the removal of foreign bodies, such as parasites or splinters. If an elderly animal is depressed because it can no longer groom itself, Crab Apple is indicated. Dogs with mange or badly matted coats are given the remedy too.

Elm. To help an animal that feels overwhelmed by its circumstances, elm is sometimes given. Perhaps its owner is difficult. Or perhaps the demands of motherhood are too much, or its work is too demanding, as in the case of some police dogs or racehorses, or too much is expected during training, or the animal must adhere to the same rigid routine daily. These animals may also tend to feel overwhelmed by illness and develop stress allergies. Elm may help restore a sense of proficiency and increase resistance. People who work with these animals should consider taking the remedy, too, as these animals mimic the problems of the people in their environment.

Gentian. This is given as a remedy for discouragement. These animals do not get enough praise from their handlers during training, performance, or competition, or they become discouraged following a domestic dispute. Gentian is for animals that, after living in a house, find themselves caged in a shelter or kennel. Or they've lost an owner or companion animal friend with whom they've grown up. These animals tend to stop eating, become sluggish, and sleep too much. Gentian helps animals to persevere.

Gorse. This one is given to restore perseverance and vitality in the utterly despondent animal that has given up all hope. It's for the mother that has lost her offspring, for animals that must remain for long periods of time in shelters, and for any animal that has lost heart. Gorse is given to alleviate symptoms that are more extreme than symptoms remedied by Gentian; the two could be taken together during the treatment of animals with terminal illnesses.

Heather. To help noisy or destructive, attention-seeking animals, try Heather, Bach flower advocates say. It's for the cat that always purrs or meows, the dog that incessantly barks for attention, or the horse that, left alone, bangs into the stable. This remedy is also recommended for animals that refuse to follow their owner's commands.

Holly. This is advocated as a help for bad-tempered animals that need to become more tolerant. These animals may have specific dislikes, such as postmen or the veterinarian, or they may not get along with other members of the pack. They tend to get intensely ill with such conditions as asthma, high fevers, and severe allergies.

Honeysuckle. For the animal that has difficulty adjusting to new situations, Honeysuckle is the Bach flower remedy of choice. The animal doesn't like vacationing with its owner or being boarded. It may long for its former owner, whether or not that person has died. The animal pines for a return to how things used to be and may become depressed, weak, or ill. Honeysuckle is said to be a cure for homesickness, and so it's given to animals newly entering the home.

Hornbeam. This remedy is said to restore vitality to weak animals. It's indicated for sick animals whose symptoms worsen in the morning and improve during the day, for animals with cancer, and for animals that need an energy boost following a bout with illness. If an animal is required to change its schedule and shift from inactivity to work—say its owner works during the week and crams most of the animal's activity into the weekend—Hornbeam could help the animal make smoother adjustments.

Impatiens. This is given, as its name suggests, as a treatment for impatience and irritability. These animals are excitable to the point of being hyperactive. They are tense, edgy, and thin, and they and don't always cooperate with their owners. Impatiens may also be used as an adjunct therapy for muscle cramps, skin disorders, pain caused by muscular tension, and digestive problems, including irritable bowel syndrome, vomiting, and colic.

Larch. This remedy is supposed to be for any animal with feelings of inferiority. So Larch might be given to the cat in the multi-cat household that is dominated by the others, or to the stray animal that has been traumatized. It's given to submissive dogs and horses afraid to jump fences. These animals may have a low resistance to illness. Larch is said to help restore confidence and the willingness to try.

Mimulus. To restore courage in animals with a fear of the unknown, this Bach remedy is given. Such animals are afraid of thunderstorms, vacuum cleaners, veterinarians, other animals, and traveling in cars, among other things. They express their fear by becoming nervous and restless, and may whine, position their ears back, shiver, or become rigid. Mimulus is also used for heart disorders. In addition, Bach proponents report, this compound can help people overcome their fear of animals.

Mustard. This is for an animal that becomes depressed for no apparent reason. The animal may lose its energy, not make eye contact, and hang its head. Of course you should keep in mind that it is rare for animals to become downcast for no reason at all, and that such a sudden change of character might be the result of a serious underlying disease. It is, therefore, important to consult your veterinarian.

Oak. To provide resiliency and restores endurance to once-courageous animals, Oak is given by Bach flower enthusiasts. The animal may keep going despite exhaustion or the infirmities of old age. Oak is said to combine well with the next remedy, Olive.

Olive. This one is used in cases of complete physical and mental fatigue. Exhaustion might be a result of anemia, seizures, long-standing illnesses, or surgery. This remedy is also for animals born weak, for geriatric animals that need to be rejuvenated, and for animals that were lost and forced to care for themselves.

Pine. This one is said to remedy guilt, and while it is debatable whether an animal actually experiences this emotion, the Pine Bach remedy is also said to help owners troubled by their own feelings of having made poor decisions about their pets.

Red Chestnut. For the animal that seems to worry excessively about others, Red Chestnut is said to be of help. The animal is overprotective of its young and puts off weaning them, or is over-concerned about its owners. Sometimes this trait is picked up from the owner, in which case the person may benefit from Red Chestnut too. This product is often combined with other remedies for fear, such as Aspen and Mimulus.

Rock Rose. One of the ingredients found in Rescue Remedy, Rock Rose is used to calm extreme fear and panic. The terrorized animal shakes and feels cold, and may be a danger to itself and others. The animal may fear open spaces and stay indoors. The remedy also helps where an animal has become sick from sunstroke or heatstroke. Rock Rose helps restore calm and courage.

Rock Water. This refers to water from a spring or to water known for having healing powers. Bach flower advocates say that this substance replaces a fixed temperament with a flexible one and helps to soften dominant or stubborn behavior. Also, animals stressed by changes in routine are said to benefit, as are arthritic animals. Rock Water is said, too, to help animals that neglect themselves take better care of their own needs.

Star of Bethlehem. This is given as an antidote for shock accompanied by great physical or emotional pain. It could be administered after a traffic accident, for example, or if the animal has been caught in a trap. The remedy is also useful for the treatment of a birth trauma or for a mother animal's shock after losing her babies during or shortly after birth. It is indicated for any enduring trauma when the animal has been neglected or abused. In such instances, Star of

Bethlehem may be needed for a longer period. Animals that become unconscious due to trauma can be brought back into consciousness, it is reported, when Star of Bethlehem is applied to their temples, nose, or gums. As we've said, Bach flower remedies should be seen as adjuncts to—not replacements for—emergency veterinary care.

Sweet Chestnut. This is used to treat intense mental torment after an animal has reached the limits of what it can endure and is ready to give up. The animal may have lived in an environment where it was cruelly mistreated or neglected. Or the animal may feel hopeless after a long bout with sickness. Sweet Chestnut is also used for animals that mutilate themselves, and for animals forcibly confined. It may also be of use to animals plagued by severe chronic illnesses or intense psychological problems, as well as animals suffering from colic or bloating. Sweet Chestnut may restore an animal's ability to strive and move forward.

Vervain. To restore control to an impulsive animal, vervain is sometimes given. This remedy is for high-strung types that never relax but are always on the go. Extremely nervous and hyperactive, they may push people out of the way. Vervain and Chestnut Bud are sometimes prescribed together in the treatment of compulsive behaviors.

Vine. This flower essence is given to the overly dominant and aggressive animal that frightens other animals and humans. The animal has extreme guarding behaviors, watching its territory to the point of not letting others near its space or possessions. Vine softens these bullies, so that their positive natural leadership qualities can shine through. Be sure to check with a holistic veterinarian to see that a central nervous system disorder or other infirmity is not the underlying problem.

Walnut. This remedy is said to ease adjustment to changes, small and great. It's for animals after a move to a new environment or a change in the present one, such as new furniture, a different diet, new people in the household, or the loss of someone familiar. If the animal has lost a part of its body or some physical function, Walnut may be of use. Walnut will help the animal that must endure a long journey or hospital stay and is sometimes given before and after anesthesia. It's also for females going through their initial period of heat, for pregnancy, neutering, teething, or weaning. Walnut, it is said, should be given to an animal about to be euthanized.

Water Violet. Proponents say that Water Violet helps to socialize an indifferent animal. While some breeds are naturally more aloof than others, individuals that seem unusually distant may begin to make more social contact with their owners and others in their environment after taking this remedy. Water Violet may help in the handling and socialization of feral cats and dogs socialized late in life. It may also help animals that withdraw when they are sick. Often, animals need time alone for healing, so a few drops of Water Violet can be added to the animal's water to gently assist in the healing process. Combined with Crab Apple, Water Violet can aid in the elimination of foreign bodies from the eyes, ears, or skin.

White Chestnut. This is used as a remedy for the restless pet that doesn't sleep well and exhibits agitated behaviors when awake. It's for the female that is restless when giving birth and that is always moving her young. White Chestnut may also remedy nervous behaviors that manifest as chronic skin problems, such as when dogs left alone get in the habit of licking or scratching themselves because of boredom or stress. Naturally you would also want to give such a dog additional stimulation and company.

Wild Oat. People use this one with the intention of restoring purpose in an animal that vacillates from lack of direction. The animal may be reacting to an owner who treats it as a show or work animal part of the time and as a pet at other times. Or the animal—an ex-racehorse, for example—may be retired from its former occupation. It is said that Wild Oat can also help animals that are not living up to their potential.

Wild Rose. This remedy may restore the will to live in an animal that has all but given up. The animal may have been abandoned to a shelter or captured and placed in a zoo. The animal is depressed and apathetic; it acts indifferent to its surroundings, and has no appetite. Wild Rose is also for critically ill animals that are cold to the touch.

Willow. This remedy is given to restore a good temper to a bad-natured animal. The animal may appear to be acting out of spite by urinating on the owner's bed or by destroying things. What appears to be spitefulness, may, in fact, be the animal's reaction to stress or a perceived need to mark territory. Again, we should note that intractable pet behavior problems can sometimes be markedly helped by an animal behaviorist.

TRADITIONAL CHINESE MEDICINE

We in the Western world have been taught to picture medicine in military terms, so we speak of a battle against germs or a war on disease, to be fought with a pharmaceutical arsenal or magic bullets. The traditional Chinese medical model, by contrast, is not combat-centered; it focuses instead upon the concepts of energy and balance. Traditional Chinese medicine (TCM) is all about keeping balance between a person or animal's heavy, cool, moist, "yin" energy, and the light, dry, active, "yang" energy. It is in cases of chronic conditions that approaches offered by TCM may be most beneficial. Sometimes there are no cures for the illness, but treating it from this different perspective can boost the body's own healing capacity, helping your pet live a more comfortable, satisfying life.

One advantage of Chinese medicine, from a holistic point of view, is that it allows the practitioner to understand how seemingly unrelated symptoms may in fact have a common underlying cause. A problem with Western medicine is that it tends to look at problems in isolation, ignoring the fact that disparate symptoms may come from the same source. Chinese medicine considers five elements—earth, water, wood, metal, and fire—and believes that each element relates to one organ, or a number of organs. Thus problems in different organs may actually be linked through one element. Each element is associated with a yin organ (the dense organ) and a yang organ (the lighter, ethereal organ) so that your dog, for example, may have a persistent hacking cough and be constipated at the same time. A Western-oriented vet would look at these two symptoms as unrelated and treat them independently of one another. But a vet familiar with Chinese medicine would recognize that the symptoms are related through the element of metal (the yin is the lung, and the yang is the large intestine in the metal element), and treat them accordingly.

A TCM treatment will begin with a comprehensive diagnosis. Diagnostic techniques may include listening to the pulse, looking at the tongue, getting a history of the animal's symptoms from its owner, and palpation. The quality of the pulse—whether it is weak or strong, among other characteristics—and the color of the tongue—its redness or pale tone—say something about what is going on inside the internal organs. Learning about the animal's history will give further insight. The owner may be asked such questions as, When does your animal feel worse? Better? Does he prefer hot or cold, or wet or dry areas? The TCM practitioner may then palpate the animal in search of weak areas. All of these assessments help uncover the source of disharmony. The practitioner will then attempt to restore balance to those areas through one or more modalities, such as acupuncture or herbs.

Chinese Herbal Medicine. A lot of Chinese medicine relies on herbal remedies, based on prescription recipes developed by Chinese doctors in ancient times, handed down through thousands of years, and still very much in use today. Different recipes contain combinations of herbs in various proportions, and each formula has its own name. A preparation may have as many as 20 different ingredients that have been found to work better in a particular combination than alone.

Two basic ingredients for the treatment of cancer are astragalus and maitake mushroom extract. Both of these are immune boosters, helping the animal utilize its own immune system to fight cancer more effectively. Astragalus, for one, increases the white blood cells and natural interferon in your pet's system. This is in opposition to Western cancer treatments, which wear down the patient's immune system with an onslaught of drugs intended to kill the cancer.

Acupuncture. Practiced for thousands of years in the Orient, acupuncture first gained popularity in the United States after former President Nixon returned home from his historic visit to China in the 1970s. Since then, Western society has become increasingly comfortable with needles, as evidenced by the reimbursement of acupuncture treatments by major health insurance companies. Acupuncture is also commonly a treatment of choice for animals that are suffering from arthritis, injury, and most any painful condition. Many qualified veterinarians have received their acupuncture training and certification through the International Veterinary Acupuncture Society.

When you think of acupuncture, you probably think of dry needles being placed at certain points throughout the body. While this is the traditional way of administering treatment, and one commonly used, there are actually several ways to stimulate acupuncture points.

GOLD BEAD THERAPY. Although it's a relatively new procedure, gold beading is quickly gaining popularity in animal health care because it can effect seemingly miraculous changes. Proponents say that gold bead therapy is practically a fountain of youth for some aged, debilitated pets. After this therapy, a lame animal can often walk with ease—and sometimes, advocates claim, even jump for joy! A veterinarian trained in the technique will permanently implant electroplated 14-karat gold beads over specific acupuncture points, which will stimulate the body's healing energy.

DRY NEEDLE ACUPUNCTURE. This is the classic, centuries-old method to effect healing. Surprisingly, many animals (although not all) take to acupuncture needles—the therapy relaxes them. One recent diagnostic technique, called hara diagnosing and developed by Japanese acupuncturists, looks at eight specific abdominal points called the eight extraordinary meridians, and treats these meridians with dry needles to bring about dramatic, sometimes instantaneous improvements.

ELECTRICAL ACUPUNCTURE. Acupuncture points can be electrically stimulated; however, unless a practitioner is attempting to reverse a severe problem, such as paralysis, this is probably not the treatment of choice. This is because the body's natural energy is subtle and may be overpowered by the electrical stimulation devices in use today.

ACUPUNCTURE WITH VITAMIN B12. In a combination of Eastern and Western approaches, some practitioners will add vitamin B12 to needles before inserting them into acupuncture points. However, at this time it is uncertain what effect the B12 has once it is injected into the site. For this reason, some practitioners prefer to use dry needles.

POSITIVE CHANGE THROUGH TELLINGTON TOUCH

Although it was first developed as a method for improving the behavior and physical health of horses, Tellington Touch, also known as TTouch, has since been widely applied to many animals with positive results. One of the pluses of this therapy is that it has no adverse side effects, so it is impossible to cause any harm by trying it out. "It can't hurt, and it might help," is what practitioners frequently say about using TTouch.

Tellington Touch is a series of circular movements that you perform with your hands and fingertips in various positions anywhere on an animal's body. The purpose of doing this is to awaken your animal's nervous system to help the animal attain better health or eliminate persistent behavior problems. Linda Tellington-Jones, a renowned horse trainer, first developed the method in the late 1970s after studying with the brilliant physicist Dr. Moshe Feldenkrais, at his Center for Humanistic Psychology in San Francisco. Dr. Feldenkrais had developed a method to help people recover from physical or emotional trauma based on the idea of "jumpstarting" parts of the brain that we don't ordinarily use. In other words, if you know one way to walk through life-long habit, and suddenly you lose the ability to walk due to an accident, perhaps you can learn to walk again by utilizing a different part of your brain to tell you a different way to do it. Feldenkrais was motivated in his work by the fact that we use only one-tenth of our brain; he was also motivated by personal practical necessity: He developed the method after he became crippled in an accident. He wanted to learn to walk again without surgery, and he succeeded.

Tellington-Jones applied what she had learned from Feldenkrais to her knowledge of horses. The development of TTouch was profoundly important to her because she felt unsettled about traditional methods for controlling horses that centered on dominance training. Through the course of traditional training, the animal learns to accept the human as being in complete control, and the animal becomes submissive. This results in conflict or tension, not the cooperative partnership that Tellington-Jones thought was necessary. Combining her belief that animals are our equals rather than lesser beings, and her idea that intuitive knowledge can sometimes be more helpful than intellect, she came up with the concept of helping horses get out of behavior or health ruts by waking up their nervous systems for new responses.

Over time, Tellington-Jones's reputation for success with horses expanded to include other animals. Today, TTouch is the culmination of years of practical research on such diverse animals as dogs, cats, ocelots, rodents, whales, dolphins, and reptiles, to name only some of the kinds of animals that have benefited from Tellington Touch. Once, while visiting the Soviet Union, Tellington-Jones even advised a small boy on how to use Tellington Touch on his pet snail. In fact, any animal with a nervous system will benefit from using this therapy.

The basic method consists of making clockwise circles of motion with relaxed fingers and a loose hand. Beginners have a tendency to stiffen their hands and fingers and should practice keeping the finger joints rounded and flexible. The practitioner's rhythmic breathing during TTouch further aids relaxation of both the practitioner and client, because an animal mirrors the body worker's breathing and releases stress as well. The first movement one learns is called the "clouded leopard." (All the 15 movements have descriptive names.) With a gently curved hand, use the pads of your fingers to make small clockwise circles anywhere on the body. You begin at 12 o'clock, make a complete circle, and continue until 8 o'clock before lifting the fingers and moving to a new part of the body. The touch relaxes while the constant movement fosters alertness. This accomplishes the goal of waking up the nervous system. You don't want to make a continuous circle in one spot because that will only lull the animal to sleep, a nice feeling perhaps, but not the goal of TTouch.

To reduce pain and swelling from injury, try the "lying leopard," which flattens the hand a bit before making circles so that a bigger area is addressed. If the area is painful, make the movements slower, and gentler, working around the injury and cupping the hands over it. If the wound is open be sure to place a sterile covering over the wound before approaching it.

The "python lift" releases tension and is wonderful for humans too (as most TTouches are). Rather than make circles, here you place both hands on either side of the legs, arms, shoulders, neck, back, or chest and use just enough pressure to lift the skin gently, about an inch-and-a-half, while supporting the muscle. The lift should be held for four seconds before you gently return the skin to its place and then release. The idea is to hold the muscle lightly so the animal doesn't hold its breath. Practice the python lift on a person you care about after a long, tense day at work. Your friend will thank you for it.

One of the greatest virtues of the TTouch method is that it not only helps the animal, but it improves the relationship between pet and owner, which is so critical in keeping a happy, well-adjusted, and well-behaved animal. Many pet owners report that once they learn the movements they almost always use them when touching their animal; they find this much superior to just mindlessly sitting and petting a cat or dog, for example. This can go a long way toward improving communication.

Remember that you can use the TTouch movements anywhere on your pet's body. Does your dog seem tense? Where are you noticing that tension? Many dogs express tension and stress through the neck, holding their heads stiffly, or holding them down due to constant feelings of shame related to training issues. If you kneel in front of your dog and perform a TTouch movement on its neck while talking to it and looking in its eye, you are letting your dog know that you care and that the two of you are in this together, even while you are performing therapy on the dog. The TTouch helps the animal unlearn poor habits, and makes positive change possible.

ANIMAL COMMUNICATORS

Have you ever connected with an animal, even for a moment, feeling as though you absolutely understood what that animal was experiencing? Perhaps you felt the animal's intense love for its newborns or its grief at a loss, its joy at running freely, or its desperation as it was caged in a shelter. If you were looking for a pet at the time, one animal might have singled you out, as if to say, "Take me!" Any sensitive and open-minded individual can communicate with animals to some degree. According to animal communicator Lydia

Hiby, this is an innate ability we have as children, but later forget: "As children we communicated nonverbally, and I believe that we can reawaken that skill, which lies dormant in most adults."[3]

Why do people consult animal communicators? Many people want to know that their pets are happy. Or perhaps the animal has an unexplainable health problem, such as the sudden appearance of seizures, that mystifies the doctors. A good communicator may tell you why the problem originated and what you might do about it. Another scenario is that the animal has a behavior problem that you want to help resolve. The communicator may be able to tell you what happened that affected your charge. Did the animal become upset after witnessing an accident? Or was a pattern of negative behavior spurred by some early-life trauma? In her work to help animals overcome trauma from abuse, veterinarian turned animal communicator Barbara Shor says, "I lead animals through a guided visualization that often seems to help clear some of these emotions." During the process, Shor can feel the animal's sadness, pain, anger, or fear. "I feel it, and if I sit with them and help them move through it, a lot of times I can feel the release." People also contact animal communicators at the end of their animal's life, when they are wondering whether the time is right for euthanasia. Moreover, animal communicators can help people understand what an animal is teaching its person. Many animals serve as mirrors to their owners. Thus the owner of a vicious dog might need to learn how to express his own anger more appropriately. One dog that Shor worked with was paralyzed for a year on the hind end. This required his owner to carry him outside, bring him in, and feed him. What the dog told the doctor was that in the process of his illness he was teaching his person how to love and care for himself as much as he cared for his dog. A well-trained animal communicator, then, is an intermediary, one who can offer much support to both animal and person.

The animal communicator usually "talks" to different species with pictures, sending and receiving visual images. Seeing life through an animal's perspective can be humbling, animal communicators say, as our fellow creatures are not just interested in survival and physical comforts, as many tend to believe, but capable of deep emotions. Many animals have the ability to love unconditionally and in so doing they help us to feel more deeply for ourselves and others.

The animal communicator works on the assumption that all life—human, animal, and plant—is energetically connected, and, thus, capable of communication.

But how do we know whether an animal communicator is really communicating with an animal or just deluding us? "A lot of the work I do is pretty controversial," concedes Shor, "and a lot of people aren't open to it." Animal communication is subjective and, therefore, difficult to validate. Since there is no objective proof to validate an animal communicator's accuracy, the whole concept is difficult for the Western-trained mind to accept. And certainly, there is room for deception. Basically, the only way to know whether an animal communicator is accurate or not is through personal experience. The practitioner says something that strikes an emotional chord. She recounts certain events that she could have had no way of knowing about (you didn't tell her). After a session, your animal starts to heal when, in the past, it was not making any progress at all. Or a behavior problem suddenly resolves. Shor speaks of dealing with information on a "soul level," and says that "for an animal to heal on that level, the person needs to be open to hearing what is said and doing something about it. If they're not, they're probably not going to work with me."

OTHER THERAPIES

The use of energy in different forms is the concept behind a variety of alternative healing modalities. Here are some that are used on animals.

Magnets. Like most alternative therapies, the use of magnets is intended to help the body heal itself, and it does that by redirecting energy flow within the pet's body. Reducing inflammation and speeding the healing of fractures are two ways magnets may benefit your animal.

Color Therapy. The idea of this modality is to use the vibrations from different colors to affect healing. Red energizes, and blue or bubble-gum pink are known to calm agitated patients, while green is a color that promotes general healing throughout the body. Advocates of this modality explain that color therapy doesn't depend on the reception of the color through sight—it's the vibration put off by the color that promotes the healing—so even color-blind animals can benefit from it. The color can be introduced through light, clothing, bedding, or anything that gets the color into the animal's environment. Color therapy works best when used in conjunction with some other type of therapy—homeopathy, acupuncture, or whatever therapy will be most effective in a given situation.

Auricular Therapy. This is a form of acupuncture or acupressure that is performed in the ear. All of the body's acupuncture points are said to be represented in the ear, so that stimulating an out-of-balance point can help the corresponding body system. The points in the ear can be treated with standard acupuncture needles or with flat needles called acupuncture tacks. Auricular therapy can be helpful in treating a lingering condition or imbalance that hasn't responded to other treatments.

Laser Therapy. Low-voltage lasers can be directed either at specific acupuncture points or at a generalized area in distress. For an injury sustained on the leg, for example, the entire calf or thigh or shin can be bathed with the laser light. Or, laser therapy can be used on acupuncture points where actual acupuncture is difficult to perform for any reason. Acupuncture points around the toes or nose, for instance, are frequently sensitive and painful during acupuncture treatment. So laser therapy is an effective alternative in such situations. Although it has been around since the late 1960s, laser therapy is not yet widely practiced in the United States, where many medical professionals consider it unproven. It is, however, an established practice in France and other parts of Europe. Because they insist on quantifiable change in a specific area—e.g., blood chemistry, or bone density—medical researchers in the U.S. aren't yet satisfied that the improvements caused by laser therapy are scientifically significant.

Laser light is monochromatic and coherent, meaning that all the individual ray's resonances are in sync with one another. Most hand-held lasers are helium neon light, which are best for treating a specific acupuncture point. Others are diode light, which work best on a generalized area. The therapy should be performed by a qualified professional only, as the misuse of lasers can have a damaging effect.

Reiki. The concept here is a transfer of energy from one place—the energy that is all around us, to another—into and onto the patient. The practitioner has been trained in how to redirect energy and may not even touch the patient, but just hold his or her hands over the afflicted area. Although it's not necessary, some practitioners are able to see the energy field around the patient. Reiki energy is said to be warm or hot when it is received.

NOTES

1. Gary Null interview with Howard Peiper, Mar. 19, 2000.
2. Gary Null interview with Susan Goldstein, Mar. 22, 2000.
3. Hiby, Lydia, with Bonnie S. Weintraub, *Conversations with Animals: Cherished Messages and Memories as Told by an Animal Communicator*, NewSage Press, Oregon, 1998, p. 158.

CHAPTER 6

Detoxing Fido

Does the following apply to you and your pet? You're feeding your animal the best foods on the market, perhaps even preparing your pet's meals yourself, supplementing with good-quality vitamins and minerals, herbs, and homeopathic remedies, and still your animal is not in peak form. If this is the case, in all likelihood the reason for your lack of success is that you are not clearing out old debris. As with humans, many of the conditions we see in animals—cataracts, arthritis, and allergies, to name a few—are really symptoms of toxicity. Dr. Lisa Newman, a Tucson, Arizona, naturopathic physician who specializes in animal care and has authored a series of books in the Crossing Press Natural Pet Care series, compares an overburdened body to a dirty engine: "…if you never change the oil, that, in and of itself, will wear down the performance of the engine, and eventually kill the car, even if you are putting in better fuel or additives."

The problem is that traditional veterinary medicine suppresses symptoms, without dealing with the more basic problem of toxicity. Sooner or later, the symptoms reappear. What's more, the chemicals used add to the toxic burden, making it more difficult for the immune system to create a curative response. Unfortunately, many supposedly holistic practitioners actually work in the same old way, treating conditions with some natural substance in lieu of cleansing the system. For instance, they may substitute the herb ephedra for an over-the-counter antihistamine, but once the herbal treatment is stopped, the symptoms return. In the long term, instead of having overcome the condition, the patient weakens. The alternative, then, is this: Rather than just treat our pets with one product or another, no matter how natural, we need to get to the root of the problem by cleansing.

Detoxification is the foundation of good health. It's what's needed first, before all the good nutrients and natural remedies can take effect. A detox program will often help reverse chronic conditions, and in some cases it may be all that's needed to eliminate them. Detoxification is a great way to help the body work from the inside out, dumping stored wastes and toxins, and letting the body start its own curative response.

Today's animals are especially in need of detoxification. They come into the world already sick from the toxic blood their mother passes on to them while they are in the womb. Once born, they are exposed to a myriad of toxins through food, air, water, and vaccinations. Veterinary journals tell us that our pets are healthier than ever before, yet they contradict themselves by lowering the age of an animal's life expectancy. Consider that ten years ago, dogs reached senior status at nine; today the number has been lowered to seven. Furthermore, animals are getting sick at younger ages. Veterinarians used to treat older animals for cancer. Now there is an epidemic of cancer in one- and two-year-olds. The reason? Too much exposure to chemicals, over-vaccination, less nutrition from foods. In short, they've got too much garbage to deal with. Our animals need to be detoxified in order to reclaim lost ground and live longer, healthier lives.

A good detoxification program can not only reverse chronic illness; it can also be lifesaving to an injured pet in that it may give an animal more power to fight infection and protect itself from internal damage. Newman provides an example: a dog bitten by a rattlesnake that showed none of the usual symptoms of shock, neurological damage, or hyperventilation. As soon as the dog was attacked its body immediately mounted a defense against the venom and protected its brain and lung tissues, two areas that are usually damaged by rattlesnake venom. The emergency clinic was able to release the dog five hours later—versus the usual three-day stay—which Newman attributed to "detoxification on a regular basis, homeopathic support, and a good clean diet with nutritional supplementation to maintain the strongest immune system possible."

Fasting for Health

Did you know that animals in the wild fast? Of course they do! They are hunters that binge after catching prey and fast when food is unavailable. In the modern world we tend to think that animals need to eat on a regular, constant schedule. We've learned that from conventional veterinary medicine and from big pet food companies. But really, animals, left to their own devices, will eat at intervals regulated by their bodily needs and success at hunting, not by the time of day.

We can help our pets by letting them skip a meal, or giving them no food for a day, only clean water, broth, and a little juice. *Important: Be sure your pet has access to plenty of liquids, especially water, during a fast.* This will release toxins from the colon and clear up all sorts of chronic illnesses that manifest as digestive, skin, joint, urinary, and other problems. Putting your animal on a 24-hour fast lets its body rest from the hard work of digesting food. That lets the animal redirect that energy into the healing it needs to do. Some of the conditions that may be helped by fasting are:

Bad breath
Behavior problems
Cancer
Cataracts
Constipation
Degenerative diseases
Diabetes mellitus
Diarrhea
Gastric bloat
Hairballs
Intestinal parasites
Lethargy
Liver disease
Malabsorption
Mucous congestion (eyes, throat, lungs, urine, colon)
Obesity
Pancreatitis
Pica
Plaque buildup
Senility

Skin diseases
Tooth loss
Vomiting

Some Fasting Guidelines. According to Dr. Newman, dogs and cats should be detoxified somewhat differently. Dogs can be fasted on a weekly basis. But cats are more difficult to fast on a regular basis because they become stressed from missing meals. Cats *can* benefit from a 24-hour fast three times a year. The spring and fall are good times of the year for this. However, Newman notes that if you decide not to fast your cat, because it is too stressful or for medical reasons, homeopathic detoxification is a good route to take. She advises use of the lower potencies—X's to low C's—of a combination product, particularly one containing the remedies Arsenicum and Nux Vomica. Actually, you can combine this homeopathic approach with fasting, and use it for dogs as well as cats.

Of course each animal is a unique individual, so before placing any animal on a fast, consult with your holistic veterinarian to be sure there are no special problems that would make going on a fast counterproductive. As a rule of thumb, you do not want to fast kittens, puppies, or geriatric pets. A sick animal might need cleansing done more slowly than the average pet. If an animal vomits or gets diarrhea during the fast, it should be stopped. Give Kaopectate every half hour to an hour to soothe and protect the intestines and stop the cleansing. Wait several days, and start once again, more slowly, perhaps skipping a meal that day. But do continue to fast the animal, even at a slower pace, since these animals are in dire need of cleansing. For the majority of animals, however, a 24-hour fast can be done without difficulty.

Newman recommends feeding your pet its regular breakfast at the beginning of the fast. Again, the pet should have free access to plenty of water to help it flush wastes and toxins out of its system. Broth (see below), as well as nonacidic fruit and vegetable juices could also be given to the animal. (Stay away from acidic juices, such as tomato or orange.) Fruit juices cleanse, while vegetables build. Overall, juices help to nourish, heal, and rejuvenate the billions of cells in your animal's body while reversing degeneration. Specifically, carrot-celery and carrot-parsnip juices are excellent aids in detoxification. Carrot-beet helps the liver and kidneys. Sprouts can be juiced, too, for their live enzymes and rich nutrient value. In addition, a little dandelion works well to move a sluggish liver and alleviate such conditions as skin abnormalities and chronic bad breath.

Don't be overly concerned if your pet, particularly your dog, is begging you for food at this time. Most of this is a psychological dependence, not a physiological need. Although your dog may be missing its regular foods, it's certainly getting plenty of quality nutrients from juice and broth during this time.

BREWING BROTH. When your pet is fasting you might try boiling sea vegetables, like kombu, to make a nutrient-rich broth. Given every few hours during the day, it will keep potassium and magnesium levels up. That, in turn, alleviates feelings of hunger. Another good broth for fasting employs a base of chicken, turkey, beef, fish, diced organic liver, or vegetables (avoid bouillon cubes; their ingredients are counterproductive to cleansing). Place the base in a large soup pot with a gallon of distilled water, cover, and simmer over low heat until the meat falls from the bone or the vegetables soften. Cool and strain off the liquid. (Freeze edible meat to be used later as pet food). If your pet is overweight, skim fat from the liquid before serving. For flavor, add a teaspoon of sea salt or kelp to each gallon of broth, and if you like, some garlic or a tablespoon of vitamin C powder. The broth can be stored in a sealed container and kept for up to a week in the refrigerator and for several months in the freezer. This broth, in addition to staving off hunger, is highly nutritional. And when your pet is not fasting, the broth makes an excellent flavor enhancer for regular food.

Another idea to keep in mind for when your pet is fasting: Try freezing a little fruit juice into cubes so that your animal can lick them at dinnertime to get a sense of eating. Moreover, you should also let your animal exercise on a fasting day to get its mind off food. Exercise has the added advantage of helping the bowels move to eliminate poisons.

This is an especially important time to brush and massage the animal's coat. You want to keep toxins moving through the pores and this will help with the elimination process.

The Healing Crisis. Don't become discouraged if, with your initial attempt to help your animal recover from a chronic disease, it initially appears better only to get worse again. Remember, the body is eliminating a lot of toxins that have, until now, been stagnant for months or years. Once the body begins breaking down stored pockets of old food, old fecal material in the colon, and old toxicity in the joints and organs, these poisons flush into the bloodstream and may cause a temporary exacerbation of symptoms, known as a healing crisis. The system is working overtime, sending blood and immune factors to each area, and this may result in the area becoming temporarily inflamed. Inflammation may resemble the disease itself, and could include such signs as a low-grade fever, runny eyes, foul breath, smelly urine, and skin-related problems.

Healing crises are familiar to people who try to "clean up their act." You stop smoking after 10 years and start to develop a hacking cough. That serves the purpose of getting tar out of your lungs. Unfortunately, most of us don't look at these healing-crisis symptoms as friends; we try to suppress them, taking suppressants to stop our cigarette cough. But nature is the true healer that puts the body back into balance, and symptoms are a part of that process.

"The healing crisis is anything but a quick fix," says Dr. Martin Goldstein, a veterinarian in South Salem, New York, and author of *The Nature of Animal Healing: The Path to Your Pet's Health, Happiness, and Longevity*. Goldstein has this perspective on the phenomenon: "A lot of times it's the make/break point. An animal or person in a healing crisis will look like they're getting worse. Unfortunately, in veterinary medicine, that's the point where the animal's either heavily drugged or euthanized." He adds that the situation is like a "Catch-22," in which the body is trying to heal, usually through inflammation. He reminds us that the inflammation is there not as punishment, but rather "to bring the healing forces of the body to the area. A lot of the drugs we've developed are anti-inflammatory drugs, which actually suppress nature's ability to heal, and the ultimate result is you wind up with cancer. Right now the Morris Foundation has reported that 47 percent of disease-related deaths in dogs in the United States are due to cancer."

As we've mentioned, you can assist the detoxification process with a combination of homeopathic Arsenicum and Nux Vomica. The Arsenicum will help the body eliminate toxins and the Nux

Vomica will reduce any nausea your pet may experience during the strenuous process of detoxifying. Give the animal three, four, or more doses during the 24-hour period, depending on the animal's condition. You can also add a diuretic, such as juniper berry, to help move things out. In addition, a few drops of Essiac tea extract will further aid the detoxification process.

Most of the time, a healing crisis is not severe; it will pass in a short time. If, however, symptoms last longer than a few days, have a blood test performed to rule out any underlying problems. In most instances, the crisis soon passes, and the animal becomes more vibrant and healthy than before.

Breaking the Fast. At the end of the 24 hours, give your pet one half of its normal breakfast, since its stomach will have shrunk during the fast. Cooked oatmeal with a little added vegetable pulp (that you saved from juicing) and broth is a good choice for this first meal, as it is easy on the digestive system. You may also give a vitamin and mineral supplement at this point. You do not want to feed your pet too much at this time; that would be counterproductive to all the cleansing work its body has accomplished. The idea is to do reintroduce foods slowly.

REVITALIZATION

Your animal is now on the road to wellness, better able to utilize nutrients for health and healing. Continue to steer it in the right direction with a regenerative diet, vitamins and minerals, and periodic fasting. Here are some ideas:

Energize Your Pet's Diet. As we've discussed in Chapter 1, cleaning up your pet's diet is all-important. You want to avoid fillers, sugars, yeast, salt, and chemical additives and preservatives—all-too-common pet food ingredients. Give your animal high-quality dry kibble along with some home-prepared foods. There are those who advocate a raw-foods diet, but, as we've mentioned, you want to be careful that bacteria-laden meat does not sicken your pet. Also, our pets are not the same creatures as their ancestor hunters; their digestive systems have changed somewhat. So breaking down and assimilating amino acids from raw meats may be difficult. You will, therefore, want to cook the food a little so that your pet can be safe and still benefit from live enzymes. Your animal's rejuvenation diet should also include some sea vegetables, grated raw fruits and vegetables, fresh juice, and a good multiple vitamin and mineral supplement.

A note about sea vegetables: They may not fit into your current paradigm of "what's for dinner" for either you or Fido, but don't let that put you off. Both humans and other animals can benefit from this excellent source of digestible protein and trace minerals; the latter are vital to health but sadly lacking in our depleted soils. Sea vegetables are also extremely cleansing, as they are able to bind with toxins, even harsh heavy metals and radioactive substances, and flush them out of the system.

Sea vegetables come in many varieties. The brown algae kelp and fucus are rich in potassium and can be sprinkled on foods as a condiment to add flavor. They will help remove strontium and radioactive iodine from the system. Red algae include gigartina, nori, dulce, and Irish moss and will absorb toxins from the digestive tract, including radioactive plutonium. The green alga sea lettuce is high in iron and cesium and will remove carcinogens. Be sure to follow package directions when preparing these.

Don't Forget Juice. Although we've already touched on the subject of juicing, this important aspect of detoxification is worth mentioning again because of its invaluable benefits. You must have noticed how, when outdoors, cats and dogs seek out bitter herbs and grasses to munch on. What they are in effect doing, in their instinctual wisdom, is extracting the purifying chlorophyll in order to cleanse and rejuvenate their systems. They may swallow the chewed plant, too, and later regurgitate the fibrous stuff. Providing your pet with a little juice instead is kinder to the system. All the animal gets is the nutrient- and enzyme-rich juice, which has already been separated by you from the plant's pulp. So whether your animal is fasting or not, be sure to make freshly squeezed juices a regular part of its diet. (See Chapter 5 for more details on juicing.)

Supplement With C. If you only give your pet one supplement, make it vitamin C for its many important benefits, particularly the ability to fight free radicals. Free radicals can injure a cell's DNA, causing harmful genetic aberrations within it. As a water-soluble antioxidant, vitamin C is in a unique position to scavenge aqueous peroxyl radicals before these destructive substances have a chance to do their damage. It works alongside vitamin E, a fat-soluble antioxidant, and the enzyme glutathione peroxidase to stop free-radical chain reactions. Vitamin C may be especially important in this day and age of widespread environmental pollution because it fights off many toxins, including ozone, carbon monoxide, hydrocarbons, pesticides, and heavy metals. Vitamin C helps the body get rid of these harmful substances by stimulating enzymes in the liver, an organ that is a major player in the detoxification process. Unlike humans, most animals produce their own vitamin C; however, when you consider the vital detoxification functions associated with this nutrient, you want to be sure your pet is getting an extra dose.

How much vitamin C should your animal be getting? Generally, a small dog or a cat will need between 500 and 1000 milligrams daily, and a medium to large dog will need between 1000 and 3000 milligrams daily to maintain optimal health. If the animal has hip dysplasia, arthritis, allergies, cancer, or any auto-immune condition, it may need more. Start with 500 mg and build up to bowel tolerance, the point *before* the animal's stool becomes loose. In other words, if your animal gets diarrhea, you must reduce the dose to just under that level. Try mixing an ester-C powder into your animal's food. Or you could use calcium ascorbate, a less expensive substitute that is also quite effective.

EXTRA DETOXIFICATION SUPPORT

Your animal is enjoying the benefits of a holistic lifestyle, fasting periodically, and following a diet that helps to support detoxification and rejuvenation processes. In many instances that's enough. However, there are times where your animal might need extra support. Now is the time to pull out your holistic medicine chest to fine-tune your animal's health.

Helping a Diseased Animal. If your animal is already diseased or on the brink of disease, it has probably long been plagued with a toxic system, and you will want to work alongside a professional, getting your animal tested to see exactly where the imbalances lie and how to proceed. Your pet's doctor can guide you as to whether or not your animal should be fasted, how slowly, and what foods and supplements it will need for optimum support.

Supporting Organs of Detoxification. Animals eliminate a lot of toxins through the skin, the largest organ of elimination. One of the telltale signs of an overburdened system is a dull or rough coat or skin eruptions, such as pimples, hot spots, greasy skin, and rashes. After your animal has fasted or skipped a meal, you can help your pet's skin and coat by feeding it oatmeal the next morning and fish for its evening meal. The fatty acids help support the skin. For cats, you will need to add vitamin E to the evening fish meal to prevent a serious disease called steatitis. Vitamins A and E, as well as zinc, biotin, and selenium, work to promote a softer, smoother, and healthier coat and skin. Add a drop of first-cold-pressed virgin olive oil to your pet's food. Olive oil contains oleic acid, which gives the skin and coat a healthy shine. Also, a juice made from a small cucumber and small amounts of beet, parsley, and ginger root is good for the skin and coat.

According to Chinese medicine, the skin is connected to the liver. If your animal has a skin condition, chances are the liver is overworked, too. To be sure, get a blood test done. That will tell you whether or not the liver's enzyme levels are normal. If the diagnosis is a sluggish liver, work with your holistic veterinarian to reverse the condition.

You may choose to create a holistic protocol with home remedies, such as milk thistle to decongest the liver and burdock root or juniper berry to flush out toxins (be sure to use herbs that promote both steps). If you prefer an already-made formula, Earth Animal carries a homeopathic product called Liver Detox. A little finely chopped watercress or parsley added to the food might help too. Repeating the blood test in a month will let you know whether your holistic protocol has taken effect and if any modifications are needed.

Homeopathic Maintenance. Naturopathic doctor Lisa Newman advocates a homeopathic approach to detoxification, not just as an alternative to fasting or in conjunction with it, as we've seen, but as a follow-up measure as well. A weekly maintenance program, with a single dose of the remedy or remedies you're using, given at bedtime, is her preferred mode of administration, and she lists the benefits as helping to process wastes, stimulating the action of the liver and kidneys, and supporting good health in general. She recommends liquid remedies as being the easiest to give, noting that if the dropper touches your hands or your pet, you should rinse it before returning it to the bottle. The most vital of the remedies that homeopaths choose for detox are Arsenicum and Nux Vomica; you'll often find these as components of the combination remedies sold. But don't think that a program of homeopathy is going to replace proper feeding of your animal, Newman reminds us. Dietary intake is always the first consideration.

Detoxification After Vaccination. Be sure to detoxify your pet after it is vaccinated to prevent vaccine-induced side effects. It's also a good idea to give your animal a homeopathic vaccine detox if he or she has been vaccinated a while ago or if you are unsure of its vaccination history.

The most commonly used formula for this purpose is Thuja (12X or 30C). The pellet is crushed and placed on the tongue an hour before or after feedings for seven days after a vaccination to help eliminate compromising effects on the immune system.

Of course, the best insurance against weakening the system is to vaccinate as little as possible. So rather than have your pet routinely revaccinated, be sure to have a blood titer done to see if antibodies to a specific disease are still present. If they are, there is no need to revaccinate for that illness. (These issues are discussed at length in Chapter 9.)

Finish Up by Cleaning Up. Finally, to really get your pet healthy, you have to clean up your house. What does house cleaning have to do with pet health? A lot. Animals are generally close-to-the-ground, or close-to-the-carpet, creatures. What's more, they tend to stay home for quite a bit of their lives. Thus, they can end up breathing in more harsh cleaning chemicals, as well as mold, dust, and pesticides, than we humans do, which is why it's important to keep your living quarters as pure as possible. Clean your house with environmentally friendly products, such as enzyme/citrus products that can eliminate urine odors naturally. You can further lessen your animal's sneezing, coughing, and scratching with the addition of a good air purifier.

Follow these simple guidelines for detoxifying your animal on a regular basis and you will increase your animal's chances for living a longer and healthier life. "That's what's so beautiful about lifestyle approaches," says Dr. Newman. "The foundation is the same regardless of the disease that you're dealing with because you're dealing with the animal's system, rather than the symptoms."

CHAPTER 7

Common Dog and Cat Concerns

This chapter looks at conditions that may afflict your pet, and at natural ways you can help your animal overcome them. Since each animal, and each circumstance, is unique, consult your holistic veterinarian as you work to regain your pet's health. Some of these problems, although common, can be serious, so professional guidance is recommended.

ABSCESSES

If you have a pet that goes outside or comes into contact with other animals, chances are you've had to deal with an abscess or two. Abscesses are holes that can start from any kind of wound—a puncture, cut, or bite. If the wound goes undetected and uncleaned it can fester and become infected. Sometimes pet owners will discover an abscess because of the swelling that comes with it; at other times the abscess may break open and begin to drain before it gets noticed. Either way, a veterinarian will probably treat the abscess by cleaning it out, putting in a drain, and putting the animal on a course of antibiotics. If the wound is severe, the vet may want to give the animal stitches once the infection is entirely drained.

If you can catch an abscess early on, you can avoid such invasive treatment and care for it at home, according to Nina Anderson, coauthor of *Supernutrition for Dogs 'n Cats*. It's fairly easy to spot an abscess once you realize this is a frequent problem. The abscess will be swollen and fleshy and tender to the touch. Before an abscess opens up, soak it in a mixture of warm water and baking soda, or apply a compress with water and baking soda to the area. This will bring the infection to the surface and cause it to pop. Then, with dogs, be sure to keep the open wound clean; in the case of cats, they will do most of the cleaning themselves. You can clean the wound with plain water and a small amount of a liquid garlic extract, such as Kyolic. The garlic will help keep the infection down. It usually takes only a couple of days for the infection to start healing.

Anderson further advises that as soon as you've spotted the abscess, you should begin giving your animal echinacea and continue doing so for 10 days. Echinacea is a natural antibiotic and will help your pet build up its own immune system; thus you may avoid the use of generally over-prescribed antibiotics. Once the abscess has started to close and the infection is entirely gone, you can apply aloe vera and calendula to it. This will usually be about a week after it first opened up. Important: Be sure to wait until it's completely closed to apply the calendula because this remedy can instigate premature healing, and an abscess needs to have sufficient time to drain completely before closing up again.

ANAL GLAND INFLAMMATION

Many people accept their symptoms of poor digestive function—flatulence, bloating, gas—as a matter of course rather than taking steps to improve their health. That's not good, and when an animal has a digestive problem, it is just as important to avoid a state of denial and to seek treatment. If your pet is having excessive bowel movements or strains when trying to defecate, it might have anal gland inflammation, and you will want to address the problem right away.

This condition is often present in obese animals, but it can occur in any animal whose digestive system does not get the proper rest. Anal gland inflammation can be exacerbated by rich or low-fiber foods, so pay attention to your pet's diet. You will want to be sure that it is eating high-fiber foods that have high nutritional value, such as whole grains, nuts, bran, seeds, fruits, and vegetables. Good nutrition goes a long way toward promoting healthy digestion, and good digestion is key to overall good health.

If your pet has anal gland inflammation, talk to your holistic veterinarian about fasting your animal. He or she might recommend a fast on water, broth, and juice for three to five days to give the body a much-needed rest. There is also a product called Gentle Dragon that could help midway through the fast. (See Chapter 6 for more information on detoxification.)

Next you will want to apply hot (but not too hot) packs to the general area or soak your animal's bottom in a tub of hot (as hot as he or she can stand without burning) water with one or two cups of Epsom salts. Do this twice a day for 10 minutes each time. At this point, you may apply *gentle* pressure—don't squeeze—to the anal area. Move with a rocking motion. You will then want to apply a thin coat of petroleum jelly or mineral oil to the anal area to soothe it.

Avoid the more conventional approaches, such as squeezing or packing, or worse, surgically removing the inflamed gland. There are effective alternatives to these harsh approaches.

You should know that anal gland inflammation may recur, so take precautions against it. Keep your animal from becoming obese, or if he or she already is, help your animal lose the excess weight. Try getting your animal to exercise more. Regular fasting can be beneficial; one or two days (at most) per week are recommended. A good diet can't be stressed enough. Finally, do not allow your veterinarian or groomer to squeeze the anal gland. It's simply unacceptable. You want to promote the natural healing process, not disrupt or interfere with it.

ANEMIA

Dogs and cats become anemic for a whole variety of reasons, ranging from simple iron deficiency to auto-immune disease to chronic liver/kidney problems, to cancer. The telltale signs of anemia are withdrawal, fatigue, paleness around the gums, and sometimes loss of appetite. If your pet demonstrates one or all of the aforementioned symptoms, it is important to have your vet determine if it is in fact anemic, and why. An animal can die quickly from this condition, and so emergency medical treatment, such as transfusions or steroids, may be necessary. After the crisis is over, you can focus on a holistic immune-building program.

If the anemia is simply the result of an iron deficiency and Fluffy or Fido has a low energy level, you can give your pet some iron (3 to 7 mg per day) and herbs, such as dandelion (1 drop of the extract per 5 to 10 pounds of body weight) to give your animal a little pep. Though it may sound like common sense, you want to avoid iron laden with additives and fillers. Essentially, you will be building up your animal's blood with the dandelion and iron. Particularly with the iron, there should be a marked change in your pet's energy level within 48 hours. If this doesn't occur, though, inform your vet.

Other herbs to consider for iron deficiency anemia, besides dandelion, are gentian and yellow dock. Sea vegetables and green vegetable juice are good too; consult your holistic animal practitioner to formulate a plan that incorporates any of these.

ARTHRITIS

Vaccines can create an auto-immune reaction in the joints, with arthritis as an unfortunate result. The holistic veterinarian will work to metabolically balance the arthritic animal, perhaps using glucosamine sulfate mixed with chondroitin sulfate to restore the proper production of joint fluid. Herbal formulas used to threat arthritis contain such ingredients as alfalfa, yucca, and devil's claw. Other herbs used to treat this condition are boneset, boswellia, and comfrey. Homeopathic treatment, specifically with the remedy rhus, tox, has yielded good results too.

Your nutritionally oriented veterinarian may also recommend other supplements. Let's look at some of these, keeping in mind that you should clear an arthritis treatment plan, and fine-tune dosages, with your vet.

Vitamin C—This is an important one for joints and cartilage, and if you combine C with glucosamine, it works even better. The total daily dose of this vitamin will be about 250 to 2500 mg for cats and small dogs, and 400 to 4000 mg for large dogs, although what you really want to do is give a bowel-tolerance dose—that is, just less than the amount that would cause diarrhea—and you want to divide that dose up throughout the day, because the vitamin works more effectively that way.

Omega-3 fatty acids—Found in salmon oil and flaxseed oil, these counter inflammation.

Vitamin E—For pain; 50 IU for cats and small dogs; 80 IU for large dogs.

Superoxide dismutase—Called SOD, this supplement, combined with vitamin E, helps increase energy, while decreasing pain and inflammation.

Vitamin A or beta carotene—For pain; 7000 IU for small dogs; 10,000 IU for large dogs; up to 5000 IU for cats
Cod liver oil

Gamma linoleic acid—Counters pain and inflammation; found in evening primrose oil, borage oil, or black currant oil, all of which are available in capsule form.

Grape seed extract—This helps strengthen collagen and the circulatory system.

Additional nutrients to keep in mind while trying to keep arthritis at bay are the B-complex vitamins and the mineral boron. A small amount of this mineral can make a difference in symptoms; consult your holistic animal practitioner on the correct dose for your cat or dog.

Juicing Helps the Joints. Freshly made organic juices can help defend your pet against arthritis. The juices of pineapple, potato, and star fruit are recommended for this condition, and you might want to try a combination juice in which you mix aloe vera, red cabbage, cucumber, dandelion, celery, mint, apple, and carrot. Also, green juices, diluted with carrot or beet juice, or with water, can be helpful. For the green elements you can use cabbage, celery, broccoli, zucchini, cucumber, kale, parsley, or spinach, adding ginger root, apple, or carrot for flavor and extra vitamin and mineral benefit. See Chapter 5 for an in-depth discussion of juicing.

BLADDER PROBLEMS

The ability to relieve ourselves is one of the many bodily functions we take for granted until, one day, we can't "do our business" without experiencing pain or discomfort. Animals are no different. If you've had a pet with a bladder problem, you know how difficult it can be. Like us, they may experience excruciating pain when trying to pass urine. Many pets become irritable and may even cry out when urinating. They hold it in as long as they can, and are more prone to have indoor accidents, to everyone's distress. Just as frustrating is the inability to "go" at all. This is not only exasperating but dangerous as well.

Bladder problems are toxicity problems. So the goal of treatment is to detoxify the body while building up the kidneys with cleansing herbs, such as horsetail. Also, juniper berry has yielded excellent results for animals with blockages.

Perhaps the most important remedy for treating bladder problems is vitamin C. Doses of up to 4000 mg per day for large dogs and between 1000 and 2000 mg per day for cats and smaller dogs are most beneficial. Not only is vitamin C extremely effective in acidifying urine and cleaning out the bladder, it is also a great preventative. Also recommended for this condition are cranberry juice and cherry juice, caprylic acid, alpha-lipoic acid, and flaxseed oil.

CANCER

In recent years, the incidence of cancer among animals has risen. There was a time when it was mostly older pets that were affected. These days, animals as young as two or three are plagued with the often fatal disease. The reason is that our pets today are toxic. Most animals eat wretched foods, drink polluted water, breathe in noxious chemicals from flea collars and other poisons in their surroundings, and are over-vaccinated and generally over-medicated. Mothers pass toxic blood to their fetuses, so animals start life with compromised immune systems. Their environments may be psychologically stressful, too, and studies have correlated stress with a weaker immune system.

Conventional therapies include surgery, radiation, and chemotherapy. Chemotherapy often makes use of platinum, which is highly toxic to cells. The problem with all these modalities is that they focus on killing or removing the cancer directly, without regard for the immune system. And without a properly functioning immune system, the animal's body cannot fight off the attacker. It's true that sometimes conventional approaches are needed; in the case of a fibrosarcoma, for instance, surgery may be necessary to get rid of this aggressive tumor and save your pet's life. Many people opt to combine conventional therapies with alternative, and if you find the right veterinarian, you can do this. Alternative modalities include immunoaugmentive therapy (IAT), ozone therapy, cryosurgery, Essiac tea and other supplements, Chinese herbs, and nosodes (homeopathic remedies made from the cancer tissue itself).

Before looking at some of the more holistic ways cancer is treated, we must note the importance of a natural diet in both the prevention and treatment of cancer. As discussed in Chapter 1, the products sold to the public as pet food are toxic, and constitute part of the problem of the increasing cancer rate in domesticated animals. You want to feed your animal foods free of chemical additives and harmful preservatives. Preparing meals yourself for your sick pet is always preferable, and if you can provide your pet with freshly made organic vegetable juices that's a definite plus, because the healing phytochemicals (or "plant chemicals") in these are immediately available for the animal's body to use. Also, for animals with cancer, protein is important, and indeed, many dogs and cats with the condition do crave it. Dr. Robert Goldstein recommends unspiced meats and raw egg yolks, preferably organic, as protein sources for animal cancer patients, and adds that if the pet's appetite allows it, the addition of whole grains, such as brown rice and millet, as well as finely chopped raw carrots, parsley, or other vegetables, is helpful. If your dog or cat does not have a good appetite at this time, getting the animal to eat anything it will tolerate is a plus, with the emphasis, of course, on the unadulterated, fresh, and organic.

Immuno-Augmentative Therapy. Developed by Dr. Lawrence Burton to treat human cancer patients, and available for that purpose in the Bahamas, immuno-augmentative therapy (IAT) is an immune-enhancing cancer treatment that has been adapted for use with small animals. The procedure involves analyzing a blood sample for its serum protein factors to determine the site of weaknesses in the immune system. Based on these findings, low- or out-of-balance factors are injected into the body, thus rebuilding immunity. Although IAT does not usually cure a condition, most of the time it is a tool for disease management. Patients are able to maintain good health as long as IAT is administered; it's similar to the situation of those who use insulin therapy to manage diabetes. The cancer remains in the body, but tumor growth either slows down or stops, or the tumor shrinks. In many instances, IAT is needed over the course of a lifetime.

Immuno-augmentative therapy has several advantages. The treatment is almost 100-percent safe, it can be administered at home once your veterinarian has taught you how to give the injections, and it effectively slows down the progression of tumors in a number of cancers. There are generally no side effects from this treatment. Occasionally an abscess will develop at the injection site from bacteria carried by the needle. But normally the immune system will destroy the bacteria, and no problem will occur. Also, small lumps may form at the injection site due to an allergic reaction. But this, too, is rare since the injected protein sources are naturally found in the body and, therefore, not perceived as foreign matter to be rejected.

There are, however, disadvantages to IAT. The therapy may be difficult for some people to administer for a variety of reasons, the first of which is that some people don't like giving needles. Nor are all animals receptive to the procedure. Cats, in particular, may be resistant and hard to hold. In addition, elderly pet owners may have difficulty wrapping their fingers around a syringe. The process is also time-consuming. During the course of treatment, subcutaneous injections are required throughout the day. In the early stages as many as seven injections may be needed five days a week, so working people may not have the time needed to tend to their animals in this way. Long-term treatment may cost thousands of dollars, which is prohibitive for some pet owners. Moreover, not all cancers are responsive to IAT. The therapy does not have a high success rate for lymphoma, lymphosarcoma, and osteosarcoma. While administering treatment will not cause animals with these diseases harm, resources might be better spent on other modalities, such as ozone therapy.

Sometimes one or more therapies are recommended along with IAT. It's best to discuss available options with a holistic veterinarian. IAT advocate veterinarian Christina Aiken explains, "Every case is individual. It's not like there is one recipe for all animals with cancer, even the same type of cancer. There are some types of cancers where it doesn't work very well. What matters, too, is what the clients are willing to do, what they are willing to spend, how intense they are going to be, and the age of the animal." Dr. Aiken lets people know what can be done, and then steps back to let them decide what to do.

Ozone Therapy. Some cancer cells cannot thrive in a high-oxygen environment, a fact that can be key in getting rid of them. Ozone therapy is a great source of oxygen that can damage susceptible organisms, including these types of cancer cells, on contact. In addition to oxygenating cancer cells, ozone therapy can attack a variety of other problems—viruses, bacteria, mycoplasma, fungi, and some parasites and yeasts.

Ozone can be administered in different ways. It can be given intravenously to kill damaging organisms in the bloodstream, rectally for a patient who is badly constipated or has lower intestinal tract disease (this will stimulate muscle contractions and circulation), orally, or topically. Also, filtered food-grade hydrogen peroxide can be administered into the bloodstream as a strong antioxidant. Since an ozone generator may cost thousands of dollars and food-grade hydrogen peroxide is inexpensive, the latter is considered a poor man's version of ozone therapy, but it is not as effective.

Unfortunately, ozone therapy is legal in only a handful of states, New York being one of these. Check with a holistic physician or on the Internet for more details.

Cryosurgery. This freezing process, which veterinarian Robert Goldstein describes as "controlled frostbite," destroys cancer cells and is often effective for removing small tumors on the body's surface or in the oral or nasal cavity. Freezing kills the cancerous cells, which then are rejected by the body. A limitation of cryosurgery is that it can't be used deep in the body because necrotic cells would have nowhere to go; trapped inside, they could cause bad inflammation and peritonitis.

Drs. Goldstein and DeAngelis have developed a special technique for removing tumors high up in an animal's nasal cavity. Such tumors are frequently found in dogs. Their procedure involves opening the nasal cavity, creating a bone flap, freezing the tumor, and then closing it again. Necrotic material will exit through the nose.

Cryosurgery is not painful and can often be performed without anesthesia. The treatment is often augmented with supplements, IAT, and other therapies.

Supplements. Consider these supplements to support your animal's immune system.

POLY-MVA. Some 35 years ago, Dr. Merrill Garnett, a dentist at the time, sought to find a gentler, more effective approach to cancer care, and formulated Poly-MVA. Today, Poly-MVA is recognized as a nontoxic cancer fighter and is currently under study by the FDA for approval as a cancer drug. This liquid supplement destroys cancer cells by interfering with their metabolism and what they use to grow. Poly-MVA is quite safe and inexpensive. It uses the metal palladium, which, unlike toxic platinum used in chemotherapy, is nonpoisonous. Poly-MVA may be administered intravenously in dogs, but not cats. Caution must be taken with IV administration, as overzealous detoxification may overwhelm the liver. Some veterinarians give vitamin C along with Poly-MVA, but, in general, it is best to avoid chelating agents or iron supplements. The latter, in combination with Poly-MVA, can cause tumor growth.

SHARK CARTILAGE. When tumors begin to form, they establish their own blood vessels. Shark cartilage contains anti-angiogenesis factor, a protein that inhibits the growth of new blood vessels. As a result, small masses never enlarge and the immune system has an easier time destroying them. Use one of the better-known brands of shark cartilage, since therapeutic qualities are easily destroyed if the substance is overheated. Two of the best known are Cartilaid and Benefin.

IP6. This rice bran extract stimulates natural killer cell activity. A good brand of IP6 is Cellular Forte.

VITAMIN C. Vitamin C will give your animal a jump-start on healing. Cancer attacks deficient immune systems, and vitamin C is the prime nutrient when it comes to immune system support. Try ascorbate or polyascorbate if your animal has a poor appetite; it is gentle on the system and not too acidic. An ester-C is also recommended. You will want to mix the powdered vitamin into your animal's food. Bowel-tolerance levels are recommended, i.e., the amount just below that which causes diarrhea, so you will want to start with moderate doses and build from there. An animal sick with cancer will generally need and tolerate much more vitamin C than a healthy animal.

ESSIAC TEA. Essiac contains sheep sorrel, burdock root, slippery elm bark, rhubarb bark, and several other healing herbs. This herbal combination will give your animal more energy, and works best in conjunction with other remedies. Health food stores carry it, or you can call Essiac International at (800) 668-4559. Follow the instructions for brewing the tea, and have your holistic vet advise you on the correct dosage for your animal.

ADDITIONAL SUPPLEMENTS. The following supplements can also help your dog or cat in the fight against cancer. Remember that since you don't want to "throw the whole medicine cabinet" at your sick pet—but rather pick out the most promising items from it—you should consult your holistic vet to formulate a treatment plan.

Vitamin A—A good infection- and tumor-fighter.

Beta carotene—Stimulates T-helper cells.

Vitamin E—Works well with selenium to rev up the immune system.

Selenium—Although it's a trace element, it's an important one for cancer treatment and prevention.

Flavonoids—These healing plant chemicals are the agents that give fruits and vegetables their bright colors. Perhaps you've heard of quercetin, rutin, citrin, or hesperidin; these are all flavonoids.

Glutathione peroxidase—This cell-defender is often overlooked.

Superoxide dismutase and catalase—Enzymes that ward off free-radical damage.

Grape seed extract—Can be helpful in slowing the cell mutation process.

Coenzyme Q10—An energy-booster and stimulant of the body's immune defenses.

N-acetyl-cysteine—Fights cancer-drug damage and helps get rid of carcinogens.

Zinc—Vital in supporting T and B cells, and in the healing process, this mineral also helps normalize appetite.

Chromium—A mineral that helps regulate blood sugar levels and, as a result, immune function.

The Herbal Arsenal Against Cancer. In addition to the above supplements, you'll probably want to consider herbs for your pet. The following are some of the herbs that have anti-cancer properties.

Hoxsey Herbs—This is a formula; it contains red clover, buckthorn bark, stillingia root, barberry bark, chaparral, licorice root, cascara amarga, and prickly ash bark, plus potassium iodide.

Ginger—Counters the digestive upset associated with chemotherapy.

Lentinan—This mushroom derivative has anti-cancer properties, and also counters the side effects of chemo.

Echinacea—Given for short periods in an on-off pattern, this herb is a prime immune-system booster.

Astragalus—An ancient Chinese herb that can be used every day to energize damaged cells.

Garlic—This often recommended herbal ammunition makes cancer more recognizable to the immune system.

Aloe vera—Containing live enzymes and essential fatty acids, it stimulates phagocyte activity, making it a disease-fighter.

Ginseng—Its components called saponins are anti-cancer agents.

Red clover—Protective of DNA.

One Vet's View. Martin Goldstein is a veterinarian who treats animals that have cancer. In his view, disease in general is just an excuse to get healthy, and cancer is the ultimate excuse. He sees cancer as the end result of a compromised immune system and likes to make an analogy involving a high school and its janitor. "The janitor gets sick, the high school gets dirty, but the garbage didn't attack the high school," Goldstein explains. "The conventional remedy for that situation is to attack the garbage, set it on fire, and burn the whole building down. The natural remedy is to get the janitor working again. The janitorial system of the body is the immune system. So cancer is the result of an immune system failure in which cells that used to be normal start to grow haywire, but it's not something that attacks the body....The proper answer is not necessarily to go in there and zap the cancer, thinking it's the enemy, but to get the body's immune system to a point that it can handle itself."

Cancer care often integrates conventional and holistic approaches, Goldstein points out. Surgery, for instance, is often necessary to save an animal's life and buy time. Drugs can buy time too. But neither approach is a cure. The animal's immune system must be strengthened to fight off the disease on its own. "We've seen animals with tumors eating through three or four of their bones. Two years later we have Cornell University's verification that not only is the tumor gone, but the bone is rehealed. We have hip joints grown back. We have brain tumors where CAT scans show half their brains are taken over by tumors and then three years later we have pictures of them being normal. We have this all verified. That's why we've gained broad acceptance. But we will use the balance of both on each individual patient."

When Your Vet Creates a Cancer Protocol. Your holistic veterinarian may want to use the following source list to create a customized cancer protocol for your pet. In my own experience with animals I have found these items to be helpful, but I have intentionally not included supplement dosages here so as not to encourage readers to give supplements to their sick pets without professional supervision. What your practitioner will do is choose a very limited number of items from the following, and then decide on proper dosage levels for each. He or she will be basing these decisions on a variety of factors, including the size, age, and condition of your pet. Then, the vet will monitor your pet's response and, over a period of months, components of your pet's protocol will be added or subtracted based on the vet's observations and judgment.

A tool that some vets use in creating a protocol for cancer—and for other chronic diseases, such as diabetes—is a blood test called the BNA (Bio Nutritional Analysis). Available to your vet from Antech Diagnostic Laboratory, it helps him or her recommend what the animal could use more of in terms of vitamins, minerals, and other nutrients. The idea is to optimize your pet's protocol for help in fighting the side effects of chemotherapy, and for building the body and immune response generally. Whatever diagnostic route your vet follows, hopefully, you and your vet working together will be able to make a real difference in your animal's condition.

NUTRITIONAL COMPONENTS
Organic vegetable juice
Cruciferous vegetable juice
Sea vegetables
Aloe
Green tea
Grape juice made from whole grapes

PRESCRIPTION COMPONENTS
Ukraine
Carnivora
Indocin
Genistein
Larch (Arabinogalactan)
Iscador

HERBS AND SUPPLEMENTS
Germanium
Shark cartilage
Thymus extract
Pancreatic enzymes
Melatonin
Ip-6
MGN 3
Alphalipoic acid

Coenzyme Q10
Citrin
Garlic
Astragalus
Bromelain
Cat's claw
Gingko
Red clover
Pau d'arco
Milk thistle
Turmeric
Selenium
Quercetin
Chromium picolinate
Flaxseed oil
L-methionine
Calcium D. Glucarate
Potassium
NAC
L-glutamine
Naturleaf (enzyme-enhanced) Plant-Sprout sterols/sitosterolins
P-Spes
MSM

CATARACTS

Imagine a world that goes from being bright and colorful—filled with varying life forms and objects of different shapes and sizes—to a blur, forever out of focus and with objects barely distinguishable. Those stairs you used to climb with little or no effort become a chore because you can't tell one from the other. Welcome to the world of an animal afflicted with cataracts.

Toxicity is a major culprit with many of the health problems our animals experience today. When the body is toxic, cellular rejuvenation is poor, particularly in eye tissues. Toxins build up, and, in an effort to defend itself, the body captures the toxins and stores them. Cataracts often result.

And while many conventional veterinarians believe that animals are genetically predisposed to cataracts, some holistic vets feel otherwise. Their approach stresses detoxification, which process helps the body attack and break down the defective tissues that make up the cataract and replace these with healthier lens tissue.

So how can you help your animal see this once colorful world with lucid images again? Start with fasting—after consulting with your holistic vet, of course. Put your animal on a 24 to 48 hour fast. Follow this up with two to three weeks of homeopathic detoxification. Silica is good for encouraging the body to reabsorb tissue, thus shedding the cataract. Arsenicum is also recommended. Build the body with vitamin E—400 IU minimally per day for a large dog and 200 IU a day for a cat or small dog. Add vitamin A at a level of 5000 to 10,000 IU/day, along with beta carotene, selenium, and chromium. Do this for a minimum of six weeks.

Positive results have been seen in animals undergoing this detoxifying and nutritional regimen. Some animals have even had 50 percent of their cataract buildup broken down within the first 9 to 12 weeks, after having been afflicted for two or three years.

DIABETES

Diabetes, a disease that usually strikes middle-aged and older animals, is rampant in the pet world, as it is in the human world, and in both it is largely due to improper diet. Empty-calorie foods and enzyme-depleted processed foods are part of the problem, as is overeating. Emotional stress is another contributing factor.

Symptoms of diabetes include excessive urination, excessive drinking, and excessive eating. An animal with diabetes either does not produce enough insulin or is unable to use the insulin it produces. Either way, the blood sugar level becomes excessively high. In an attempt to lower its sugar level, the animal drinks a lot of water. But the sugar stays high and the animal simply urinates more. Usually sugar, in the form of glucose, supports the muscles and brain, but with this condition there is not enough insulin to push glucose to the cells. Thus the animal loses energy; Rover or Puff will stop running and jumping. In traditional Chinese medicine, diabetes is known as a thirsting, wasting disease.

If your animal experiences excessive thirst, weight loss, a voracious appetite, and excessive urination, it's important to take it to see your veterinarian to get a blood test. If your pet is diagnosed with diabetes it will usually be put on insulin and have its urine tested to monitor insulin levels so as not to overmedicate.

But a holistic veterinarian will take additional measures to help your animal. A different diet may be suggested, as well as antioxidants and other vitamins and minerals to bolster the immune system. When your pet is placed on a good immune-boosting program, its dependency on insulin may dissipate in time.

Dr. Gerald Johnson is a veterinarian who treats his diabetic animal patients holistically in order to get them on the lowest amount of external insulin possible. In many cases, he has had excellent success. In fact, many of the cats he has worked with no longer need insulin. Dr. Johnson's protocol consists of an improved diet, a mild exercise program, acupuncture, and herbs.

Supplements. Herbs helpful in treating diabetes include dandelion root, eyebright, blueberry leaves, and ginkgo biloba, which helps the condition by increasing circulation. Vanadyl sulfate is a mineral supplement that may help; consult your vet about the proper dosage of this and any other supplement for your pet.

DIARRHEA

In humans, diarrhea can be uncomfortable, but it is often a temporary state that soon passes. When an animal has diarrhea the condition is more dangerous, even life-threatening, if not addressed and corrected right away. So be sure to consult your vet if this problem develops.

As with many other conditions, toxicity can be at the core of this problem. Our pet's body is trying to say that something is terribly amiss, that an imbalance is occurring somewhere, somehow. You may not be able to pinpoint the cause right away, but you and the vet will want to address the immediate problem. Sometimes, if the problem is severe, fluids and electrolytes are administered intravenously to counteract dehydration. But there are also natural remedies that can be administered orally—placed in your animal's food or water or directly in its mouth.

The homeopathic formula Arsenicum is sometimes used to help

NATURAL PET CARE

143

restore energy after fluid loss. Next you will want to build your animal's immune system with vitamin C. Garlic is often used too because it is both antiseptic and fortifying.

EAR PROBLEMS

Ears are one of the body's eliminative pathways. If you are fasting an animal, the ear will produce a lot of wax during that time. Problems often develop in an animal's ears because the ears don't have good circulation. Bacteria and fungi tend to develop there.

Sometimes a good nutritional protocol is all that's needed to help free the ears of trouble. At other times the problems are more persistent. Many topical preparations for the ears are available at pet stores. If these fail to work, it's best to consult a doctor for a conventional medical treatment to gain stability, and then follow up with a holistic veterinarian's advice. Chinese herbs work well for some animals with ear problems. So does diluted apple cider vinegar; the acid medium kills yeast and fungi. Three quarters of a teaspoon of the apple cider vinegar can be diluted into half a cup of water and carefully applied in the ear with a Q-tip or eyedropper.

A common problem for animals, particularly cats, is ear mites, an annoying condition, that, if left untreated, can result in inflammation and hearing loss. Mites love finding homes in the ears of animals and staying put. Once they're settled, it takes effort to evict them. But it can be done.

If your animal grabs its ear and scratches furiously, it just might have ear mites. Often the ear becomes so inflamed that herbal preparations may not be strong enough to deal with the problem. This would be one of those rare times when conventional medicine might be more effective. Veterinarian Robert Goldstein feels that "in some cases, [the herbal approach] can cause more damage or inflammation than it's worth. So, generally, with ear mites, I just bite the bullet and say, 'Listen, use the medication for seven to ten days to get rid of it, and then we'll make sure that the ear stays healthy.'"

How do you ensure that your animal's ears stay healthy? The best safeguard against ear mites and other infections is to keep your pet's ears clean. Watch out for excessive wax production. Try an herbal combination made by Halo or an herbal wash from Noah's

Kingdom. If you are unsure how to clean your animal's ears, consult with your veterinarian or pet groomer.

EYE PROBLEMS

The eyes are the gateway to the body. They can reveal if something is wrong inside. Sometimes, then, eye problems are not a primary, but rather a secondary, problem. In Oriental philosophy, there's a close correlation between the eyes and the liver. In fact, some acupuncture points for the treatment of chronic eye problems are on the liver meridian. Dr. Martin Goldstein relates an unfortunate story of a dog with glaucoma that had his eye removed surgically. "A year later the dog developed liver cancer. Looking back at the dog's history I found that three years before that the dog's liver values were not normal. That s when it should have been addressed." Vitamin A is great for vision, he says, but a lot of its benefit is directed toward the liver, not so much the eye.

There are homeopathic remedies for chronically irritated eyes, as well as herbal formulas that contain such eye-regenerative herbs as bilberry and eyebright. The formulas are administered as eyewashes or taken orally.

FLEAS

Don't be alarmed just because your pet is scratching. Itchy animals are not necessarily fighting fleas. But if you do identify a problem, you will want to nip it in the bud, and you can do so, in many instances, using nontoxic products, including those you can prepare at home.

First, since prevention is the best medicine, make sure your animal charge is eating a good diet, as fleas are attracted to sick animals and tend to leave healthy ones alone. Avoid low-grade commercial foods and home-prepared products that make your pet more appealing to parasites. Fleas are attracted to animals that eat sugar, animal fats, and refined flour, so I'd advise avoiding:

White, refined flour
Refined sugar
Pork
Bacon and cured meats
Meat or chicken fat

Also, every pet owner should own a flea comb, a thin-toothed comb that will pick up fleas and their eggs. If you should notice insects, don't panic. They may not be fleas but rather some other more benign creature. Learn to recognize a flea problem by educating yourself about flea characteristics. Flea excrement is a tiny black speck that changes to a brownish-red color when placed on wet tissue paper. Flea eggs are small and white and hatch into larvae that grow into adults several days later.

If you notice fleas you will need to develop a treatment plan that kills and repels the critters naturally whenever possible, heals damaged skin, and strengthens the animal so that future attacks are avoided. Poisonous products appear to solve the problem fast, but in the long term they are detrimental to an animal's immune system and organs. They are also harmful to humans, having been associated with cancer, nervous conditions, reproductive problems, and other conditions. In the long run your goal should not be to destroy all "bad" insects—every living being has a purpose; parasites, in particular, were designed to weed out the weak—but to keep your pet strong and thus safe from parasite attacks.

When you notice fleas early on you will have an easier time getting rid of them. You can take simple measures such as adding garlic oil and nutritional yeast (or 5 mg of thiamine) to your pet's food each day, or brushing the coat with the essential oil of fleabane, a natural product that repels fleas. You could also apply a natural flea powder, such as diatomaceous dust, to the coat, although some animals may be allergic to this. Other natural skin rubs that have been proven effective include brewer's yeast, ground cloves, raw lemon slices, and garlic oil. Additionally, there are natural flea collars made from a combination of plant oils. Moreover, you will want to shampoo your pet with an herbal shampoo or add between 1/4 and 1/2 teaspoon of citronella oil to the regular shampoo followed by a cream rinse or oil. While the water alone may be enough to kill fleas, the herbs will serve to destroy new fleas as they hatch from their eggs.

If the flea population has grown to moderate proportions, in addition to the foregoing measures you could spray the coat with a natural flea and tick spray, being careful to avoid your animal's eyes and other sensitive areas. In the most severe cases, you will be tempted to turn to harsh poisons, and indeed, if the situation has reached life-threatening proportions this may be the only measure to take. That said, if your pet is not yet anemic and you are patient and concerned about your pet's welfare, stick to natural measures a bit longer. You may very well succeed.

In addition to all the steps just mentioned, you could sprinkle a powder made from garlic powder, brewer's yeast, or diatomaceous earth onto carpeting, furniture, and sleeping quarters or use a pre-made powder, like the natural product from Flea Busters that is said to work for one year (see Appendix). Use the herbal flea shampoo frequently—every two to three days—until fleas disappear. Make sure your pet is wearing an aromatic flea collar made from citronella and eucalyptus. Pennyroyal is also highly effective, but too much could be poisonous. Vacuum your entire home each day to remove fleas, eggs, and pupae, and change the bag after each cleaning. Powder should be reapplied throughout the house after each vacuuming. In addition, you will need to wash bedding in very hot water, or destroy it. If all else fails and you must resort to a bomb spray that contains insecticides, be sure that all living creatures are removed from the home for many hours. Finally, you should brush your animal's hair each day and follow with a vigorous massage to remove dead debris and increase skin vitality.

After the parasite population diminishes your dog or cat may still be suffering from the ravages of flea infestation. At this point you must establish a plan for resistance to insect attacks, and at the same time heal raw, damaged skin that can cause pain to your friend. Initially, you will need to remove all eggs, excrement, and other detritus from the skin because that can cause severe suffering in animals. Find a shampoo designed for this purpose such as the one made by Allergroom. Next you will need to renew damaged skin by soaking it in a rich oil for 5 to 15 minutes. Good choices are sesame or baby oil. Other skin treatments can be made at home. Brew a strong goldenseal root tea and after it has cooled apply twice a day to raw skin. Or dilute one of the following and apply: vinegar, witch hazel, onion juice, rosemary, or blackberry tea. A good home-opathic remedy for getting rid of leftover fleas and healing the skin is Sulphur. To prevent future flea problems, you might use Earth Animal's natural internal powder.

NATURAL PET CARE

HEART DISEASE

People usually associate heart disease with older folks who consume a lot of greasy foods, but animals can suffer from heart problems too. If your pet has a dry, hacking cough in the middle of the night, he or she may have a cold, but it could also be a sign of a failing heart. Similarly, a distended belly could be from fluid buildup, not weight gain. So if your animal is overweight without overeating, you should suspect a heart problem. Other signs of heart disease include loss of appetite and energy, reluctance to climb stairs, depression and lethargy, fainting, or lack of coordination. Heart disease can strike animals as young as five or six years old, and since heart disease can be fatal, prevention and early detection are vital. One way to detect heart disease early is to take your pet to a holistic veterinarian annually for a complete physical exam. At these exams, the vet will assess your animal's overall health and may run routine blood tests that will give an early indication of heart disease or some other physiological problem.

Possible causes of heart disease are poor diet, over-vaccination, exposure to toxic substances, and over-breeding. If your animal is diagnosed with heart disease, don't lament just yet. While conventional veterinarians may not be terribly optimistic about managing heart disease, other options exist. Sufficient daily doses of vitamin E (between 200 and 800 IU depending on your animal's size), L-carnitine (250-750 mg), and coenzyme Q10 (25-200 mg) will ensure that your animal gets the nutrients it needs to promote fortification of the heart; talk to your vet about exactly what your animal requires. Taurine is given to cats, with cats under five pounds given 250 mg daily, and those five pounds and over getting 500 mg. Also, some vets recommend garlic concentrates as being good for purifying the blood, lowering blood pressure, and improving circulation. Cats and small dogs get a half a tablet daily, with the dosage ranging up to two or three tablets, depending on weight, or you can add one to two chopped garlic cloves to the food.

Going Beyond Garlic. In addition to garlic—considered by many to be the herbal superstar—there is a whole spectrum of herbs that can help fight heart disease and strengthen circulation. As you scan the list, a caveat: In the wilds, your pet's ancestors probably knew instinctively which of the many plants available they should munch on to feel better. Today, though, the wilds have been replaced by the health food store, and since you don't want to bombard your ill animal with too many remedies, you should consult with your holistic vet about which of the following are right for your particular pet's condition.

Ginger
Turmeric
Hawthorn berry
Bugleweed
Gingko biloba
Mistletoe
Tansy
Wild yam
Alfalfa
Arjuna
Indian snakeroot (Rauwolfia)
Black cohosh
Bilberry
Butcher's broom

Creating a Heart Disease Protocol. If your animal is lucky enough to have a holistically oriented veterinarian, that practitioner can use the following supplements to tailor a heart disease protocol for your pet. The idea is to choose one or two supplements to begin with, gradually building upon that in stages over a period of three to four months, while monitoring the animal's response. I have purposely not included dosages because these must be determined by your vet as he or she takes into account your animal's species, size, and condition.

Coenzyme Q10
Calcium
Magnesium
Garlic
L-carnitine
Lecithin
Phosphatidyl choline

Citrin
DMG
TMG
Max. EPA
Potassium
Selenium
Vitamin E
Melatonin
Vitamin B complex
Vitamin C
Ginkgo biloba
DHEA
Hawthorne
Flaxseed oil
Naturleaf (enzyme enhanced) Plant-Sprout sterols/sitosterolins
MGN 3

HEARTWORM AND OTHER PARASITES

Spread by mosquitoes, heartworm is one of the most common diseases in dogs in the U.S. Cats can get it too, if they're outdoors a lot. Unfortunately, unless you test for it, recognizing heartworm is not always an easy task, and many cases go undetected until severe symptoms develop. Indications include an increased appetite, weight loss, a cough, and exercise intolerance. Once the disease progresses, the heart enlarges. The obstructed arteries of the heart give rise to a forceful pumping action that increases blood pressure. Consequently, the lungs become filled with fluid. Unable to keep up with the pace, the heart eventually fails.

Conventional treatments present a significant risk to the dog. Animals are usually treated with arsenic, which is very toxic. Permanent damage can occur to a dog or cat's heart and surrounding arteries while leaving the animal disabled. In addition, treatment is often expensive and lengthy; therefore, prevention, through a blood test, is key.

There are some natural remedies you can use, though. The essential oils of oregano, cinnamon, peppermint, and clove are a good treatment for heartworm and other parasites. These are given in capsule form. Also, C.J. Puotinen, author of *Natural*

Remedies for Dogs and Cats, describes an anti-parasite powder made of equal parts of dried wormwood, cloves, the Indian herb neem leaves, and rue. These are ground and the resultant powder mixed in with a substance the animal will eat, or the mixture can be encapsulated. Black walnut hull tincture, and the aptly named wormwood are other tried-and-true natural anti-parasitic remedies. Chaparral and pau d'arco are sometimes beneficial too. Useful in fighting intestinal parasites are garlic, coarsely chopped pumpkin or citrus seeds, and diatomaceous earth. For hookworm, which can be a big problem for newborn puppies and kittens, Dr. John Heinerman, author of *Natural Pet Cures*, mentions the herbal remedies aloe, carrot, catnip, garlic, papaya, tarragon, white oak, wild plum, and wormwood.

Black and green teas (cooled), are recommended heartworm fighters, says Heinerman. And cooled boiled cabbage juice, a carrot/parsley or carrot/wheatgrass juice mix, dandelion root tea, or boiled corn or potato water can help as well. For animals with difficulty breathing, Heinerman recommends peppermint tea. Of course you'll want to consult your holistic vet about serious problems, and to zero in on those remedies that will best aid your pet's fight against parasites. Following is a list of anti-parasitic herbs that your vet can help you choose from:

Green black walnut hulls
Western wormwood
Cloves
Quassi chips
Mullein leaf
Fennel seed
Cascara sagrada
Pumpkin seed
Garlic
Cramp bark
Capsicum
Thyme
Sweet Annie
Cinchana bark
Goldenseal root
Elecampane root

HIP DYSPLASIA

Walking is one of those things most of us take for granted. We constantly walk, as do animals, and, like us, animals depend on their hips and legs to perform this vital function. But when an animal has hip dysplasia, walking doesn't come easily.

Hip dysplasia is the result of weak tendons and ligaments. When the body does not get the nutrients it needs—B12, B6, biotin, and ascorbic acid, to name a few—collagen production suffers, and, as a result, tendons and ligaments do too.

If you should spot a stray dog that is limping or cannot even stand, it's likely that that animal is suffering from a nutritional deficiency. Proper diet with sufficient minerals, vitamins, and live enzymes cannot be emphasized enough. Such therapy has been known to reverse hip dysplasia, and it has the added advantage of creating a stronger system that staves off other problems too.

Hip dysplasia usually affects dogs, although other animals are becoming increasingly affected. Cats and even horses are now being diagnosed with the condition. Some cases of the ailment can be attributed to genetic predisposition, often due to over-breeding. When animals are over-bred, the weaker genes of body structure become more dominant. Thus, the dog that at one point walked on its foot pad now walks on its hock, all because some breeder wanted it to look a certain way.

The best thing you can do for your pet is to feed it the proper wholesome foods and supplement its diet with vitamins and minerals. If your dog has a limp or cannot stand up, consult with a holistic veterinarian.

INFLAMMATORY BOWEL DISEASE

We all know how debilitating an upset stomach can be. We cannot do much of anything besides rest or try to focus on something other than our troubled belly. If your animal vomits after meals, has lost its appetite or much weight, or has a weak stomach, you want to clear up the problem as quickly as possible. Your pet may be suffering from inflammatory bowel disease, or IBD. Depending on the animal, symptoms may be different, with cats more prone to vomiting and dogs more prone to diarrhea. (That's because cats are generally affected in the upper portion of the intestinal tract, while dogs are more susceptible to inflammation in the lower portion of the bowel.)

Many veterinary textbooks attribute IBD to unknown causes, yet clear links exist. For example, animals that drink contaminated water may get parasites, such as Giardia and whipworm. These can lead to chronic infection and IBD. A simple fecal sample test can tell you if your animal is infected with parasites. Another potential culprit is vaccinations, which can compromise the immune system in their effort to strengthen it. With IBD, as with many conditions, bolstering of the immune system is necessary. Note that animals that live in stressful environments, where fighting occurs, and animals that eat a poor diet, are more susceptible to the disease.

Left untreated, IBD can lead to a degenerative condition requiring extensive medical attention and hefty veterinary fees. One of the problems is that your animal may lose proteins; get a blood test to look at albumin and globulin levels. Albumin is especially important in maintaining osmotic pressure, ensuring that blood does not leak out into the tissues. Moreover, any levels above or below normal can indicate disease or malnutrition, so have your animal tested.

Conventional therapies incorporate cortisone to block and suppress possible auto-immune effects, but this suppression only drives the symptoms deeper and, in the long run, makes the animal sicker.

Holistic protocols for this condition focus on whole food sources, such as unadulterated lamb or chicken, whole brown rice, tofu, or cottage cheese. Naturally occurring fiber, which cleanses the intestinal tract and promotes proper bowel conditioning, is critical. Your aim is to limit the number of foods traveling through the inflamed intestinal tract while giving your animal the nourishment it requires. If your dog has inflammatory bowel disease, start him on a potato-based diet, using cooked sweet and white potatoes, as well as some cooked meat and turnips. Your holistic animal practitioner can help individualize the diet for your animal. If the condition is induced by parasites, use garlic to help get rid of the parasites and tincture of goldenseal to fight infection.

For acute conditions, try Kaopectate from natural clay or use the herb slippery elm. Both are good for soothing the stomach and intestines. Try a bland diet with white rice, boiled beef or chicken, and mashed carrots until the symptoms become controllable.

For chronic conditions, again, use goldenseal. In addition, the herb licorice works like the natural cortisone manufactured by the adrenal glands in helping to suppress the auto-immune effects of IBD and reduce inflammation. While using goldenseal and licorice may help your animal overcome IBD, you will not want to use these herbs over an extended period. If you are concerned about the delicate membranes of your animal's intestines or stomach—and in most cases, you will be— be sure to pick up the homeopathic remedy called Gastroenteritis that works specifically on these membranes.

Once your animal stabilizes from the effects of IBD, it is important to replenish its immune system. Incorporate garlic into the animal's diet to cleanse the intestinal tract of decaying material. Add yogurt to the meal to replenish beneficial bacteria. Weekly fasts or skipped meals will allow the animal's intestinal tract to detoxify and recoup. A supplementary product similar to Gastroenteritis is Acetylator, which works to protect the lining of the stomach and intestines. It is available only from licensed veterinarians, so consult with your holistic veterinarian for more information and to obtain the product.

KIDNEY DISEASE

Kidney failure is a common condition in older cats, whose kidneys appear to weaken as they age. Part of the problem may be low-protein foods fed to senior animals. We feed our cats these formulas, believing they are easier on the kidneys. But when the body does not have enough amino acids to replenish tissue growth it may start breaking down other systems. This is what may happen to the kidneys. High-protein foods, on the other hand, may hurt the kidneys, too, if the quality of that protein is poor. Indigestible protein becomes a waste product that contributes to the body breaking down its own tissue, and one of the first places to be affected is the kidneys. If your cat should fall victim to this life-threatening condition, see a holistic veterinarian right away.

Of course each case is individual, but if your animal has a bad case of kidney failure, the doctor will probably place it on a low-protein diet. Without good kidney function the animal might not be able to cope with all the work needed to break down protein. Actually, if you correct for some of the imbalances in kidney failure, you can feed the animal a fair amount of protein. You can help your animal regain that balance with plenty of fresh water and fluid therapy, which your veterinarian will probably recommend for this condition. Extra fluids delivered subcutaneously help prevent dehydration and uremia and thus prolong life. Your veterinarian can teach you how to administer fluid therapy at home—using approximately 200 cc's of fluid every other day—to avert kidney failure. Some vets also recommend adding salt to the diet to encourage the animal to drink more water. But this can lead to other serious problems, such as heart weakness, because the salt can create edema (fluid buildup) around the heart. You don't want to substitute one serious condition for another, so do not give salt to your animal.

The benefits of fluid therapy may be augmented when it is used in conjunction with homeopathic remedies. A homeopathically trained physician may prescribe phosphorous, sulfur, nux vomica, or arsenicum album, depending upon the needs of the animal. The combination of fluid therapy and homeopathic treatments will usually have a palliative effect; that is, they won't necessarily cure the problem, but may well help the animal to live a better life than would normally be expected.

Some vets use Eastern modalities—acupuncture, and even chi gong—on animals. Veterinarian Henry Pasternak uses this latter form of energy medicine on many of his patients. He reports much success, including one case involving a 17-year-old cat with kidney failure. After treating the cat with acupuncture, he started using chi gong. The following day, he received a call from the cat's ecstatic owner, who reported that the animal's condition had improved from listless and lethargic to lively and involved. The cat was once again able to run and eat its food.

Supplements for Kidney Disease. There is a whole range of supplements that a holistic vet might use in creating a protocol for a dog or cat with kidney disease. Following is a list of these, from which your vet would choose up to two items to give at a time. The idea is not to bombard your pet with supplements, but rather to see what works and build on that, in carefully observed stages, over a period of several months.

> Cranberry extract
> Acidophilus
> Lecithin

Vitamin C
L-arginine
L-methionine
"Vital K" (for potassium)
Green tea
Ginkgo biloba exract
Evening primrose oil
Parsley/cornsilk tea
Burdock root tea
Echinacea extract
Dandelion extract
B complex
Vitamin B2
Vitamin B6
Beta carotene
Vitamin E
Flaxseed oil
Calcium/magnesium
Zinc
Buchu tea
Hydrangea
Uva ursi
Marshmallow tea

LYME DISEASE

We hear a lot of warnings about deer ticks and the need to take precautions in wooded areas, but we generally think in terms of protecting humans. While the incidence of Lyme disease is lower in animals than in humans, it does exist. Lyme is more difficult to detect
in animals because there is no rash or redness around the bite area,
a symptom that often appears in humans. Many animals will
become lethargic in the early stages, and later on they may develop
arthritis. Periodic lameness is a red flag for Lyme in animals.

If you suspect that your pet has Lyme disease, see a veterinarian as soon as possible and get a blood test done. If the Lyme titer
is high and clinical signs of the condition are present, the conventional treatment will be a course of antibiotics over several weeks. A
holistic veterinarian might try natural antibiotics, or conventional

antibiotics, if need be, to resolve the problem. But he or she will probably also do a detailed nutritional analysis of your animal in order to customize a nutritional program for it. The idea is twofold—to support the immune system and offset any deleterious effects of the medication your pet is receiving. The oils of oregano, cinnamon, peppermint, and clove, in capsule form, are all helpful in countering Lyme disease.

Beware of the Lyme vaccine, as it may provoke symptoms of the disease itself, such as arthritis.

MOTION SICKNESS

If your cat meows and howls relentlessly when being transported, it may be because of motion sickness, a problem that affects about a fourth of companion animals. Symptoms of motion sickness are excessive salivation and or vomiting in dogs and prolonged crying in cats. If your animal is prone to this problem, it should travel on an empty stomach. Make frequent stops. And give your pet a flower essence or homeopathic formula before the ride. You might have to experiment with different ones until you discover the remedy that works for your animal. Bach's Rescue Remedy, a flower essence found in health food stores, is a popular one for this purpose. You can also try Calm Stress from Dr. Goodpet (call [807] 222-9932 to order).

NEUROLOGICAL PROBLEMS

In the wake of all the inbreeding and over-breeding that our animals, particularly dogs, have gone through, it is amazing that some animals survive at all. With each new generation we see compromised body systems and malfunctioning organs. Neurological problems are one unfortunate manifestation, and seizures, in particular, are often upsetting to behold. To see our animals convulsing and losing control of their bodily functions is not a happy experience, nor is it something we can stop once an episode occurs. However, with proper care, seizures and other neurological problems can be managed.

Vitamin B complex yields remarkable results in animals with neurological problems. If your pet takes at least 100 mg of high-grade B complex, its neurological condition should stabilize. This dose is usually safe for any size animal. Some animals even show signs of reversal within 24 to 48 hours if they are taking higher doses, such as 150 mg or more daily.

Be careful not to overdo it. If you are using B and other water-soluble vitamins in high therapeutic doses, your animal should be fine, but if you should, however, incorporate fat-soluble vitamins in the mix, you are putting your animal at a greater risk of retaining those vitamins, which can cause toxicity after prolonged use—i.e., several weeks, or even only days in some cases. So do be careful. As always, to be sure you are on the right track, consult with your holistic veterinarian before attempting to treat such a serious problem on your own.

Your pet may also benefit greatly from energetic healing. Acupuncture or homeopathy can make your animal stronger and more resistant to further neurological problems. Acupuncture, the placing of needles along specific points in the body known as meridians, can improve energy flow and help correct the underlying problem. Marcie Fallek, D.V.M., a certified animal acupuncturist from Fairfield, Connecticut, claims to have broad success in the treatment of paralyzed animals with this modality. She attributes her excellent results to the release of chi, the Chinese term for energy, as energy blockage is seen in traditional Chinese medicine as the root of all problems.

Similarly, homeopathy can yield good results, says Dr. Fallek, who stresses that the remedy used for an animal will be individualized according to a wide array of symptoms. As she explains, "When I prescribe a medicine for a dog with paralysis, as important, or more important than the paralysis is the fact that it has a certain skin condition around its mouth, the fact that it is very needy, the fact that it drinks a lot of water, the fact that it had a sore toe. You take everything about the animal, you put it together, and you select the homeopathic medicine, out of the 1500 that are available, that addresses the whole animal."

PARVOVIRUS

Does your dog seem lethargic? Have bloody diarrhea? Dehydration? Sudden-onset vomiting? Fever? While these symptoms may indicate a number of conditions, you definitely want to rule out parvo. If you notice one or more of these symptoms, don't wait. The parvo virus strikes with the speed of a hawk attacking its prey, and can result in a painful death days later.

The disease is usually spread through infected fecal matter, although direct or indirect contact with other excretions can spread it as well. Parvovirus is found in parks, kennels, pet shops, dog shows, humane shelters, and other places where dogs assemble. People can contribute to its spread by carrying infected fecal material from place to place on their shoes.

Unfortunately, the parvo virus is quite resilient and can withstand extreme temperatures. It can survive for up to six months in cages and soil. Extreme cold prior to snowfall will kill the virus, though it can survive under a blanket of snow with temperatures as low as 25 degrees. Bleach has been used as a disinfecting agent to kill the virus. Should you decide to use this approach, dilute the bleach in a ratio of 9 parts water to 1 part bleach, and keep your animal clear of the area, as you don't want your pet inhaling this chemical.

In treating your animal, you will want to strengthen its immune system, in addition to treating symptoms with antibiotics and antiemetics to lessen signs and aid in the control of dehydration. More recent conventional treatments for parvo include antitoxins and antiparvo serum in conjunction with hospitalization. Naturopathic remedies include high doses of vitamin C, echinacea, and goldenseal.

If you should have the misfortune of losing your dog to parvovirus, wait at least six months to a year before purchasing a new puppy, as your environment may still be infected, even if you have disinfected it. If your animal is lucky enough to survive parvovirus, it will most likely develop immunity to it and not be infected again.

PREGNANCY

Pregnancy is generally a time for celebration, but it has its discomforts and dangers. Animals cannot communicate directly how they feel, but speak to us in subtle ways. It's our job to pay attention to their cues and take the necessary precautions to ensure that our pregnant animal delivers safely. Consult with a holistic veterinarian who will guide you through this process.

Be especially careful of herbal formulas you might be giving your pet, as some can be dangerous for an expectant mother. Pennyroyal, for example, is great for controlling pests, but it can cause spontaneous abortions in pregnant animals. The best way to safeguard your pet from potentially harmful herbs during pregnancy is to do research. The general rule is that if an herb is not safe for humans during pregnancy, it is not safe for an animal either.

If your pet has a weakness, chances are that problem will manifest during pregnancy. Learn to pay attention to the subtle signs of something having gone awry. You might even want to take notes, keeping a daily journal of your pet's activities and eating habits. In monitoring your pet's eating habits, it is important to note what she eats daily (as you remember, of course, to feed her a wholesome, balanced diet). If you find that your animal has not eaten for a day, this is fine; just continue to monitor your pet. But when your cat suddenly skips two days of eating and is lethargic, you should suspect that something is wrong. A homeopathic detoxification protocol might be warranted here. Homeopathy is usually very safe for pregnant animals, but do consult your vet. A little arsenicum or nux vomica may be recommended.

Some vets recommend that to prevent eclampsia, you give your pet a calcium supplement (ground eggshell or oyster is good). Start this about two weeks before the due date, and continue for six weeks beyond the birth.

RABIES

Of all the conditions that an animal can have, rabies is probably the scariest. Most of us have heard horror stories about pets dying or becoming incorrigible. Sadly, both are possibilities. Rabies is not a condition you should attempt to manage yourself. If you suspect your animal has rabies it needs to be under a veterinarian's care to ensure that the animal is not going to bite anyone.

Rabies is a fatal disease caused by a virus that is contracted from the bite of an infected animal. Any warm-blooded animal is susceptible. Wild animals, such as raccoons, skunks, foxes, and bats, are commonly infected with the disease. A domestic animal that is not vaccinated against rabies, and that comes in contact with a wild or stray animal, is at risk for picking up the disease.

In the early stages of the disease, animals may show a slight change in mood or behavior. Once the disease progresses, your pet may have the tendency to roam or eat things it normally wouldn't. It may become restless and hyperactive. The animal may even drool excessively or have trouble swallowing. Often the animal will become vicious. Convulsions may occur, and these are usually fatal. If the animal survives convulsions, it usually suffers paralysis of the lower jaw. "Dumb" rabies usually occurs shortly. Paralysis spreads across the entire body, and death follows.

To witness some or all of this in your pet can be heartbreaking, to say the least. So if you at all suspect that your animal has the disease, be certain to have your pet under the care of your holistic veterinarian.

Note on Vaccination. Because rabies is such a horrendous communicable disease, rabies vaccinations are required by law as prevention. As discussed in Chapter 9, the general population regards vaccines as safe, and has no qualms about recommending yearly or bi-yearly shots. But this overzealous use of vaccinations is not wise. While you will need to vaccinate your pet, take measures to prevent vaccinosis, a vaccine-induced condition that can mimic symptoms of the disease itself. Don't vaccinate routinely, but rather, when it's time to revaccinate, have your doctor perform a blood titer to see whether the antibodies are still present (if they are, revaccination is not needed). Have your doctor give the vaccine alone, not with other vaccinations. Never vaccinate an animal that is sick. And always follow with a homeopathic nosode to detoxify the animal's system.

SKIN AND COAT PROBLEMS

In over 75 percent of animals, skin and coat problems are symptoms of a toxic lifestyle and are intimately connected to an over-burdened liver. Cleaning up the diet and detoxifying your pet is the foundation of better health and appearance. Step two is to consider a high-quality vitamin and mineral supplement to help improve the skin and coat. Try vitamin E, zinc, and biotin to make the coat softer and healthier looking. If after a few weeks on this protocol the coat remains brittle, add some extra biotin for a month. Most animals will respond to that. Then return to a maintenance dose of 50 micrograms daily. Also consider liver detoxification with herbs, such as milk thistle and juniper berry. Be sure to use good-quality supplements, as the fillers in lower-end products can cause drying skin.

THYROID PROBLEMS

Hypothyroidism. Hypothyroidism is an auto-immune disease; in other words, the body perceives its own thyroid gland as being diseased and develops an immune reaction to it. The number-one cause of hypothyroidism is vaccinations, especially in dogs. Initial inflammation causes the thyroid to become hyperactive. Then it tires and a hypothyroid condition results.

Conventional doctors often give a dog suffering from hypothyroidism a synthetic thyroid hormone replacement. But replacing the body's own function with a fake may make the body dependent on the substance and may, over time, cause the body to shut down. Holistic physicians will generally try to get the thyroid to function again. They work to balance the pituitary gland, the adrenal glands, the liver, and the thyroid gland, with the aim of getting the thyroid working again.

Hyperthyroidism. Hyperthyroidism is being seen in cats in epidemic proportions. It is one of the documented side effects of vaccines. The problem is also believed to be related to chemical additives found in some pet foods that may stimulate the overgrowth of the thyroid gland. This is one of the reasons to keep your pet's diet as pure as possible.

UPPER RESPIRATORY VIRAL INFECTIONS

Symptoms of an upper respiratory infection include nasal discharge, fever, lethargy, and anorexia. These symptoms actually help fight the virus in the animal's body. What we need to do for our pet is to give it extra tools to win the fight sooner.

Vitamin C is a great place to start building your pet's immune system. Give your animal high levels (500-5000 mg per day, depending on its size and bowel tolerance levels) for two weeks. Couple that with echinacea (1-10 drops per day depending on size) for ten days. On the eleventh day, stop the echinacea. You may need to restart on day 20 for another 10 days. This time add goldenseal for extra strength. For dogs—but not cats, please note—garlic (Kyolic works well) will also help the plan. Hot steam with eucalyptus oil for 30 to 60 minutes, once or twice a day, will be effective for congestion; take care to avoid burning accidents. A wet cotton ball is good for removing discharges from the eyes or nose. Keep your pet on a low-food, high-liquid diet.

Be sure to monitor your pet throughout this process for any changes in temperature, breathing, appetite, and discharges. Maintain contact with your holistic veterinarian to keep him or her abreast of any new developments.

VOMITING

Vomiting is one way the body cleanses itself. Through vomiting the body gets rid of toxins and creates time to rest and heal. Overeating, and the absence of fasting, are two culprits that weaken an animal's stomach and intestines. Then when your animal meets a trigger, such as grass or food on the street, or even stress, its digestive system will react violently, usually in the form of vomiting.

Sometimes vomiting can be indicative of serious problems, so it is important to monitor your animal carefully. Watch out for persistent vomiting, blood in the vomit, and the presence of fever or pain. If any of these symptoms occur, take your pet to an animal hospital or holistic veterinarian as soon as possible, as your animal will require blood tests and quite possibly x-rays. In extreme cases, exploratory surgery may be indicated.

If serious problems are not involved, you may be able to treat vomiting with a simple herbal cleanse. Do not feed your animal any solid foods for a few days. Instead, give it water and broth for up to three days (see Chapter 6, on detoxifying). On day two of the fast, give your pet a dose of Gentle Dragon.

Once the fast has ended, you will want to restructure your animal's diet. Start by adding more fiber to the diet. Fruit, vegetables, rice, and oatmeal are examples of foods high in fiber. You will also want to add green foods, such as grated salads, to your pet's diet. Greens are rich in cleansing chlorophyll. Introducing regular fasting is another component in restructuring your animal's diet, so incorporate that into your plan as well. The long-term goal is to build up the digestive system while sustaining it, and proper diet, inclusive of appropriate food volumes and frequency of feedings, will ensure that this occurs.

EMERGENCIES

In addition to overcoming illness and optimizing general health, you will want to steer your animal clear of sudden, unexpected dangers. A little knowledge of pet hazards will go a long way toward protecting your animal from needless harm. Familiarize yourself with the facts; learn about substances that are dangerous to animals, and keep them out of your pet's environment. The following are common hazards you should know about.

Protect Your Pet From Poison. By now, everybody knows the importance of childproofing one's home, but people don't always consider taking precautions to protect their pets. It is essential that you pet-proof your home by keeping substances toxic to Fido or Fluff out of the home or out of their reach. From chemicals to chocolate, you've got to be aware of what your pet could get its paws—and jaws—into.

HOUSEHOLD CHEMICALS. Just closing the container isn't enough to keep a curious animal away from cleansers and other chemical products kept at home. A bored or lonely dog might amuse itself by puncturing a can or chewing on a plastic container until the toxic ingredients pour out and drench his feet and fur. Sometimes a small exposure is all it takes to poison a pet. Be sure to place a latch or lock on the cabinet door or keep these substances high out of an animal's reach. Cats are much more cautious, but still in danger of being poisoned if exposed to even small amounts of household products. Also, make sure to keep insect and mouse traps in places that your pet can't get to.

MEDICATIONS. Child-proof bottles might be insufficient protection when a determined dog decides it would be fun to break into a container, so follow the advice given above and store medications safely away in a latched or locked medicine cabinet. Note: Never give a cat Tylenol or another painkiller, as the ingredients can prove deadly.

ANTIFREEZE. *Antifreeze is highly lethal.* That's why you must never leave an uncovered container of antifreeze within an animal's reach. Also, be sure to clean up any spills immediately, as your animal might walk through the green puddle and lick the stuff off its fur. All it takes is a teaspoon of antifreeze to kill a cat and less than a tablespoon to kill a 20-pound dog.

"FOR DOGS ONLY" LABELS. Never give a cat a product geared strictly to dogs. Flea products labeled "for dogs only," for instance, contain more toxic chemicals than a cat's sensitive system can process. Many of these products are not good for dogs either, but they probably won't kill them right away. Cats, however, may have a sudden lethal reaction to the stuff.

COMMON FOODS. There are many foods that you must keep away from pets. If you are a "chocoholic," your main concern is probably limiting the amount of chocolate *you* eat to avoid extra calories, but the consequences of your dog or cat eating chocolate can be far more serious. If a small dog were to eat a small bar of chocolate, that little bit could actually be deadly. Chocolate contains the stimulant theobromine, which can be toxic to dogs' hearts. So be sure to hide your Valentine's chocolates from Fido. Other foods not to feed dogs and cats include onions, onion powder, alcoholic beverages, yeast dough, coffee, coffee grounds and beans, tea, macadamia nuts, hops (used in home beer brewing), tomatoes, tomato leaves and stems, and rhubarb leaves. One would think this goes without saying, but let us say it anyway: Never let your animal eat cigarettes, cigars, snuff, or chewing tobacco. And do not feed your animal moldy or spoiled foods. Your pet is not a garbage can! Moldy foods contain a toxin that dogs and cats can't tolerate. Also, keep avocados away from birds, mice, horses, cattle, and dairy goats. They could have a lethal effect. Some people give salt to a dog to induce vomiting, but salt is lethal to their systems too.

PLANTS. Some common household plants are deadly to animals when eaten. They include azalea, oleander, castor bean, sago palm, Easter lily (cats only), and yew and yew-plant-material-based medications.

Animal Poison Control: (888) 4ANIHELP

Should you suspect that your pet is poisoned—common signs of poisoning include fatigue, diarrhea and vomiting, a severe tremor, or seizures—it is imperative that you get the animal treated immediately. Call the National Animal Poison Control Center at (888) 4ANIHELP. This hotline is open 7 days a week, 24 hours a day. You will also need to visit your veterinarian as quickly as possible so that the doctor can assess the seriousness of the situation and advise you on managing it.

A Pet First Aid Kit. You will want to be prepared for any emergency, so, in addition to posting your veterinarian's phone number near the telephone, as well as the number of a 24-hour animal hospital, stock your medicine chest with the following:

Thermometer—the proper temperature for a dog or cat is about 101 or 102 degrees F. Below 100 degrees F is too low.

Lubricating jelly—to more easily insert the thermometer

Aconite—to bring down a fever before you get to the vet

Pedialyte—mixed with a little honey and given by mouth, this helps prevent dehydration and shock

Heating pad

Eyebright solution—as an eyewash this will remove foreign substances and decrease the chances of infection

Bandages

Peroxide and alcohol—wound cleansers

Goldenseal or calendula—antibacterials for treating infections, open wounds, sores, or hot spots

Rescue Remedy—for treatment of shock, trauma, emotional upsets

Arnica—for acute trauma, bruising, shock; works well with Rescue Remedy

Kaopectate and slippery elm—either remedy can help diarrhea and intestinal problems

SICK ANIMAL WARNING SIGNS

Long before a full-blown disease appears in an animal there are usually subtle warning signs that indicate a problem is brewing. By noticing early signals and taking corrective action right away, you can restore your animal's health more easily than if you wait for a crisis. Look for these signals, any one of which could indicate that something is amiss:

> Loss of enthusiasm for normal activities
> Lack of affection
> Loss of appetite
> Coarse or dull coat
> Foul body odor
> Excessive thirst and urination
> Rapid weight loss
> Rapid weight gain
> Hyperactivity
> Sudden aggressiveness
> Dull eyes
> Loss of response to verbal cues

As with children, when your animal stops acting like his or her normal self, something physical may be wrong. Should you notice that something does seem wrong, seek confirmation from a veterinarian. Testing will probably be done to see whether or not your suspicions are correct. If your pet is indeed ill, your holistic vet will guide you in taking the proper action, reviewing your animal's diet, adding live enzymes to the food, making sure the water is pure and always available, and adding vitamin C, a good multiple vitamin, and perhaps a glandular and the herb astragalus for immune support. A nutritionally aware veterinarian can advise you on the specifics needed to help your pet.

CHAPTER 8

Other Animal Friends

BIRDS

Birds delight our senses with resplendent colors and brilliant songs. On a deeper level, their ability to gracefully soar to great heights speaks to our longing for freedom, happiness, and peace. Bird fanciers relate well to Emily Dickinson's eloquent lines, "'Hope' is the thing with feathers— That perches in the soul—" No wonder we seek these elusive creatures in the wild, buy special feeders to attract birds to our gardens, and invite them into our homes for companionship.

If you think about it, it becomes clear that pet birds have to make one of the biggest adjustments to living arrangements of any domesticated animal. Most pet birds are domestically raised and therefore not accustomed to total freedom. Still, these creatures are free-spirited by nature and must be made comfortable living in some form of confinement. It's easy to see why stress and anxiety are such common problems for birds living in captivity.

If your bird seems anxious or stressed, it may be because it is alone. Birds in the wild almost always live in pairs or groups. Or it may be that its housing, food, or routine may not be appropriate for the species of bird you own. Let's explore some ways to minimize the stress in your pet bird's life.

Housing. While no bird was meant to live in captivity, some will adjust better than others. Check with an expert to make sure that the accommodations you're providing are the correct ones for the kind of bird you have. Bigger birds need bigger cages and even small birds need adequate space for flight. Cages should be free of toxic paint and metals (such as zinc and lead). The ideal cage is made of stainless steel. Also, all birds need the opportunity to exercise outside their cages, in a safe environment (either in your home or in an enclosed space outside), where they can be protected from other pets, as well as predatory animals and birds. It should be remembered that wild birds can carry diseases and parasites harmful to domesticated birds.

Birds need about 10 to 12 hours of sleep a night and, to recover from sickness, they may need additional rest and quiet time. To foster restful sleep and quick recovery from illness, you can cover the cage with a towel or blanket.

Stress can sometimes be caused by a change in the environment. When a modification is necessary, try to introduce the change gradually. Basically, anything new, especially other animals, new housemates, and children, is stressful to a bird. Try to keep excess noise down around your bird.

Provide your bird with safe, durable toys, ones large enough to eliminate the possibility of a choking hazard. (You should know that birds sometimes like to take things apart, so bear this in mind when screening toys for choking hazards. Bells are not recommended for this reason.) Be sure your bird's feet will not get caught in the toys. Keep in mind, too, that toys should be free of harmful dyes and toxic metals. It's a good idea to question a pet shop manager or breeder about toy safety.

If you would like your birds to breed, you will need a nesting box, as birds require privacy. Be especially careful around your bird when it is breeding; this is especially important with larger birds, which may become temperamental and think nothing of snapping at you with their beak. While most birds will use their beaks in playful ways, when threatened, some birds may be capable of snapping off a finger. Note: Never allow the beak to be around your face or eyes.

Is Your Bird Food for the Birds? Poor nutrition is one of the leading causes of illness in birds. Commercial bird feed is generally not as healthy as other, natural fare you can provide. In fact, store-bought food with artificial colors and preservatives can be detrimental to your bird's health. Furthermore, many stores sell products that have been sitting on the shelf for a year, rendering them nutritionally worthless. One exception to the commercial food situation, according to avian veterinarian Arthur Young, of Stuart, Florida, is a brand of food called Harrison's, developed by bird expert Greg Harrison of Lakewood, Florida. According to Young, if you feed this food to birds, "70 percent of their problems will not occur."[1]

Another good option is to feed your bird a diet consisting of fresh fruits and vegetables, grains, legumes, and seeds. "Anything that is healthy for humans, basically, is healthy for your parrot," in the words of bird expert Alicia McWatters, Ph.D., who is not an advocate of feeding birds a pelleted feed. McWatters, author of *A Guide to a Naturally Healthy Bird: Nutrition, Feeding, and Natural Healing*,[2] notes an exception to the "anything healthy for humans" rule: the fruit avocado, which has been found to be toxic to some birds.

Parrots can be finicky about food. If you present a parrot with a bowl of mixed nuts and seeds, for example, the parrot is likely to pick out only its favorites. To trick parrots into eating a more balanced diet, McWatters has created the "mash diet," a blend of various fruits, vegetables, legumes, grains, and seeds run briefly through a food processor. The end result should be a mixture that is chunky or minced rather than pureed.

Beans and grains for the mash diet should be presoaked in the refrigerator for 24 hours; frozen vegetables have been blanched before being flash-frozen, and no cooking of the food is necessary. Once you have prepared a batch of the mash diet, you can keep it frozen for 10 to 20 days. After that, the ingredients' nutritional value starts to decline. A variation of the diet, thinned to the consistency of a broth, may be hand-fed to newborn baby birds.

Although all birds require the same basic nutrients, different species may need more or less of specific nutrients, calories, protein, or fat. For example, birds that need fewer calories from fat include Amazons, pionus, and Quaker, cockatiel, and budgie parrots. Some long-tailed parrots, such as macaws or conures, usually require more fat than other species.

For all birds, change the water once to twice daily to keep the supply clean and free of feces and food debris. Ideally, birds should drink filtered water. Their body weight is many times smaller than that of a person, and they're more susceptible to the harmful effects of fluoride and other pollutants.

Also, realize that an irregular feeding schedule is another factor that can cause stress for your bird. Birds in the wild forage for food early in the morning and in the afternoon. It's best to imitate this schedule as closely as possible for pet birds. If they haven't finished all of their first meal when it's time for the second, be sure to clear away the leftover portion. Fresh foods, used in the mash diet, spoil quickly. Four to six hours is about as long as fresh food should be left out.

Additional Treatment. A good diet is the basis for keeping your bird healthy and happy. However, conditions may still arise that need treatment by you or a vet. If your bird becomes ill, be sure to take it to a certified avian vet. You can check with the Association of Avian Veterinarians for a list of certified avian vets in your area. [Their phone number is (303) 756-8380.] Symptoms that will require a trip to the vet may include difficulty breathing, diarrhea, constipation, vomiting, listlessness, fluffed feathers, excessive sneezing, loss of balance, nasal discharge, refusal to eat or drink water, listlessness, or broken wings or legs. Also, a healthy bird should not require a beak trim. An overgrown beak might indicate liver damage and require immediate attention.

Birds in captivity require a regular wing trim to keep them safe from harm. Exceptions to this rule are birds kept in a spacious aviary where there is plenty of room for free flight. A wing trim will prevent your bird from flying into a wall or window, two of the leading causes of death in pet birds. Wing clipping will also keep a bird from escaping out the door, possibly never to be seen again. Once your avian veterinarian or another experienced person has shown you how to trim wings properly, you can do it yourself.

Your bird has ten primary wing feathers, and six to ten of these should be clipped. Secondary wing feathers must never be clipped. The feathers on both wings should be clipped evenly. Once its primary wing feathers are clipped, your bird will not fly upwards but glide safely downward, without injury.

Supplements for Birds. Vitamins A, B, D, E, and K, plus many minerals, are essential to your bird's diet. A deficiency in any of these can lead to disease. If you are going to give your bird any supplements, such as calcium and magnesium to balance the phosphorous in the mash diet, McWatters recommends buying a natural supplement in liquid form and adding it to your bird's food. She generally does not recommend putting anything a bird can taste into its water because, with their notorious fussiness, birds are likely to refuse water with anything mixed into it.

Herbs. A bird that seems anxious, and whose anxiety doesn't respond to a simple change in living conditions or diet, may respond well to calming herbs such as passionflower, chamomile, valerian, or oat straw. Dosages depend both on the species and the symptoms, so get advice from a professional before treating your bird with herbs. Too little won't correct the problem, and too much can be toxic. Once the correct dosage is determined, a bit of the liquid or powdered herb can be added to your bird's food.

Flower Essences. You may want to treat your stressed bird with flower essences, which you can purchase at a health food store. Flower therapy is based on the principle that disease is caused by disharmony between body and spirit. Birds, being so sensitive by nature and prone to stress-related disorders, have been observed over the years to react favorably to flower therapy. People experienced with this therapy recommend adding one to two drops of a flower essence remedy into your bird's drinking water; they report that most birds will ingest it that way because the remedy imparts no noticeable taste change to the water. If your bird is unusually tame and trusting it might permit touching. In this case, you could add two drops of the flower essence to a 1-ounce bottle of water, shake well, and rub the remedy on your bird's head or under its wings. Don't feel slighted, though, if your bird does not allow this, as many won't. An alternative is to put the flower essence and water into a mister bottle and spritz the bird.

Homeopathic Remedies. You can use homeopathic remedies for first aid at home in cases of trauma, injury, bruises, or swelling. Homeopathic remedies come in tablets that you can grind into a powder with a mortar and pestle. Then you mix this with a little bit of distilled water and give it to your bird in a syringe. Never touch the tablet itself with your fingers, as it will lose its effectiveness. If your bird appears to have injured one of its wings, be extremely gentle when trying to examine the bird or hold it. Struggling with the bird may aggravate the injury. You can bandage a sprain yourself, first positioning the wing correctly and then applying, not too tightly, a gauze bandage and vet wrap. (If your bird is stressed because of the injury, which is likely, this is a good time to administer one to two drops of a special flower essence, the Bach flower Rescue Remedy. Homeopathic Arnica should be used for injuries, such as a broken wing, followed by Symphytum after the wing has been set.

Homeopathic Euphrasia (also known as eyebright) can be given as an internal remedy, but the herb euphrasia can be made into a tea for external treatment of eye irritations or infections like conjunctivitis. Once the tea has cooled, dip a cotton ball into it, and apply it to the eye. The problem should clear up in a day or two.

Homeopathic Belladonna can be used to treat heat exhaustion if a bird has accidentally been left outside on a hot, sunny day. How do you know if your bird is overheated? Since birds don't have sweat glands, an overheated bird will hold its wings away from its body, and its mouth may be open. Besides administering homeopathic Belladonna, the owner of an overheated bird should help the bird gradually cool down by spraying it with water from a mister bottle, a few sprays at a time, for half an hour to an hour, or until the bird has recovered. Be sure to always provide your bird with shade and cool drinking water when taking it outside on a sunny day.

The Tellington Touch for Birds. Originally developed to promote healing and communication with horses (see section, below, on horses), Tellington Touch massage has been expanded to include all animals, and can help to quiet and calm an overexcited bird. How do you massage a bird? you may wonder. Because bare hands might be perceived as threatening, touching is done with bird feathers as extensions of the hands and arms. The feathers should correspond to the animal's size (smaller birds need smaller feathers) and be stiff enough so that contact is felt. A warm-up technique lightly strokes the bird with two feathers, one on either side of its body, to promote a sense of calm. The back is never touched, as that will incite fear of being attacked. Sessions are initially short, about five minutes, and later lengthened to 10 or 15 minutes. The more frightened the bird, the shorter the session. A few repeated sessions, spaced anywhere from a half hour to two days apart (more trusting birds require less of a break) can begin to calm even the most panicky bird. As confidence builds, the feathers can slowly be rotated down to the chest and under the wings. Strokes should be performed slowly and accompanied by deep, rhythmic breathing on the part of the masseuse, because the bird will begin to mirror this and become more serene itself. Tranquil music can be used as an aid. Once relaxed, a bird might lift its wings, allowing you to lightly massage the area with your fingers. At this point, you may want to try other Tellington Touch (also known as TTouch) techniques. These easy-to-learn methods can be of great benefit. The development of the process, the actual techniques, and the rationale for why they work are well explained in *The Tellington Touch: A Revolutionary Natural Method to Train and Care for Your Favorite Animal*, by Linda Tellington-Jones,[3] or you can call (800) 854-TEAM for more information.

Keeping Your Bird Happy. Domesticated birds sometimes develop behavioral problems, such as biting, screaming, and aggressiveness. Aggressive birds are irritable, and they may lean toward you as if about to attack. Often problem behavior can be eliminated with behavior modification techniques. First, be sure you do not encourage unwanted behavior by offering attention or a dramatic response to it. Instead, remain calm, and give special attention only to a bird that is behaving well. This is the time to praise it. If you need extra help in molding your bird's behavior, speak with a behavioral consultant. They are listed in avian publications or may be found on the Internet or through personal recommendation. In general, be sure to give your pet bird sufficient attention. It may surprise you to learn that birds love human attention and require a lot of it, sometimes even more than dogs and cats do. If you cannot do this, a lone parrot may need a companion. A neglected bird will become neurotic and resort to feather plucking, a common behavioral problem encountered by bird owners. Herbal remedies and other natural methods may be helpful for resolving these issues in conjunction with creating an environment that is peaceful and calming. But remember that, for any unusual problems or behaviors a bird is exhibiting, you will want to consult a certified avian vet for a definitive diagnosis. Birds' symptoms can be subtle and difficult for the layperson to correctly interpret. When you are selecting a bird, too, you will want to get recommendations for reputable, reliable breeders. Providing your bird with a healthy environment, as well as an optimal diet, are key to a happy pet.

RABBITS

Rabbits can make wonderful pets, but they do present unique challenges for their owners. The most common mistakes well-intentioned rabbit owners make relate to housing and diet.

Where Will Your Rabbit Live? If you've heard that rabbits can be housebroken, believe it! Just like cats, rabbits can be litter-trained and can live roaming freely in their owners' houses or apartments. This eliminates the need for cages, apart from special situations where your rabbit may need to be temporarily kept in one place. Cages are unfairly confining, and can make rabbits easy prey for dogs that can bite through the wire. Nesting boxes or wooden hutches are preferable to wire cages. If your rabbit does need to be in a cage, and it is outside, make sure it has lots of shade and protection from bad weather. Rabbits are quite susceptible to heat—a temperature as low as 80 degrees F can bring on heat prostration.

The Rabbit Diet. As for diet, commercially prepared rabbit pellets are actually not healthy for rabbits. They're too low in fiber and dense in calories. A rabbit's diet should consist of low-moisture vegetables such as dark leafy greens, carrots, and some grass hay. This is closer to a rabbit's natural diet than are the pellets. An exception to these guidelines would be providing extra protein for a nursing mother rabbit, and pellets specially formulated for nursing mothers are available. If you're not sure whether your rabbit is getting enough nutrients, you can supplement its diet with a multiple vitamin for rabbits.

Health Challenges. Another challenge for rabbit owners is that rabbits' immune systems are not as developed as those of many other animals. A pet rabbit's lifespan is going to be about seven years. This is why rabbits reproduce in such famously large numbers—in their natural state, through frequent reproduction, rabbits can survive as a species even though they don't have great defenses against disease. For the owner of a domesticated rabbit, rabbits' poor immune systems mean being on the lookout for the chronic conditions to which rabbits are susceptible. The most frequent rabbit complaint is Pasteurella, a bacterium that can turn up anywhere in a rabbit's body, causing a variety of problems, including abscesses, liver trouble, imbalance in movement, and pneumonia. Abscesses in rabbits must be treated by a veterinarian because a rabbit's pus is solid, with the texture of cottage cheese, and therefore can't drain by itself as it does in other animals or people.

Pneumonia can be caused by Pasteurella or other bacteria or viruses. Here again, for suspected pneumonia, a trip to a conventional vet is necessary, but the inflammation of the lungs may also be reduced by acupuncture or by treatment with vitamins C and E, or coenzyme Q10. These can supplement, but not replace, antibiotics, if antibiotics are called for to treat the pneumonia.

If you are treating a rabbit at home for anything, be aware that a rabbit's mouth does not open wide enough for you to force a pill down its throat. So whether you're giving it supplements, herbal medications, or other medicines, it's preferable to work with a liquid or powder for your rabbit. Some rabbits will voluntarily drink a supplement mixed with carrot juice or something else sweet. With other rabbits, you will have to squirt the mixture into their mouth.

Another common rabbit health problem is frequent or chronic diarrhea, stemming from a variety of sources. One cause is parasites. Rabbits are prone to parasites, including one called a "rabbit bot," which lives underneath the skin. According to rabbit veterinarian and natural pet care advocate Nancy Scanlan, D.V.M., parasites are "… one of the cases where most natural treatments are no longer as good or as safe as medical treatments…. So, this is one of the few times that I actually do recommend Western medicine over traditional herbal remedies."[4]

FERRETS

Although ferrets are frequently thought of as exotic pets, they've actually been domesticated for thousands of years—almost as long as dogs or cats. In ancient Rome it seems that ferrets were used as hunting animals, with their keen sense of smell and ability to wriggle into tight spaces serving them well.

Nowadays, these weasel relatives are becoming increasingly popular as household pets. If you are considering purchasing a ferret, however, check first to make sure it's legal to own one in the area where you live. Because of the misapprehension that ferrets are exotic, many governments, from local to state, ban ferret ownership under the umbrella of laws against owning any exotic animals.

First, Ferret Out the Facts. Ferrets may not really be exotic, but they are a unique species, and owning a ferret is different from owning a dog or cat, with its own rewards and drawbacks. For this reason, it is important to do research about living with ferrets before making the commitment to bring one into your household. Although ferrets are cute and cuddly-looking, weighing only one to three pounds, resist the temptation to buy one on the basis of its good looks alone. Read books about ferrets, or visit ferret-related sites on the Internet. Check for ferret clubs in your area, and, if they exist, attend meetings and subscribe to their newsletters. Talk to ferret owners to learn about the day-to-day aspects of living with one. Maybe you could even visit a ferret-owning household to get an idea of what it's like. You might find their musky odor to be something you would rather not live with. And although the incidence of allergic reactions to ferret dander in people is much less than it is with cats or dogs, you may have allergies to these animals. This you would discover only after being exposed to a ferret for quite some time. Other factors to consider are the age of your children and whether or not you have other pets in the house. Very young children must be supervised at all times around animals, but can be taught proper handling by the time they are six or seven. Puppies and kittens that have been raised around ferrets often do well together, but dogs or cats unfamiliar with the ferret might cause harm.

If you do decide that a ferret is for you, it's best to obtain one from a reputable breeder, so that you will have an idea of its background and temperament. A ferret may cost anywhere from $100 to $200. Ferrets do fine on their own, but if you have the time and energy, you may decide to adopt two, and the pair should get along fine.

Ferret-Proofing Your Home. Ferret experts disagree on how safe it is to let these frisky critters roam freely in a house or apartment. Some believe that a ferret should never be left alone in any room without human supervision because it's just too easy for the animal to cause damage to itself and its surroundings. Whenever the ferret is unattended, they say, it should be securely locked in its cage. Others believe that certain types of rooms are safe for ferrets without a person watching them. Either way, before you let your ferret out of its cage, you must ferret-proof any room or area it will be allowed into.

Just like child-proofing for a toddler, ferret-proofing involves securing and covering up anything that may be dangerous. Ferrets are more curious than cats, and with their small, wiry bodies, they can squirm into the tightest of spaces. They can climb and scurry out of reach easily, and are amazingly agile. For example, ferrets can open drawers or cupboards—and do you really want your ferret exploring in your dishes or underwear? Ferrets can also wiggle under closed doors. You will need to block this avenue of escape with a rolled-up towel or something similar. A collar with a bell will help you to locate your ferret should it slip out of sight.

Also be sure to clear the space of dangerous potential edibles, as ferrets will consume anything they can chew or swallow, including rubber, sponges, and chemicals. For your ferret's safety, you will need to make sure it has no access to nondigestibles, including children's plastic toys, or poisons such as household cleaners. I can't stress enough the issue of ferret-proofing your home to prevent terrible accidents. Sadly, an acquaintance of mine opened her dishwasher one morning only to discover that her beloved ferret had crawled inside and—when the dishes were washed—had drowned.

Litter Training. Now, with your ferret running all over your house or apartment, where will it go to the bathroom? Fortunately, ferrets can be litter-trained. Unlike cats, however, ferrets do not take to litter boxes instinctually, so you will need to work with your ferret to get it in the litter habit. Ferrets also tend to forget about their litter box if it's out of sight, unlike cats, which will remember and return to whatever part of the house their littler box is in. With ferrets, you might have to make a box available in every room where the ferret might go, and again, you'll need to train it to know the locations and use all the boxes you have put out for it. You can save time litter training by purchasing a ferret that has already been in the habit of using a box.

Your Ferret Needs Friendship. While your ferret is out of its cage, it will want to play with you. Like dogs and some cats, ferrets can learn to come when called by name, and they love to play fetch— just make sure that your ferret doesn't try to eat the ball or toy! Safe toys are easily found—empty rolls from toilet paper or paper towels, empty orange juice cans minus their metal edges, shoe boxes, ping pong balls. Ferrets can also be taught to walk on a leash, and, most important, most ferrets love to be handled and cuddled. Baby ferrets that are petted, played with daily, and taught not to nip, become excellent pets. You can easily carry your trained ferret on your shoulder or in a carrying bag as you go about your household chores, and spend companionable time with your ferret as it sits on your lap while you watch TV, work at your computer, pay bills, or talk on the phone. Except for the occasional independent-minded ferret, a cuddled ferret is a happy one.

Housing. Your ferret's cage could be plain or fancy. Minimally, you will want your ferret to have several feet of space, at least enough room to move about comfortably to get to its food and water on one side and to its litter box on the other. Or you might choose a more fancy enclosure, one with enough height to house a ferret "condo."

Food. Food that has been specifically formulated for ferrets is available at good pet supply stores. Don't make the mistake of feeding dry cat food to a ferret, even though the two animals' foods look alike in texture, shape, and size. Ferret food needs to meet the nutritional needs of this unique species. Ferrets need meat protein, not plant protein. The food you provide for your ferret should be 32-38 percent meat protein, and it should have a fat content of 18-22 percent, according to Geraldine Bucsis, author of *Training Your Pet Ferret*. Ferrets need that much fat to keep their wiry, athletic bodies going. On a diet that's deficient in protein or fat, a ferret will be undernourished no matter how much it eats. Ferrets can self-feed, and they like to eat every three to four hours, so you should keep their food constantly available to them. Just be sure to change the food and clean the food bowl and water bowl frequently.

"People food" is not really good for ferrets, but you can give your ferret an occasional healthy treat, such as small pieces of fresh vegetables or fruit. Ferrets love the taste of dairy products and sweets like cookies or candy, but they cannot fully digest these foods, so try to avoid these types of treats.

Additional Treatment. When it's time for a trip to the vet, you will need to make some calls and find one who handles ferrets regularly and is knowledgeable about ferrets' unique needs. A veterinarian will notice if the ferret is getting enough nutrition from its food or needs a change in diet or extra supplementation. Fish oil, for instance, might be recommended if the skin is not healthy. Ferrets should never be declawed. Their claws are not designed like cats' claws, which can be (but also should not be) removed. Once a qualified vet has shown you how to do it, you can clip your ferret's nails at home, yourself. Ferrets, like other pets, are required by law to be vaccinated against rabies. Some ferret experts believe that a canine distemper vaccination is also a good idea, although ferrets are susceptible to reactions to distemper vaccine. Any other vaccinations should be given only after you have discussed it with your veterinarian. The risks of overimmunization apply to ferrets just as they do to dogs and cats.

A ferret needs to have a checkup at least once a year, including a physical exam and feces test for parasites. Ferrets are not as susceptible to parasites as are other animals, such as rabbits. If parasites are found, they can be treated conventionally or herbally, but if you choose to use an herbal treatment, do it under the guidance of a ferret vet, because wrongly administered herbal cures can be lethal to ferrets. A ferret reaches middle age at around three or four, so at that point you may want to increase its checkups to twice a year. Ferrets also need to have their teeth cleaned once a year. The most common serious health problems for ferrets are diseases of the adrenal glands, which can be treated by removing cancerous adrenal glands, by glandular therapy, and with nutritional support. A change in weight, or any abnormal behaviors, can be symptoms of illness in your ferret. If these occur you should contact your vet right away. Ferrets are also able to contract and spread human flu, so watch out for flu symptoms in your ferret, for its sake and yours!

Unfortunately, many ferrets in the U.S. die prematurely, of

cancer. In other countries, ferrets tend to live longer lives. Researchers who have compared the American and European ferret have correlated the problem with neutering and spaying, which appear to weaken the ferret's system. American-born ferrets undergo the procedure at 6 weeks and develop cancer 3-1/2 to 4 years later. In Europe, when ferrets are neutered or spayed as adults, they also develop tumors 3-1/2 to 4 years later. When the operation is performed at age 4, they tend to get cancer at 7-1/2 or 8. It would seem, then, that neutering and spaying should be delayed, but a complicating factor is that if a female ferret is left unspayed and is not bred regularly, she will be in heat for prolonged periods and will develop anemia, which can be severe enough to be fatal. At present, there needs to be more study of the spaying/cancer connection. On a positive note, there are ferret specialists who say that with good medical care, proper nutrition, and a safe, loving home, your ferret may share almost a decade of life with you.

FISH

Fish ownership is controversial when it comes to tropical fish, endangered by capture and over-harvesting by unethical fish traders. PETA, People for the Ethical Treatment of Animals, advises against owning any tropical fish at all, so as to avoid supporting international dealings in these beautiful, fragile creatures. However, you may already have a tropical fish, or one may come into your life as a gift or as a hand-me-down from someone who can no longer keep it. Also, some fish enthusiasts do point out that there are species that have been domesticated for so long that they no longer resemble their wild ancestors. You could purchase this type; examples are Siamese fighting fish and guppies.

If a tropical fish is already in your life, don't try to re-introduce it to its natural habitat. Tropical fish cannot just be dropped off anywhere; individual species, such as the beautiful fish that hail from the lakes of Africa, come from isolated parts of the world and must be returned to their home waters. You should also be aware that fish in captivity can pick up and become carriers of diseases that do not exist in their natural habitat. If re-introduced to the sea or lakes, a fish can bring along new diseases, wreaking havoc on the native fish population. (Ecologists also advise us not to attempt returning aquarium plants to the wild, and not to flush them down a toilet. We don't want species "taking over" habitats they were not meant to be in.)

After reading and educating yourself about the controversies involved in keeping a tropical fish, you may decide to purchase one from a respectable dealer, under circumstances you are certain are beneficial to the fish. Not all fish experts advise against owning tropical fish, but all agree that if you do, you must take special care to respect your fish's existence as a creature from another world, the world under water.

Aquatic Arrangements. Your first responsibility as a fish owner, then, is to do everything in your power to make its life in an aquarium as healthy and stress-free as you can. Give your fish as much room as possible in your own living arrangement. For each inch of length that your fish measures, allow 12 inches of water surface. Make sure that the water in the tank is properly treated. Check with a tropical fish expert before treating tank water, to make sure you have the correct chemical balance for the species housed there. Before you place any fish in your new aquarium, let the water filter (necessary to remove waste particles) and pump (necessary to provide oxygen) run for two weeks. There are two types of filters, inside or outside the tank. Each has advantages and disadvantages, and after talking with a fish expert you may well end up with a combination system incorporating features of each.

Don't keep just one fish if you have room for more. Fish enjoy companionship. But make sure that the different types of fish are compatible and thrive in the same aquatic environment before mixing species in your tank. For example, different types of fish may require different pH levels in their water. Also, different fish carry different diseases, and illnesses such as white spot may be introduced by a new fish in the tank. Fish need a constant water temperature of 68 to 78 degrees, depending on the species. Keep a thermometer in the tank to monitor the water temperature. You can easily attach an aquarium thermometer to the glass with a suction cup. Your fish tank needs to be cleaned regularly, probably twice a week or so. But never change all of the water at one time. Fish like familiar water. Exchange 10 to 25 percent of the water at each cleaning. Give your fish live plants for shelter and protection, instead of plastic plants, which do not provide oxygen for the tank. Besides live plants, driftwood, rocks, and ceramics make good hiding and playing areas for your fish. Rocks are especially good for territorial fish, such as cichlids or red-tailed black sharks, which need hiding places. You can build a cave for your fish out of several small or mid-sized rocks. Make sure that all rocks you place in your aquarium have smoothed-off edges. Fish can injure themselves on sharp edges. Avoid metal objects, which will rust and are unhealthy for the fish; rocks or stones that contain lime; coconut shells; and seashells.

Deep-Six the Stress. As you can tell from these guidelines for tropical fish, owning any fish is a commitment of time and energy. Many people mistakenly think of aquariums as aesthetically pleasant and fish as pretty "things" to look at that don't require much maintenance other than dropping in some dry food every now and then. In reality, home aquariums need to be in an area where the external environment, as well as the environment within the tank, can be controlled. Sudden changes in light levels—as happens when overhead lights are switched on and off—can startle fish, as can sudden loud noises or vibrations from stereos or televisions. The temperature around an aquarium needs to be controllable and fairly consistent, just as does the water temperature. Direct sunlight or exposure to drafts from vents, windows, or doors, can change the water's temperature. Different fish can tolerate different levels of light around their tanks, and many tropical fish need to be surrounded by as low a light level as possible. Do not locate a home aquarium in an area that will undergo sudden, unpredictable changes in light, such as a space next to a window. Also, fish are susceptible to environmental pollution from outside their tanks. Smoke and fumes from cigarettes, cleaners, kitchens, or work areas can make their way into your aquarium and compromise your fish's health and well-being. Fish may feel threatened if they are housed in a well-traveled area such as a hallway or the space next to a door. You have to understand that fish are easily stressed, and that stress is one of the leading causes of illness in aquarium fish. So everything you do for your fish should be based on this consideration. The best location for a home aquarium is one that is relatively dark, quiet, and unvisited. You need, in short, a place where your fish can just be... a fish.

When you are buying an aquarium, don't cut corners on cost. Investing in a high-quality aquarium will pay off for you in the quality of your fish's life. You will need to cover the floor of your aquarium with something in which plants can take root. Your bottom covering may also contribute to the aesthetic design of your aquarium. Fine-sized quartz gravel is one attractive and practical choice. Large gravel can bring too much dirt along with it, polluting your tank. Gravel must be neutral, meaning free of lime, so as not to disturb the water's pH balance. The quartz should also not be too light-colored; otherwise, it will reflect light inside the tank, making the water too bright for your fish. Although quartz may be pre-washed when you buy it, it's a good idea to wash it again before adding it to your tank. Mix in an aquarium fertilizer when you first put the gravel in the aquarium. You may also press tablets into the gravel later, if you need to, to support plant growth. Sand is not a good bottom cover, but some fish like to "root" in a sandy bottom and will appreciate a small sandy spot in the gravel. Corydoras and barbs are examples of these fish. Check with your supplier to learn if one of your fish is a rooter.

Allow yourself enough time to set up the aquarium properly. Making a mistake along the way means you'll have to start over from scratch. You can avoid time-consuming and expensive mistakes by proceeding slowly and deliberately from step to step. Allow yourself at least one complete day; a weekend off is even better. Patience is the rule when setting up an aquatic environment and adding fish to it in your home. Just think of the millions of years it took to create your fish's natural habitat. It's important to remember that once the pump and filter have been installed and are functioning, you should wait two weeks before introducing any fish. Fish placed in unconditioned water can become seriously ill. Never put a fish in cloudy water.

During those two weeks you can select and purchase the fish for your tank. So many types of fish are available that trying to choose can be overwhelming. Your guiding principle should be to select fish that will be comfortable in your aquarium, depending on the size and location of your tank. When buying different species that will live together, you need to create a balanced community of compatible fishes. Some species cannot be successfully housed together. You also want to avoid, at all costs, overpopulating your tank, which will create undue stress for your fish and can lead to serious out-breaks of disease. When you are mixing species, don't put all the fish in at one time. Add a few from one species, then more of another species a few days later, and so on. Even within species, some fish cannot be mixed. Territorial male fish, for example, will not tolerate sharing an aquarium with another male of the same species. They will fight to the death. Siamese fighting fish are an example of this type of fish.

Some fish are top dwellers, some middle dwellers, and some bottom dwellers. In mixing species, take advantage of all the living space in your aquarium by having some fish from each category. Just be sure to get expert information on species that can or cannot be housed together—before move-in day.

Only buy fish that you are certain have come from clean, healthy, and well-maintained aquariums. Before you purchase any fish, check them for symptoms of disease, including frayed fins, dull skin, white, granular spots, cottony white patches, or drifting. Drifting is a warning sign that a fish may be dying. Flying foxes are one good fish to start out with because they are algae eaters that will actually help you keep your tank clean.

The transition from store or source aquarium to home aquari-um is a difficult one for sensitive fish. To ease the stress of this change, first place the water-filled plastic bag that the fish comes home in inside the aquarium. When the temperature inside the bag matches the water temperature inside your aquarium, open the bag and let the fish swim out.

It's rare, but occasionally tanks do burst or develop leaks. Before purchasing an aquarium, add it to your contents or home-owner's insurance, if possible, and find out if you have coverage for water damage, or can add it to your existing policy. Whenever you buy an electrical accessory for your aquarium (lights, filters, pumps, heaters, etc.), make sure it has been approved by the Underwriters Laboratory (abbreviated UL). Equipment that goes inside the tank must be explicitly labeled as meeting underwater safety require-ments. Between the current source and any electrical accessory to your tank, attach a "fault current protective switch." This will inter-rupt the power supply immediately in the event of a defect in appli-ances or electrical cables. Always unplug electrical accessories or appliances before working in the aquarium or removing appliances from the aquarium. Never attempt electrical repairs yourself. Hire a qualified professional. Here, too, your investment will pay off—in health and safety!

Feeding Your Fish. Once your fish are home and acclimated, you will, of course, face the responsibility of feeding them. Your fish need a varied menu of dry food, frozen or freeze-dried live food, and actual live food. Dry food is fine as the basic source of your fish's nutrition, but live or frozen food add variety and flavor. The best thing about live food is just that it is alive. Since it moves, it attracts your fish and interests them more than dried or frozen food. Back in the old days, home aquarists could catch their own live food in the form of insects, larvae, water fleas, and other tiny tidbits, at a nearby pond or creek, using a net. But nowadays this is neither healthy, due to heavy pollution of natural waterways, nor, in many cases, even legal, due to wildlife conservation laws that protect tadpoles, for example. Nonetheless, you can still provide your fish with live food ordered through an aquarium supply store or directly from a manufacturer. Here again, you will not want to cut corners on cost. Some live foods, such as tubifex worms, can carry pathogens if they have been raised in polluted conditions. Make sure that any live food you purchase has been raised under the cleanest conditions possible.

Dry food, in tablet, pellet, or flake form, can be a healthy basis of your fishes' diet. Tablets are good for bottom dwellers, since they will drip straight to the bottom of the tank. Flakes are good for top dwellers. Whether you are feeding your fish dry, frozen, or live food, the fish should eat quickly—most of the food should be gone within five minutes of adding it to the tank. Stay and watch your fish after you feed them, to make sure they are eating properly. If the food isn't consumed quickly, you're giving too much, or it's the wrong kind of food, or there's another problem that needs to be identified. Not eating at all is a sign of disease in fish. Remember that underfeeding is better than overfeeding in the case of fish, which can easily bloat and become constipated. Note, however, that if you have baby fish, they'll need to be fed frequently, every few hours. If you have to be away on vacation or for an extended period, automatic food dispensers are available. But remember that automatic feeding will deprive you of the opportunity to observe your fishes' eating behavior. As a beginning aquarist, do not give your fish leftovers of "people food" except as an occasional special treat. The food you eat can cause many problems for your fish, such as the introduction of unhealthy-for-fish bacteria into the tank. More experienced aquarists develop a sense of what's appropriate, and how much, to give a fish from a human diet. In general, fish need to eat only tiny amounts of food. They cannot handle large chunks of leftovers.

Waste products (excrement, decaying food, and plant parts) are not a problem as long as you maintain a clean tank and as long as sufficient oxygen is present in the tank. If your fish refuse to eat or come to the surface and gasp for air, they may be suffering from hypoxia, poisoning due to lack of oxygen caused by excessive waste in the tank. If this happens you will need to add oxygen to the tank continually for two to three weeks to get the balance right again. Change one-third of the water immediately upon noticing the symptoms of poisoning, and one-third every week for the next three weeks. Clean the filter immediately. Do not feed the fish for three days. Remember, you can avoid such emergencies through good routine cleaning and tank maintenance.

Controlling and Treating Illness. Because disease spreads quickly throughout an aquarium's population, it is important to get help for a sick fish as quickly as possible. Besides behavioral symptoms such as gasping for breath at the surface, refusing to eat, or not moving at all, physical symptoms to be on the lookout for include dull or bulging eyes, white film around the mouth, reddened or faded gills, bloating, or anything that seems out of the ordinary to you. Fish are especially susceptible to internal and external parasites and bacteria. There are fish veterinarians, but a qualified one may be hard to locate. For faster help with a sick fish, turn first to a qualified fish dealer or expert. In case a sick fish needs to be quarantined, you will need to set up a "hospital tank" to keep it in during its illness. A hospital tank is similar to a regular aquarium, but less elaborate. It still needs a filter and a pump, however. Make sure your hospital tank has plenty of oxygen to support your fish's healing process. It is also likely that all of your fish will need to be treated if one becomes ill, since disease spreads quickly through aquarium populations. In this case, you may still want to keep the fish with the symptoms quarantined away from the rest of your fish.

As you can see, the proper care of fish is somewhat involved, but once these splendid creatures are a part of your environment, you will probably find that it is well worth the effort.

HORSES

Why do people love horses? A horse is expensive, it is not a house pet, nor is it a creature that will be with you most of the time, a companion for day and night. Yet a horse *is* a companion—a huge, strong friend, an athlete in its own right, whom you will enter into partnership with if you intend to ride. Pleasure riding is the major motivator for most people buying horses, and so it is the best place to start when thinking about what's involved in horse ownership. The challenges and conditions of horse ownership are far different from those facing the owner of smaller, house pets. Since your horse will not live under the same roof as you, you may not be your horse's only—or even primary—caretaker. If you are fortunate enough to have enough property for a corral and stable, and live in an area where those things are legal, that's great—you will be involved in your horse's daily life. If you are planning to own a horse that will be boarded somewhere other than your own property, you will need to know and trust those who will be feeding, grooming, and tending to your horse when you're not around. Taking care of a horse is a big responsibility, and it has to be done properly. Good care for horses can be expensive, so budget has to be another primary consideration when buying a horse. Boarding a horse can cost anywhere between $300 and $1000 per month.

Learning about Horses. Before you consider purchasing a horse, you need to familiarize yourself with the highly specialized world of horses, trainers, and all those who will be caring for your animal. First take riding lessons for at least six months—or even better, a year—to get thoroughly comfortable with handling horses. This period will help you get to know horse breeds and horse personality types and eccentricities so that you can make an informed choice about what kind of horse you might want to own. Don't just ride during your lesson time, but get to know the nuts and bolts of horse care, and the equipment involved. You will need to learn how to tack and untack a horse (this is the lingo for saddling up and unsaddling a horse), bathe and clean it, pick out and clean the hooves, inspect the shoes for loosening and excess wear, and of course feed it. You will need to hang around a stable when you're not riding so that you experience different aspects of the horse's existence. Through this immersion, you will gain knowledge about how a horse exhibits its moods, what a horse looks like when it's sick, and so on.

Before you make a purchase you also need to know what you want from your horse. Assuming that you will ride, which most owners do, are you planning to ride just for pleasure, or do you have dreams of competing, or jumping, or showing your horse? If you plan to compete, you'll need to spend hours every day practicing and taking lessons. So depending on your wishes, you will need to make a greater or lesser time commitment to being with your horse, and to buy a more or less expensive horse.

Once you've made the decision to buy, and you are at the shopping stage, spend enough time with your potential horse to get to know its temperament. Each horse is unique, and a horse's innate personality will remain the same no matter what the training, so you will want a horse that is sweet-natured and kind. Ideally, you and your potential horse should just take to each other. Remember, you're going to be working and playing together.

You also, of course, want to buy a healthy horse. Check its eyes for good, strong, uncloudy brown color (although some types of horses do have a blue eye) and very little white visible around the eye. Have a vet do a checkup and give you a clean bill of health. Colic is an extremely common, and dangerous, condition for horses because they have a "one-way-only" digestive system, notes Susan Travellin of Woodside Farm Dog and Horse Training in Califon, New Jersey.[5] That is to say, horses cannot throw up. They also have extremely long, twisting intestines, and so it's easy for a horse to develop a blockage in its intestines. Many horses will experience colic at least once in their lifetime. The easiest symptom of colic to spot is bloating in the horse's belly, so when you are horse shopping you certainly want to make sure no bloating is present.

Veterinarian Nancy Scanlan stresses the importance of having a vet check out any horse you are contemplating buying, noting that you want to make sure that the animal doesn't have a condition that could result in permanent lameness. Also, if you're interested in breeding a mare, the vet can check her for breeding soundness.

Housing Your Horse. Horses are by nature walkers, wanderers, and grazers. In the wild, horses walk and run and munch outside all day long. The only time they look for shelter is in cases of inclement weather—extreme heat as well as rain or snow. It stands to reason, then, that one of the major stresses for the "domesticated" horse is having to spend most of its time in a stable, or otherwise confined.

In choosing boarding for your horse, look for a place with as much open, outdoor space as possible, and a groomer or trainer who will take your horse outside regularly—every day, for hours, if possible. This will go a long way toward keeping your horse happy and healthy. Horses need proper exercise, fresh air, sunshine, and an opportunity to see the outside world without having to look out over a high wall. (In the wild, whenever a horse raises its head it means that it's alarmed.)

One of the physical consequences of over-confinement is an increase in the number of horses suffering from arthritis. Another is stress, which can lead to ulcers. Keep your horse moving to help avoid this!

Grooming. Horses also need to be groomed every day that they're ridden, and it's a good idea to check their feet and shoes every day, no matter what. Make sure none of the shoes are loose, and that the horse doesn't have any rocks caught in its feet or shoes. Horses love to roll in mud, but it isn't good to leave mud caked on them, so your horse will need to be bathed, or at least cleaned off, whenever it rolls.

Dental Care. Dental care is a most important part of horse maintenance. The stress associated with tooth problems is highly misunderstood and responsible for many a death from some related complication. Loss of balance, lameness, and other profound problems may stem from this portion of a horse's anatomy.

Horses, like guinea pigs, rabbits, and rats, are grinders, and because domesticated horses are fed concentrated foods they aren't given the opportunity to grind as much as they should. As a result their teeth often develop sharp points, which can cut their tongue or cheek. To keep teeth healthy, a qualified veterinarian or dental technician will need to grind down the sharp points, which is called "floating." Teeth should be floated at least once a year, sometimes more. Later in life, horses may need to have the incisors or their front teeth shortened because they don't get the kind of wear they would in the wild nipping grass and scraping roots of plants in sandy soil.

Hay!... What's for Dinner? Horses are natural foragers who, by nature, will munch on food all day long. If a horse does not eat for four or five hours its stomach may become irritated and an ulcer may develop. This is why horses should have hay available at all times and not rely on finely ground, concentrated feeds that are given two to three times a day.

Although commercially produced horse feed is of generally good quality, the more fresh, organic food you can give your horse the better. A quality, grass-mix hay is a good basic diet, commercial or fresh. Horses love carrots, apples, and all fruit as treats. Many trainers like to give them alfalfa, especially in the winter, for its extra protein and calcium. Plain oats, barley, and corn of a good quality are healthful, too; they should be rolled so as not to cause excessive wear on the teeth. Note that heavily muscled breeds, such as quarter horses, do best with as little grain as possible. An alfalfa hay is a prime food choice for performing horses that need some extra protein. Timothy hay seems to get mixed reviews—some trainers think it's a good basic ingredient, but others feel it is nutritionally weak. Not surprisingly, processed and pelleted foods should be avoided. Such foods can cause intestinal problems such as ulcers.

Some people feed young horses high-protein diets to get them to grow quickly so they will be ready for competition sooner. But baby horses are not supposed to grow too fast. Their bones should grow at a relatively slow rate. Otherwise, their bones may become too soft and their ligaments too weak to hold up the horse's weight. That can result in serious bone, muscle, neurological, and joint problems.

Supplements for Horses. Horses can benefit from well-balanced integrated vitamin programs. High-performance horses and older, arthritic ones might do well on chondroitin sulfate, glucosamine, and MSM, but used as preventatives in young horses these may interfere with the body's ability to take care of normal wear and tear on its own.

Vaccinations. Some immunizations may be important to protect against such painful and fatal diseases as rabies, and particularly tetanus, to which horses are susceptible. Other vaccines, however, may not be necessary unless your horse is at high risk for that particular condition. Routine revaccinations should be avoided too, unless a blood titer is done and reveals a loss of immunity. Over-vaccinating an animal may compromise its immune system and cause auto-immune problems. To minimize this possibility, some veterinarians accompany allopathic vaccinations with homeopathic ones called nosodes. (See Chapter 9 for an in-depth discussion of vaccinations).

Other Veterinary Considerations. To maintain good health and resolve special problems, you might consider a visit to a chiropractically trained veterinarian. Chiropractic adjustments align the skeletal system, which, in turn, releases blockages in body passageways. Once freed of congestion, the nervous system can operate smoothly. This is important as the nervous system promotes healing and keeps an already sound body fully functioning. "What we do with chiropractic care," says Judith M. Shoemaker, D.V.M., of West Grove, Pennsylvania, "is get the hardware straight so the software can run."[6]

When chiropractic care is performed correctly, that is, with a light touch of the hands and accurate technique, horses look forward to their chiropractic treatments, which they find relaxing and comfortable. Look for a qualified practitioner, one certified by the American Veterinary Chiropractic Association (AVCA). To locate a chiropractic veterinarian in your area, call the organization at (309) 658-2920. For maintenance a horse should be adjusted about three times a year, and for special problems on an as-needed basis. Maintaining mechanical balance will help a horse live healthily for many years.

Acupuncture is something you may want to look into for your horse; very good results have been seen with this therapy for lameness and chronic colic. Another thing to be aware of is that horses need to be wormed regularly in order to prevent possible damage to major blood vessels.

Avoid Unnatural Manipulation. Some people will take extreme measures to make their horses suitable for competition. Horses may be bred for certain traits, such as color, shape, gait, or head shape. In the process, though, other problems may develop. Certain breeds, Arabs, for instance, are prone to immune system disorders. It's better not to "play God" by breeding for arbitrary characteristics. Also, mechanically, horse owners manipulate through tail setting, breaking the tails and putting them in tail sets to produce a higher set tail. This has the unfortunate effect of altering spinal cord function. Horses are also given inappropriate shoes or toe grabs, which are supposed to make a racehorse grip the track better with its front feet. In actuality, toe grabs increase the rate of breakdown injuries. Such manipulations are not just inappropriate, they're destructive and unnecessary.

Talking—and Listening—to Your Horse. Sam Powell, the man now famously known as the "horse whisperer," can teach us a lot about building a relationship with a horse. Powell's fundamental insight, and one shared by other holistic trainers, such as Linda Tellington-Jones, whose "Tellington Touch" we will discuss below, is that horses are smart, not dumb, as many people mistakenly think, and that they need to be talked to, as opposed to trained. Or, even better, as Sam Powell says, "… it's not the art of horse whispering that I'm trying to teach people. It's the art of *listening*." The lines of communication need to be kept open between horse and human because, when a horse "misbehaves" or acts out through aggressive, antisocial behavior, the real problem is not in the horse's nature but in the fact that the horse doesn't understand what is wanted of it. The human has failed to communicate by trying to dominate rather than understand the horse. In the wild, Sam Powell points out, horses are prey for other animals, such as mountain lions. Therefore, horses have great survival instincts. And when a human tries to dominate a horse, those survival instincts kick in. This can cause many of the behavior problems seen in some horses, such as head throwing and resisting capture for saddling.[7]

A healthy horse should have a lifespan of 20 to 30 years, although it may not be strong enough to ride past its 20s. It can still have a happy life, and be a friend to you.

The Power of Touch. Linda Tellington-Jones, working from her experience as a horse trainer, has given us one of the most revolutionary and successful methods of dealing with "problem horses." In order to understand why her method, called the Tellington Touch, is revolutionary, and why it can so drastically change the relationship between a horse and its trainer/rider, perhaps it's best to review a bit of the thinking about horses.

The relationship between people and horses is unique in the spectrum of pet ownership. True, other animals have been domesticated as long as horses (dogs, goats, even ferrets used for hunting in ancient Rome). True, other animals have been used for work (herding dogs, sledding dogs). But there is something special about the work relationship between people and horses, and something unique in the partnership. Sometimes—perhaps even usually—this is a beautiful, meaningful relationship, and in fact Linda Tellington-Jones herself is an example of a person whose life has revolved around horses and their care. As Susan Travellin says, there are such things as "horse people," and horse people pretty much don't talk about, or think about, anything much besides horses.[8] So a person like Tellington-Jones, or Travellin, or Sam Powell, has come to understand a lot about traditional approaches to horse training, which are generally based on the assumption that horses are "dumb" and that they need to be dominated into submission.

Linda Tellington-Jones grew up in western Canada, in a world full of animals and close to nature. Early on she became a horse trainer and began to realize that horses are not "lesser beings," but sentient beings, like us, that need to be trusted, respected, and communicated with for an effective relationship. Years later, Tellington-Jones found herself studying with the celebrated physicist Dr. Moshe Feldenkrais, learning his Feldenkrais Method of Functional Integration at the Humanistic Psychology Institute in San Francisco. The aim of Dr. Feldenkrais's method is to reintegrate the mind and body following any sort of imbalance, such as injury, illness, or undue stress. The method is used by athletes, dancers, or anyone else in peak form wishing to reach a fuller physical and mental potential. The technique involves a series of nonhabitual, gentle movements and manipulations all over the body. After studying this for several years, Tellington-Jones combined the principles she learned with her understanding of horses. Her goal was to help humans teach horses by encouraging rather than dominating. Thus, tensions between horses and humans that made the animals resistant to learning could be eliminated, and the learning potential of horses could be expanded. The system of training and bodywork for horses was termed Tellington Equine Awareness Movements (TEAM) and the principles underlying the application of circular movements for horses, and later for all animals, became known as TTouch.

When you are doing a series of TTouches on your horse or other animal, the point is not to stimulate muscles, but rather to stimulate the nervous system. Therefore, the touches may be very light—especially if you are working on a small animal or an injured large animal—and still be highly effective. Achieving the right touch takes some practice; when starting out, practitioners tend to automatically switch into massage mode, which actually illustrates a key factor of the Tellington Touch: the nonhabitual aspect. The point of using the TTouch on a horse is to help the animal break destructive cycles or bad habits that it has fallen into. In order to "wake up" your horse you will be touching it and stimulating it in ways that are new and different. The idea is to energize your horse, make it more aware, and make it more responsive. So stay at the surface to communicate with its nerve endings.

Most Tellington Touches are clockwise circular motions, and any of them can be performed on any part of the horse's body. Does your horse seem tense? Where is it holding that tension? You might want to start there. Or start around the neck and face so that you can talk to your horse as well. Since horses are prone to colic and digestive problems, the belly can be a good place to start. One of Linda Tellington-Jones's first experiences with healing a horse in a holistic manner, before she developed the TTouch, was working on a horse suffering from severe colic, which doctors did not expect to live. By staying with the animal all night, working over its ears and stomach, she helped the horse pass the blockage in its intestines, and the horse made a full recovery. One thing that Tellington-Jones took from this experience was that ears are a receptive part of the body, something that is also known to acupuncturists and other holistic practitioners.

There are 15 basic TTouches, and each one has a name. Starting out with your flat hand somewhere on the horse's body, and pushing the skin around in clockwise circles, is called the "abalone touch." This is a good one to start with. Then lift your fingers so that only your fingertips are touching, and again turn your fingers in a circle. This is called the "clouded leopard." And so on. The movements are performed in conjunction with rhythmic breathing—the practitioner's—in order to increase the practitioner's focus and relaxation. This then helps the horse tune into the person, enhancing communication between them. The technique is simple as well as effective, so, instead of petting or patting your horse pointlessly you might get into the habit of always doing one of these moves. It could improve your relationship dramatically.

The Tellington Touch method can be used on any animal, and is discussed in Chapter 5.

RODENTS

Hamsters, guinea pigs, gerbils, mice, rats… they're small, they don't take up much room, and to many people they barely seem like pets at all but more like a novelty, or a toy, to keep in a little cage somewhere or anywhere, with very low maintenance.

Wrong! A lot of us have misconceptions about domesticated rodents. Rodents are living beings with their own needs. And probably their biggest need is for their caretakers to realize this. Just like other furry pets, they require attention and care, and, at base, respect for the creatures that they are. Sometimes parents buy rodents for young children, thinking they will be easy pets for kids. But there are many facts to be aware of before you buy a rodent as a pet for your child. First, many rodents are nocturnal or crepuscular, meaning they prefer to be active at night or during the twilight hours of early morning or late evening. (Examples: chinchillas or hamsters, and rabbits too, actually, although they are able to adapt to human schedules more easily than other rodents). At night, the little hamsters will be awake in their cages, running in their wheel while the kids they share a room with are trying to sleep. This is one reason that families sometimes abandon rodents that were bought with good intentions. If nighttimes aren't the problem, children may insist on making the hamster's playtime coincide with their own, after school or all day on weekends. This can be incredibly stressful for a rodent, since it drastically interferes with the animal's own body clock.

Not only are many rodents nocturnal, but they can be biters as well, making them problematic for young children. Gerbils are also a problematic choice for a child's pet because gerbils like to stay busy constantly with their own building projects. They do not like to be interrupted to be held or played with, and they can simply refuse to be held by children, squirming their way out of a child's grip and scratching the child in the process.

This doesn't mean, however, that rodents should just be left alone. Like other domesticated mammals, rodents want their owner's attention, and some playtime is good for them. Paying attention to your rodent will help it avoid health problems.

Housing. Rodents need a cage that is large enough to be comfortable, and they need litter in the cage that is safe. Shredded newspaper, which nowadays is mostly lead-free, is a good choice, as is clean newsprint. Some people use rabbit pellets as litter substrate, because the pellets look like grass and so are aesthetically pleasing. This is okay, because if your rodent eats the pellets it won't hurt it. Pine shavings have received a mixed review for safety—problems have cropped up, but they don't seem to be the norm. Still, with some rodent experts advising against them, pine shavings should probably not be your top choice. For the animal's health and safety, don't use anything that has a strong aroma. Your pet will urinate in the litter, and the mix of urine and strong wood vapors can cause an array of dangerous respiratory problems. Worse yet, cedar or chlorophyll vapors, when mixed with urine in the litter, can actually rot your hamster's feet over time, leaving the animal helpless and near death. Occasionally, inattentive hamster owners will experience this unhappy outcome. Whatever type of litter you choose, it needs to be changed every other day. This can be a lot of work, but the chore creates time you will spend with your pet on a regular basis. In short, understand your rodent when shopping to fill its needs, and when home be sure to check in with it regularly. These two habits will go a long way toward avoiding big problems.

Food—Remember the Fresh. Feeding rodent pets also requires some time and thoughtfulness. Although commercially produced pellets can be the basis of a rodent's diet, these animals do need some fresh foods every day in order to stay healthy. As far as the pellets are concerned, just check the package for freshness before making a purchase. Don't buy pellets in a box—if you can't see them, chances are that they are old, discolored, and have lost most or all of their nutritional value. Many manufactured rodent foods are packaged and then shelved for months. Different species have different nutritional requirements, so check with your vet or a rodent expert to find out what's best to provide fresh for your rodent. Guinea pigs, for example, need vitamin C, so you might want to give a pet guinea pig small pieces of freshly sliced oranges, or red pepper. But hamsters do not need vitamin C added to their diet. For all species, make sure the fresh food is raw, not cooked. A couple of slices of carrot are good additions for any rodent, and easy for you to add. Slices of uncooked yam are another good offering. You can help your rodent even more by rotating, or changing, its daily fresh food. Rodents by nature tend to get stuck on eating just one or two favorite foods, but if you trick yours into eating a more varied, nutritious diet you are doing it a big favor. You may be familiar with this "food rut" problem if you own parrots, which like to pick out only their favorites from a selection of seeds. As with all living beings, a good diet is fundamental to rodent health. Unfortunately, the life expectancy of most rodents is only about three years, but you can make your rodent's short life happy, and reduce trips to the vet, by keeping it on a solid, nutritionally rich diet.

Health Concerns. If, in spite of your best efforts to keep your pet on a healthy diet, a hamster or guinea pig starts being constipated or having loose stools or diarrhea, for immediate treatment you can give your pet a commercial probiotic, or a small amount of plain yogurt or cultured buttermilk. You should, however, take your pet to a veterinarian so that it can be checked for parasites or bacterial infections, two common causes of rodent digestive upsets. Diarrhea is a serious problem in rodents. If your pet does have parasites, many holistic vets will recommend treatment with conventional medications because natural treatments, such as garlic, will simply not kill off the parasite, which has to be your first goal. You may augment this medication with herbal treatments or homeopathy in order to boost the animal's immune system, but without medication the parasites are likely to return, causing further problems. Remember, paying attention to your little guy will help you ward off a lot of problems that can crop up in ignored rodents—or any other pet.

SNAKES

This book has repeatedly emphasized that pet owners need to understand their animals' experience of the world in order to be good caretakers for them. The wilder a species is—the further it is from human existence—the truer this maxim is. Whenever you are considering buying a so-called exotic pet, you are thinking about bringing into your home a creature that was not created for living in a human world. Dogs, cats, horses, and goats have been domesticated for millennia, and co-existing with humans is part of their essence. But other animals are simply not designed or intended for living in houses or apartments. Fish are an example of this. As we discussed in the section on fish in this chapter, the responsible fish owner needs to create a water world that is separate from, and protected from, the contaminants and noise of our human world. To be responsible pet owners, we must respect our animals by understanding each one's needs.

Snakes, like birds and fish, live a natural life far away from human contact. Being domesticated puts snakes under a great deal of stress, just by virtue of their being captive in an unnatural environment. The wild snake slithers when it wants and rests when it wants (in fact, many species of snake, such as the python, are extremely placid in their natural state), lives on the ground or climbs trees, and, being cold-blooded, moves under shelter when it needs to escape extremes of hot or cold. Since snakes are mostly tropical creatures, they prefer and are healthiest in temperatures of around 80 degrees. Now, proceeding from a snake "mindset," imagine being forced to live in confined, cold, mammal spaces—no wonder domestication is stressful for a snake!

Housing—and Hiding—Your Snake. The name for a snake cage is an herpetorium. The herpetorium you provide for your snake must be roomy enough for it to move around in, and you need to put some branches in it for climbing, as well as a place to hide, such as an upside-down box with a hole cut out for an entrance. Giving your snake a hiding place is especially important. In the wild, snakes have rocks to slither under, or holes to retreat into, whenever they want. The lack of a proper hiding place is extremely stressful for a housebound snake. It will express this stress by being unusually restless and hard to handle. Snakes like to decorate their own spaces in captivity, so don't be surprised if you put a box in your snake's herpetorium, only to find it moved to a new corner a couple of days later. Leave it where it is if this happens—your snake is happier with its own interior design. Since snakes thrive in warm temperatures, be sure to keep your herpetorium in an area that is properly heated and away from drafts. Use heat lamps, if necessary, to provide extra warmth. Your snake's herpetorium should be lined with newspaper that you change frequently. Also, make sure, as with any pet, that your snake has constant access to clean water.

Food. One risk for pet snakes is inadequate nutrition. Actually, this is true with any type of pet because often, the people pets live with, however well-intentioned they may be, do not understand their animals' nutritional needs. In the case of snakes, snakes eat rodents as a basic part of their diet. So snake owners go to the pet store and buy mice for their snakes to eat. But those mice are themselves mal- or undernourished because they have been thoughtlessly overbred and poorly cared for. In this way poor nutrition works its way up the food chain, to your snake. And now your malnourished snake is at risk for health problems it otherwise might not have. Unfortunately, there isn't really a solution for this large problem, but do try to provide your snake with rodents from a reputable dealer, and preferably one you know well.

Treating and Avoiding Problems. If your snake does become ill, it can be treated by a veterinarian just as any other animal can. Snakes are prone to mouth rot, which is caused by an organism called aeromonas. They are also prone to improper shedding and to pneumonia. These conditions can be treated with conventional or alternative therapies. Homeopathic remedies are available for most snake ailments, and for stressed-out snakes, some people report that Bach flower remedies can be helpful. You can easily apply Bach's Rescue Remedy when your snake seems stressed, they advise, simply by letting one or two drops fall on its back.

The Tellington Touch has been applied to snakes, as well as to our furrier friends. This approach takes into account the fact that snakes have unique physical structures that may suffer from domestication. Did you know that a snake's lungs are almost half as long as the snake itself? A snake can develop lung trouble if it's confined to its cage for too long a period; the snake can't stretch fully and so lung congestion results.

This is where T Touches, such as the "belly lift," can help. To use this technique, slowly lift the belly of the snake off the ground, hold, and then release. Repeat the movement down the snake's belly. You can also try the "python lift" to relieve tension and spasm in the neck area (it's good for humans, too). Place your fingers on the back of the snake, just below the head. Lift the skin and muscle an inch or so. Hold for a few seconds, and then slowly release. Do not put too much pressure on the muscle; that will cause the snake to hold its breath.

NOTES

1. Gary Null interview with Arthur Young, V.M.D., May 10, 2000.
2. Gary Null interview with Alicia McWatters, Ph.D., Mar. 10, 2000.
3. Tellington-Jones, Linda, with Sybil Taylor, *The Tellington Touch: A Revolutionary Natural Method to Train and Care for Your Favorite Animal*, Penguin Books, 1993, pp. 129-142.
4. Gary Null interview with Nancy Scanlan, V.M.D., Mar. 17, 2000.
5. Gary Null interview with Susan Travellin, August 2000.
6. Gary Null interview with Judith Shoemaker, August 2000.
7. Gary Null interview with Sam Powell.
8. Gary Null interview with Susan Travellin, September 2000.

Controversy in the Kennel: Issues in Pet Care

Just as with human health, the field of animal health is filled with unsettled—and sometimes unsettling—issues. Is it okay to declaw a cat? What kind of flea control is best for a dog? How can we tackle the animal over-population problem? And are we over-vaccinating our pets? This last question is probably the most controversial one right now, so let's start by looking at the vaccination issue.

THE PROBLEM OF OVER-VACCINATION

Imagine your doctor saying, "Today you'll be getting vaccinated for measles, mumps, rubella, smallpox, hepatitis, and tetanus. And, while you're here, why not get your flu shot as well?" You'd probably drop your jaw in disbelief. Yet many people think nothing of subjecting their companion animals to multiple vaccinations year after year. Our puppies and kittens start life with four or more initial shots, followed by a five-in-one or seven-in-one booster each year for the next 10 to 15 years of their lives. Animals are vaccinated and revaccinated against a whole slew of conditions—far more than we humans are. This use, or overuse, of vaccines is a cause of great concern.

Not just the alternative, but the conventional veterinary community as well now link overzealous vaccination protocols to numerous problems. One particularly disturbing side effect is a kind of fibrosarcoma—an aggressive vaccine-induced tumor—sometimes seen in cats following a rabies or feline leukemia vaccine.

The condition, named vaccinoma, develops at the injection site in 0.3 to 0.7 percent of vaccinated cats, which is an unacceptably large percentage considering the severity of the disease. One researcher, Dr. Dennis W. Macy, professor of oncology at Colorado State University, estimated 22,000 such cases in the mid-1990s, and found that more cancer developed when vaccines were repeatedly given at a particular site over time.[1] In addition to cancer, many veterinarians believe that chronic degenerative diseases, including heart disease, thyroid disorders, skin problems, intestinal disease, and arthritis, are at times associated with vaccines.

In recent years conventional veterinarians have become increasingly aware of the problems stemming from over-vaccination. A leading professional publication, the *Journal of the American Veterinary Medical Association*, has been reporting on the controversy; in one article entitled, "Are we vaccinating too much?" several veterinary experts conclude that the need for annual parvovirus and distemper boosters has not been established and that the practice of administering weekly parvovirus vaccines to young puppies is unnecessary and possibly harmful.[2]

Fortunately, a new trend in veterinary medicine is to vaccinate less frequently. Instead of automatically revaccinating each year, some doctors are choosing to inoculate animals every three years. Veterinary organization guidelines are changing; veterinary teaching hospitals at Colorado State University and the University of California-Davis, for example, are encouraging veterinarians to vaccinate adult dogs against rabies, parvovirus, adenovirus, parainfluenza, and distemper every three years instead of annually. Additionally, the American Veterinary Medical Association is reconsidering annual vaccine guidelines, and the American Association of Feline Practitioners already encourages the three-year approach. These new official guidelines, combined with an insistent, knowledgeable public that demands greater caution, could influence more veterinarians to be conservative in their vaccination protocols.

The Homeopathic View. Homeopathic medicine finds the whole concept of vaccination, as it is conventionally understood, to be problematic. This is a point of view worth examining.

In allopathic medicine, vaccines are believed to immunize against disease by imitating the disease process. With the introduction of weakened (attenuated) or killed viruses or bacteria into the body, the immune system is fooled into producing protective T- and B-cells against the foreign invaders. In the event of a future exposure to the virus or bacteria, the cells are supposed to remember their former encounter and respond by producing appropriate antibodies against the disease.

But the homeopath would argue that the conventional vaccine does not guarantee protection and that it may not help at all. (Actually, the only way to truly establish life-long immunity is to survive a disease.) Rather than protect, vaccines interfere with a living organism's vital energy (a force called chi in Oriental medicine). Disease symptoms may be suppressed, only to resurface years later with a greater vengeance or to manifest as some other disease. Many believe, for instance, that the deadly parvovirus is a mutation of feline distemper, another fatal disease, because it first appeared shortly after widespread inoculation against distemper.

Homeopaths attribute life-long problems to conventionally practiced vaccination. The term for these vaccine-induced illnesses is vaccinosis. Vaccinating a dog against canine distemper, for example, may suppress acute symptoms of the disease, such as vomiting, diarrhea, and loss of appetite, but at the same time initiate chronic gastritis, hepatitis, pancreatitis, and appetite disorders. Similarly, administering a rabies vaccine may foster the continual expression of restlessness, uneasiness, apprehensiveness, and viciousness characteristic of the disease. You will not see the original diseases—distemper or rabies—but you will now have distemper vaccinosis or rabies vaccinosis, chronic vaccine-created illnesses. (This is not to say that you should forego vaccinating your pet for these two particular diseases, as we shall discuss later.)

In some instances, vaccinosis may even contribute to death from the disease a vaccine was designed to prevent. When a vaccine creates a chronic illness in an animal (or person) who is highly susceptible to the disease, a later exposure to the natural form of the disease may result in the natural disease combining forces with the established disease to create an illness more life-threatening than the original illness.

When vaccinosis is present, treating symptoms of a disease homeopathically may fail unless the original cause of the problem—the vaccination—is treated first. Richard H. Pitcairn, D.V.M.,

Ph.D., a veterinarian practicing classical homeopathy, concluded that this is more the rule than the exception after discovering that many hard-to-resolve cases improved only after the use of Thuja, an anti-vaccine remedy.[3]

Homeopathic physicians believe that problems arise because of the way vaccines are given. When you inject a virus or bacteria you bypass the body's natural filtration mechanisms. Usually, the mouth and respiratory system are the first lines of defense against communicable diseases. In the article "The case against immunization," Richard Moskowitz, M.D., argues that when we vaccinate we short-circuit these very important primary responses to disease. He explains that "by cheating the body in this fashion we have accomplished precisely what the evolution of the immune system seems to have been designed to prevent: we have placed the virus directly in the blood, and given it free and immediate access to the major immune organs and tissues without any obvious way of getting rid of it."[4]

Vaccines introduce substances in addition to viruses or bacteria that the body must now fight off. They contain antibiotics or fungicides used to protect the vaccine against bacterial contamination, and aluminum sulfate or mercuric oxide added to carry viral particles into the body in the injection procedure. Also, the medium in which the vaccine is grown, such as chick embryo or fetal bovine serum, enters the body and can trigger adverse reactions.

Looking at the big picture, many homeopaths wonder whether the widespread use of conventional vaccines is suppressing natural disease to such a degree that it will have serious consequences to the health of future generations. Many would agree with Dr. Moskowitz when he says, "... I have always felt that the attempt to eradicate entire microbial species from the biosphere must inevitably upset the balance of nature in fundamental ways we can as yet scarcely imagine."[5]

Nosodes. In the ongoing controversy surrounding vaccinations for pets, some members of the anti-vaccine side have advocated what are called nosodes as an alternative. Nosodes are homeopathic remedies that have been made from a diseased agent or from tissue that has been affected by a specific disease. For example, a nosode for parvovirus would originate in a bit of a dog's intestine that had been infected by the virus, while the raw material for a heartworm nosode is actual heartworm larvae. These samples have been diluted to the point where there are no viral particles left in the nosode solution itself, only the "molecular energy memory of what was in there before," as Dr. Jean Dodds explains. Dodds was named the 1994 holistic vet of the year, and although she urges caution in the use of vaccines, she believes that, at present, nosodes are not really an acceptable alternative to all vaccinations.[6]

The reason for Dr. Dodds's reservations about nosodes is the lack of reliable studies done on their effectiveness against disease. The only studies done so far, conducted in England, were not well controlled. One nosode trial, conducted in the U.S. against parvovirus, one of the most lethal diseases that can strike dogs, showed that the nosodes did protect the puppies in the trial against the disease. But this one case study alone does not constitute enough evidence to make generalizations about the use of nosodes, and questions about these substances as an alternative to vaccines are still unanswered. Anecdotally, there are cases where people have treated dogs with nosodes instead of vaccinating them, and the dogs have not gotten sick. But in such uncontrolled circumstances there is no way of knowing whether the dogs were actually exposed to the diseases that the nosodes were intended to protect against. More research on this vaccine alternative needs to be done.

However, there is another way to use nosodes that has been proven effective. These substances may be administered to a dog or cat, before or after vaccinating it, as a preventative against adverse reactions to the vaccination. In these circumstances, the use of nosodes is entirely safe and runs virtually no risk of side effects. Nosodes can also be administered after a dog is known to have been exposed to a disease such as parvo, and in these cases nosodes are known to help the dog's condition. These are sound alternatives to the risk of using nosodes in lieu of all vaccinations.

A veterinarian with extensive experience around the issue of nosodes is Dr. Charles E. Loops, a conventionally trained veterinarian who now practices homeopathy almost exclusively. Dr. Loops believes that the most important factor in prescribing nosodes in lieu of vaccines is simply the feelings of the pets' owners. After you have researched the vaccination question extensively, you may decide that your pet is not likely to be exposed to the common diseases that vaccinations are intended to prevent, and that you simply do not want to run the risk of vaccinating your animal. In this case, says Dr. Loops, "There is a place for using nosodes to help in case there is an exposure to one of these diseases." However, Dr. Loops shares Dr. Dodds's concerns about the lack of studies conducted on nosodes. The result of this lack of evidence is that, at present, nosodes are used randomly, without a body of knowledge to guide their application to specific diseases. Their effectiveness has not been proven—sometimes they seem to work, he points out, but at other times, they don't. Using nosodes, according to Dr. Loops, "… is the sort of thing where you have to look at the situation, and look at the individual nosode before you use it. It's not a straight-forward subject."[7]

A Conservative Approach. Whether or not to vaccinate is an individual decision, and deciding what to do can be a difficult choice. So it was for Richard Palmquist, V.M.D., of Englewood, California, who had stopped inoculating animals altogether after a dog he had just vaccinated died of anaphylactic shock, "… and a few animals paid the price with their lives." That difficult lesson convinced the doctor to re-evaluate his stance and conclude that "… vaccines have a definite place."[8] While some veterinarians and owners refuse to vaccinate altogether, many others take a middle ground. They inoculate against only the most life-threatening conditions, give one vaccination at a time, and detoxify the animal afterwards. Here, in more detail, are sensible guidelines to follow:

You may want to vaccinate only for the most important communicable diseases. Because of the dangers associated with vaccines, many holistic veterinarians encourage pet owners to take a long look at the risks and benefits of each vaccine, and to choose only the ones most needed. When two or more are necessary, space shots two to three weeks apart or rotate vaccines so that the animal is not getting several every year. Three vaccines that most holistic veterinarians recommend for dogs and cats are those for rabies, distemper, and parvovirus.

The rabies vaccine is high-risk—as mentioned earlier, it will cause vaccinosis in a small percentage of cats—but it's necessary as it is required by law for all dogs and cats in most localities. To minimize side effects, the rabies vaccine should be given by itself, and homeopathic antidotes—discussed later—should be given at the same time.

Distemper is a cruel, fatal disease striking both dogs and cats that can be easily controlled with a vaccination, which has been around since the 50s. Before the vaccine was developed, distemper was an epidemic that took the lives of thousands of animals. Since the advent of the vaccine the incidence of distemper in vaccinated, domesticated cats and dogs has fallen dramatically.

Parvovirus is another lethal canine disease, which first appeared in the 1970s. Since a vaccine was developed in the late 70s, the incidence of parvovirus in domestic dogs has also been slashed. In the opinion of many holistic vets, then, canine and feline rabies, canine and feline distemper, and canine parvovirus are the only vaccines that should indisputably be administered to all pets.

With regard to other vaccinations, each case needs to be considered individually. Feline leukemia is a disease against which cats are routinely vaccinated, and yet the vaccine is not all that effective. Not only that, but there are problems. As mentioned earlier, feline leukemia is one of the vaccinations to which cats may have serious adverse reactions, including injection-site fibrosarcoma tumors, which must be surgically removed. In light of this, the owner of an indoor-only cat, who is not likely to come into contact with any other cats, including other cats brought into the household, may feel confident in not giving the feline leukemia vaccine to his or her pet (only 1 percent of indoor-only cats manifest the disease). On the other hand, the owner of an indoor-outdoor cat, or outdoor-only cat, who will run a greater risk of exposure to feline leukemia, needs to seriously weigh the risks and benefits of the vaccine before making a decision (30 percent of outdoor cats develop an acute form of the disease). By the way, if your cat tests positive for the disease be sure to test again in three weeks to be extra certain that the first result was not a false positive reading.

Try to avoid vaccines of lesser importance, especially when there are other, less drastic ways to treat the condition. For the average, healthy pet, the corona virus is not a significant disease; it just causes a bit of orangy diarrhea that will go away in a few days when the animal is kept warm. A less healthy pet might succumb to this infection, though even here the usefulness of the corona vaccine has not been established.

Boarding kennels will only take animals that are inoculated annually with the bordetella vaccine. A problem with the procedure is that kennels will take animals the day after they've been vaccinated, long before immunity to the disease has had a chance to develop. In fact, after a single vaccination of bordetella, you need to wait two to three weeks and then follow with a booster before getting any sort of immunity at all. Also, the vaccine is not really necessary, according to retired veterinarian Lester Morris of New Jersey. "To me, it's like a human being getting a cold," he says. "You get over it."[9] If your animal has had the shot once and its immunity is proven via blood titer, have your veterinarian write the kennel a note so stating, along with results of the titer for proof. As an extra precaution, supply your pet with extra vitamin C and echinacea during its stay. When deciding whether or not to vaccinate, consider whether your pet is exposed to other animals (in or out of your house) and what diseases are prevalent in your part of the country.

There is quite a bit of concern about animals, especially those in Northeastern states, contracting Lyme disease. While this fear might be somewhat overplayed (only 5 percent of dogs that are bitten by ticks contract the disease), you will still need to take preventive measures; however, vaccinations are not the hoped-for solution. In fact, both short- and long-term effects of the Lyme vaccine are proving to be as devastating as the disease itself, or even more so. Soon after the inoculation pain, the animal may have local reactions such as swelling, pain, and even an allergic reaction leading to breathing difficulties. Later on deeper difficulties may develop. These include immune suppression and autoimmune reactions in any number of body systems. Thus, your dog or cat may develop seizures, arthritis, dermatitis, or thyroiditis. Repeating the Lyme vaccine annually could prove devastating with the development of kidney or liver disease, or even cancer. The best line of defense against Lyme is to examine your dog (or cat) after a walk, especially around the eyes, in the ears, between the toes, above the shoulders, and under the neck. Should you spot a tick, pull it off with tweezers, making sure the head is intact, and flush it down the toilet. In addition, you should check your animal's Lyme titer yearly. Should the disease be present, take appropriate measures needed to fight the disease while at the same time building up the animal's immunity.

In addition to administering only the most important vaccinations at sensible intervals, there are other important considerations.

Before vaccinating, always consider the health of your animal. Is your pet lively and vigorous, or does it have symptoms of an immune system that is already compromised? If your pet is fighting cancer, for example, or experiencing a flare-up of a chronic health problem, it's best not to further disrupt its immune system with a vaccine. Although vaccine labels clearly state, "for healthy animals only," some veterinarians will vaccinate sick animals regardless of the warning unless an informed owner insists the animal not be vaccinated at that time.

If the animal is undergoing another medical procedure, such as spaying or neutering, your pet's doctor might think that this is an easy time to vaccinate, but you should never allow it. Multiple procedures, anesthetics, and medications will place further stress on the immune system and at the same time may lessen the effectiveness of the vaccine.

Never vaccinate an animal that is younger than 6 weeks old. Preferably, shots should begin at between 9 and 16 weeks. Youngsters acquire a natural immunity through the antibodies in their mother's colostrum, the first milk feedings. This protection may last as long as 14 to 16 weeks. When vaccines are given too early, maternal antibodies may interfere with immune response. Here's a good beginning vaccination schedule for puppies and kittens, developed by Robert Goldstein, V.M.D:

PUPPIES
9 weeks—distemper, modified-live vaccine (killed not available)
12 weeks—parvovirus, killed vaccine
15 weeks—repeat nine-week immunization
18 seeks—repeat parvovirus, killed vaccine
21 weeks—rabies, killed vaccine (three-year, if possible)

KITTENS
9 weeks—feline distemper/rhinotracheitis/ calicivirus vaccine (combination only)
12 weeks—repeat nine-week immunization
15 weeks—rabies, killed vaccine (three-year, if possible)[10]

Vaccines should be given singly. (This is especially true of the rabies vaccine.) Avoid combination vaccines, which may be convenient to use but are detrimental to the health of your pet. Ask your veterinarian to order individual vaccines (although for some vaccines, this is not possible) and to give just one shot per visit. Additional vaccines should be spaced at least one week apart, or preferably two or three weeks apart. Also, use killed vaccines, when these are available. Modified-live vaccines are banned in Scandinavia because their abilities to replicate and mutate make them far more dangerous.

Detoxification after an inoculation is essential. To offset possible negative side effects from vaccines, many holistic veterinarians give their patients the homeopathic remedy Thuja, which is considered the most important antidote for preventing or reversing vaccine-induced illnesses. Realize, however, that Thuja, like vaccines, is not a panacea, and that the best approach is to vaccinate as little as possible. Thuja can be bought in health food stores in a 12X or 30C potency, or ordered from Boericke and Tafel at (800) 876-9505. While this remedy is best begun the day after the inoculation, if Thuja is administered at a later date, it will still work to detoxify the animal. One to two pellets (depending on the weight of the dog or cat) should be given daily for seven days. As with other homeopathic remedies, Thuja should not be touched with the hands but placed on the crease of folded white paper, crushed with the back of a spoon if too large to swallow, and poured into the animal's mouth. This procedure will maximize the remedy's effectiveness. Another vaccine antidote is Viratox, which can be ordered through veterinarians from Homeo Vetix at (800) 521-7722. A teaspoon of this remedy is taken daily for two weeks, beginning on the day of the first shot.

Because the correct approach to vaccinating is so essential to the well-being of your beloved cat or dog, it is well worth a review:

Initially, vaccinate only for the most important communicable diseases.

Before inoculating for other conditions, weigh the risks and benefits.

Do not automatically vaccinate each year. Request an annual blood titer to determine whether or not boosters are necessary.

If more than one vaccine is needed, spread them out as much as possible, giving one every two to three weeks. This is especially important for rabies. Another option is to rotate vaccines so that the animal doesn't get too many shots in one year.

Never vaccinate an animal that is sick, pregnant, on corticosteroids, or undergoing surgery or some other medical procedure.

Whenever possible, use killed vaccines rather than live-attenuated vaccines.

Do not vaccinate at the same site each time.

Always detoxify with remedies such as Thuja or Viratox to counteract potentially harmful vaccination effects.

YOUR CAT NEEDS HIS CLAWS, BECAUSE...

...basically, because he's a cat. That's why, in the controversy about whether or not you should declaw your cat, I come down squarely on the side of those who say, "Don't do it."

Let's go back 50 million years. Paleontologists have discovered that an early ancestor of the cat that lived at that time, called Miacis, was like the cat of today in that it had beautiful fur and retractable claws. Since earliest times, a cat's claws have been one of its most exceptional features. Indeed, they're a vital part of its anatomy—in essence, what makes a cat a cat. Your cat depends on its claws to walk, run, sprint, climb, and stretch. Removing a cat's claws is not only painful, it's also damaging to your cat's physical health and psychological well-being. In fact, in the U.S. and abroad, pet shows recognize declawing as an inhumane procedure and ban declawed animals from participating.

A cat's claws serve many functions, the most important of which is protection. A cat uses its claws to climb to safety when escaping trouble, and to scratch an enemy when cornered. It will claw surfaces to condition its nails and to visually mark its territory. A cat's claws give it the footing it needs to get around. Cats will also claw for relaxation and entertainment, although when the object of the entertainment is the family sofa, pet owners can get peeved.

Indeed, destruction of furniture is a prime reason some owners and veterinarians view declawing, or onychetomy, the surgical removal of the claw, as an option to be considered. Fortunately, though, this point of view is becoming less popular, and for good reason. Declawing upsets a cat's physical health and causes great psychological distress. Removing a cat's claws is like amputating the ends of our fingers—it's very painful. Claws also contain energy meridians, which means that their removal results in disrupted energy flow, and, therefore, diminished vitality. During its long period of recovery, the cat will walk with great difficulty. For the rest of the cat's life, its balance will be shaky, increasing the risk of injury from a fall. Also, the cat's muscles will gradually weaken after the procedure. What's more, a poorly performed surgery might result in a post-operative infection, hemorrhaging, bone chips, the accidental cutting of the foot pad, nerve damage, pain, or the regrowth of deformed claws.

An important consideration is that without claws, cats lose their ability to climb. Cats minus their claws feel helpless, and the profound stress they experience makes them more receptive to diseases of the immune system, including feline leukemia. In addition, a cat that feels threatened might start to bite. To mark its territory, the cat might begin to urinate around the house or apartment. A declawed cat can never leave home. If it should get out through some unforeseen circumstance, its life may be in peril. It's important for cat owners to realize how essential claws are to a cat's physical and emotional health and, conversely, how detrimental it is to remove them.

Another surgical procedure to end scratching is the tendonectomy, in which the tendons to the claws are cut. After the procedure is performed, the cat still has its claws, only it is unable to use them properly. While this approach is less invasive than the onychetomy, it will nevertheless scar the animal physically and psychologically and should, therefore, be avoided as well.

A More Humane Approach. With a little time and forethought you can preserve both your possessions and your cat's claws. When applied consistently, behavior modification techniques yield good results. Buy a scratching post, or, better yet, since different cats have individual preferences, make your own using materials your cat likes to scratch on, such as a tightly woven fabric similar to the one covering its favorite armchair. Cats also like carpeting and sisal rope. Or you can attach the rough bark from a log onto a sturdy base. Your homemade post should be no less than three feet tall, and higher is better. If you have the time, build more than one. Then sprinkle the post with catnip, and place it next to the cat's favorite clawing spot.

Train your cat to use the post by placing its paws on it and moving them. Kittens will catch on more quickly than older cats that are already in the habit of clawing household items. If your cat returns to its old ways, don't give up. Redirect your cat by picking him up and once again placing him next to his scratching post. If the trouble persists, the next time you catch your cat clawing the carpet, squirt him with a little water.

Cats also love their own furniture, such as "cat condos" and other objects to climb into and onto. Designate one part of your living space the cat's corner, and fill it with scratchable objects. Again, through behavior modification techniques, your cat will learn where clawing is appropriate and where it is not.

Trimming your cat's nails on a regular basis will cut down its need to claw (see Chapter 3 for how to do this). And when all else fails, buy Soft Claw, a product recommended by veterinarians. In addition, when decorating, look for items that have the least claw appeal. Furniture made of a smooth wood is less enticing to a cat than furniture with a coarse finish. Also, consider short-pile carpets or hardwood floors rather than deep carpets that cats can easily grab. You might finish windows with attractive blinds or shades instead of long drapes.

INSECT REPELLENTS: THE NATURAL, AND THE NOXIOUS

Whenever dogs and cats return home from time spent outdoors they run the risk of bringing back unwelcome guests. Some animals—the less healthy ones—are more susceptible to parasites than others, and certain locales present greater challenges. Flea infestation is especially rampant in Southeastern states, where, in the worst-case scenario, their vampire-like attacks deplete blood faster than it can be replaced, and sometimes result in the need for a blood transfusion. Fleas also carry diseases—they can transmit haemobartonella to cats—and they can promote allergies.

Because parasites can be extremely destructive we want to annihilate them through any means possible. For several decades we

NATURAL PET CARE

have looked to chemicals to do the trick, but the results have been less than perfect. While fast-acting insecticides may initially prove effective, resistant strains always win out in the end. As history reveals, the fittest survive, and we become plagued by even more powerful super-bugs. "Insects become immune, so companies have to double whatever the chemical is to try to get through another few generations," observes herbalist Janette Grainger, author of *Natural Insect Repellants for People and Plants*.[11] Of course, retaliation with harsher and harsher chemicals is no solution, since ultimately it is impossible to outwit nature. At the same time, we are poisoning the very animals we are trying to protect.

We should not attempt to obliterate a part of nature that's lived for millions of years even if we do not understand its purpose. What we should realize, however, is that when an insect population is out of control it means that something in the environment is out of balance. Similarly, when a dog or cat is covered with fleas the animal's immunity is weak and not in balance. Of course a few fleas or ticks on a dog or cat is normal, and, believe it or not, even healthy. Consider that research on horses raised in an atmosphere completely free of parasites showed the animals to become much more susceptible to parasite-induced diseases when confronted by these insects later in life. The immune system is actually strengthened by the presence of some parasites. In the same way, an occasional flea or tick will strengthen your dog's or cat's ability to withstand future bites.

This is not to say that fleas and ticks do not present problems, such as allergies and disease, that must be dealt with. Left unchecked, they can multiply at a rapid rate and wreak havoc on your pet and in your environment. As a first line of defense, it is generally preferable to use natural remedies. There may be times, however, when natural products cause adverse reactions, and occasions when an animal is so compromised by a parasite that a quick chemical intervention may be necessary. Consider your animal's state of health and then select the best option. Whatever the choice, be sure to simultaneously build your pet's health with good food, herbs, and supplements, so that it will become strong enough to fend for itself in the future.

Holistic treatments work especially well as preventatives. Start with a strong foundation by providing your pet with healthy basics:

a good diet and vitamin and mineral supplements. That alone will provide basic protection, as hearty animals have a strong natural immunity to fleas and ticks. They may pick up a few parasites during a walk in the woods, but these pests are less likely to thrive and more apt to leave and pursue a less sound host.

For extra support give your dog a supplement containing brewer's yeast (or blood-building vitamin B12) and garlic. (But note that cats do not tolerate garlic well.) Brewer's yeast rubbed into the skin will also act as a natural repellent. In addition, a drop of apple cider vinegar added to the animal's water bowl daily will discourage fleas and ticks while building the pet's immune system.

Many holistic vets guide their clients in the use of herbal methods of flea and tick control. Whether these products are eaten or sprinkled, the herbal scent will linger on the skin, but don't wash it away too soon because the odor acts as a natural insect repellent. When you do clean your dog, use a shampoo containing tea tree oil. (Again, cats do not do as well with this.) If you're applying the oil directly, be sure to dilute with water, as full-strength tea tree oil, if licked off and ingested, might cause some GI-tract irritation. Other herbs that will deter insects include eucalyptus, rosemary, sage, bay, basil, lavender, pennyroyal, and citronella. One good product, Earth Animal's Internal Powder, contains high-quality vitamins, minerals, and herbs, and can easily be mixed into an animal's food. Some people also report good short-term results with Avon's Skin So Soft.

Groom your pet every day, especially in flea and tick season. Fleas like matted hair that they can crawl into. Brush the hair the wrong way, and then back to the way it should be. When you're finished, sprinkle your pet with a powdered herbal repellent or spray on some diluted oil, being careful, of course, not to spray the eyes. To dilute, use a tablespoon of the essential oil in a pint of water. This is good to do for temporary protection, for instance, just before a walk in the park. Try a small amount of pennyroyal (highly effective, but dangerous if too much is used) or eucalyptus, or, to be extra effective, combine two or three oils, such as eucalyptus, rosemary, and sage.

When a multifaceted holistic approach is followed consistently, natural remedies can also diminish, and sometimes even eliminate, a flea population that's already settled in. To begin, you will want to bathe your pet in an herbal bath with anti-flea ingredients. Or try bathing the pet in salt water. Either method will kill many pests. Water alone will drown the pests, but the addition of herbals will kill flea eggs as they hatch. As we've mentioned, certain herbs can be ingested as well. Two formulas to consider are available through Earth Animal: One is called No More Fleas, and the other No More Ticks. Herbal flea collars will help decrease the flea population on a small pet.

Rather than pollute your house with poisonous insecticides and chemical fogs, sprinkle a boric acid formula or a diatomaceous herbal powder on your carpet. Straight boric acid may be too concentrated and, therefore, dehydrating and harmful to your pet. [A good formula can be ordered from Flea Busters at (800) 353-2786.] Let this sit for a day before vacuuming. Along with the powder you will pick up dead and dehydrated fleas. Any eggs that hatch at that time will not survive. In the yard you can sprinkle tobacco dust, although beneficial organisms may be destroyed along with the fleas. A safer alternative would be a nematode that has been developed to eat flea larvae and eggs. These can be purchased at organic nurseries.

Some people who work with animals say that because physical disturbances reflect disharmony on the emotional and spiritual planes, flower essences can be of benefit, too. They believe that balancing the emotions releases the animal from the fear and anxiety that give parasites the incentive to attack, and spiritual balance increases the animal's vibratory rate so that physical and emotional problems will not manifest. One flower formula designed to discourage fleas is Anaflora's Be-Gone. This 12-flower formula contains windflower, said to stabilize mood, temperament, and physical vitality; lilac and wisteria to balance the nervous system; and even a flower called fleabane.

Chemical Solutions. When should you use synthetic chemical solutions for insect control? I would follow the advice of those vets who recommend using them only as a last resort, when your dog or cat is chewing itself alive, already anemic, and intensely ill from fleabites. Should this be the case, choose the least toxic topical application, one that is directly applied to the animal's hair and skin, and that kills fleas directly by poisoning the insects' nervous systems. And remember that it's only since the Second World War that Americans have been using synthetic chemicals for pest control. In that short period dosages have been increased in order to destroy newer more resistant strains. These poisons take their toll on your pet's liver, and are one of the reasons animals live shorter lives today than they used to. Today we think that a 15-year-old cat has lived a long life, but in the 1940s it wasn't unusual to have a cat for 20 or 25 years.

There are incredibly harmful substances on the market that you want to avoid at all costs. Some of these formulas contain highly noxious nerve gases, but because small amounts are administered, these products have earned FDA approval. What is not taken into account, however, is the fact that these toxins' effects are cumulative, so that ingesting a little each month can eventually have devastating effects. Also, oral medications should be avoided, as these products poison the system and work on the ludicrous supposition that an animal's blood can be used to deliver toxins to fleas. And be aware that chemical flea collars found in supermarkets and pet stores may pose serious dangers. Reactions may include rashes around the neck, and fur and hair falling out in these same areas. Many of the aforementioned products carry labels that advise purchasers to wash their hands after use and not to breathe in the dust. One has to wonder: Are not dogs and cats living, breathing creatures too?

Realize that even the best topical chemicals are not completely safe. Everyone is raving about one popular brand on the market today, but its application with gloves and placement at the back of the neck where the animal can't lick it off say something about its toxicity. In a short time, the insecticide works its way all over the body, and although the label says it does not penetrate the skin, at least to some degree it must.

The fact is that three years after introduction of this product, the first signs of its not being so safe are becoming apparent. While some animals appear to have no bad reaction, the veterinary literature contains numerous accounts of such side effects as severe rashes, vomiting, diarrhea, and loss of appetite. Adverse reactions are seen more often when the product is used frequently, that is, more than once a month.

So use these products judiciously—for one or two consecutive months only. If a bad reaction should occur, scrub the animal well to remove the product. And even if your animal has no apparent problem with the product, it's still wise to build your pet's strength with good food and flea-prevention supplements. As Dr. Robert Goldstein explains, the best antidote is sound health: "You want to get to the point where the fleas are no longer interested in the animal.... Using an insecticide kills fleas, but it doesn't change why the flea was in that animal to begin with. You have to change that animal, and that comes with boosting its immune system and changing its diet."[12]

SPAYING AND NEUTERING

Watching a cat or dog tend to her newly born infants may be delightful, but finding good homes for the average puppy or kitten can be a difficult task in a world overpopulated by animals. Animal shelters everywhere are on a mission to educate owners about the importance of spaying (the removal of a female's ovaries) and neutering (the removal of a male's testicles). If performed at the right time in an animal's life, the operation will not only prevent reproduction but also promote better health, behavior, and safety.

Neutering is a simple surgery that involves making a small incision in the ball sacs, removing the testicles, and putting some powder on the wound. Older puppies sometimes need a few stitches. Spaying is more involved; it requires making a small incision in the belly and removing the ovaries. Every veterinarian trained to work with small animals is qualified to perform sterilization. It is considered a safe procedure, and since the patient is completely anesthetized, it is painless as well.

Timing is all-important. Because young puppies and kittens require smaller incisions and have less tissue to be removed, shelters tend to spay animals extremely early in life. Sometimes the animals are as young as two or three weeks old. This is terribly wrong, as invasive surgery is severely stressful to an animal just starting out in life. It requires exposure to heavy doses of anesthesia for 25 to 30 minutes—the average length of time it takes to spay—and afterwards to high doses of antibiotics to counteract any bacterial infection that might occur. As antibiotics destroy helpful intestinal flora along with unfriendly bacteria, the ability to assimilate nutrients becomes compromised. These animals tend to weaken and become sick. An animal should never be spayed or neutered at less than six months of age. Performing the operation between six and eight months, just before the first heat, is wise. At this point in the animal's life, some hormones are beginning to kick in, which keeps the animal in better balance. Some people prefer to wait a little longer. They feel that if you can keep your dog or cat away from other animals it's best to sterilize after the first heat so that even more hormones are released. (Females should never be spayed in heat. As the organs are larger and more active at that time, the operation may result in complications.) Older animals are able to keep themselves cleaner, too, minimizing the likelihood of infection. The age of the animal when it is spayed or neutered will make all the difference as to whether the results of the procedure are destructive or stabilizing.

When performed at the correct time, spaying or neutering will help an animal enjoy a better quality of life. Nervousness, irritability, and aggressiveness—the type of stress that leads to health and behavior problems—will be gone. Neutered males have a lower incidence of prostate cancer, and spayed females have less mammary and ovarian cancer. The animal will exhibit calmness year-round, and your relationship is bound to improve as he or she focuses less on other animals and shows a greater appreciation for you. A spayed or neutered animal is also a safer animal, in that it is less likely to run away and get hit by a car, get into a fight, or eat objects it should not eat but otherwise would due to its natural urge to forage.

Some people feel that sterilization is an unnatural procedure and prefer to keep their cat or dog segregated from other animals during heat. But this is difficult to do, as an animal will continually cry to attract a mate, and will escape at any opportunity. In light of an overpopulation problem of astronomical proportions, why take chances of contributing to that problem? Consider that every unneutered animal in the world could be accountable for the birth of thousands more. This is no exaggeration: In one year, an unspayed dog could produce 16 puppies; in two, she and her offspring could produce 128; in three, the number could increase to 512; in four, you could see 2048; in five, 12,288; and in six years you could have 67,000 puppies! For cats, the numbers are equally staggering. With so many facilities willing to spay or neuter at a low cost, there is no reason not to do so. If you would like your children to witness the birth of a litter, instead of adding to the numbers crisis, rent a video. You will be teaching your children how to act responsibly and at the same time doing a great service for animalkind.

EUTHANASIA

Euthanasia of a terminally ill or critically injured animal as a last resort is an act of compassion, but what of the 12 to 20 million healthy companion animals that are "put to sleep" in animal shelters each year? In a world flooded with surplus animals, is ending their lives a necessity or mere convenience? Do other options exist? What does the easy and widespread disposal of companion animals say about our attitude toward animals and, on a larger scale, our sense of morality?

People who do not take animal adoption seriously may discard an animal for any number of reasons. The animal may be more difficult than anticipated. They may discover that it chews the furniture, tears the drapes, soils the carpet, barks excessively, or is overly aggressive or too territorial. Or it may no longer fit into the owner's lifestyle. A baby is about to arrive, for example; a fiancé doesn't like animals; the new apartment does not permit pets; the cat might destroy the refinished furniture. There are dozens of reasons people let their animals go.

One person who knows firsthand about unwanted pets is Valerie Angeli, director of public information at the New York-based American Society for the Prevention of Cruelty to Animals (ASPCA). Angeli receives many calls from frustrated owners anxious to give up their cats and dogs and reminds us that "… adopting an animal is a responsibility much like adopting a two-or three-year-old child that is totally dependent…. If you had a child who had behavior problems you wouldn't think of putting it up for adoption. Once you make a decision to get rid of an animal, you're saying something very serious and kind of tragic."[13]

People may drop off an animal at a shelter hoping for the best, but in reality there is little hope left. Giving an animal to a shelter is generally synonymous with putting it to death. Most animal shelters are animal control facilities whose purpose is to get rid of the excess animals in society. Due to severe overcrowding at these institutions, the cat or dog deemed adoptable will have from two days to a couple of weeks to actually get adopted before being killed. Death usually comes in the form of a lethal injection of sodium pentobarbital, although other, inhumane methods are used in some places. They still club animals to death in certain shelters in the south and Midwest, Angeli sadly reports. The larger tragedy is that most of the animals that are killed are perfectly healthy, and would make good pets. It's just that there are not enough good homes. With millions being dumped into shelters annually, Angeli states, "It's a fantasy to think that all these animals get homes. It's just not true. There is an absolute crisis of pet overpopulation in this country and all over the world."

There are many who believe that euthanasia of surplus animals, though a great tragedy, is a compassionate last resort for an overflowing animal population. One argument would be that animals are dependent on humans, and when there is no quality of life in the natural world—no guarantee of food, shelter, companionship, and safety—it is an act of caring on our part to end their suffering. It is more merciful to end an unwanted animal's life in a relatively painless way than to subject it to a world replete with danger— abuse, neglect, starvation, and isolation. Most animal shelters wholeheartedly believe this to be their mission and take pride in never turning an animal away.

But opponents of euthanasia question the ethics of killing surplus animals. They believe companion animals have the same right to walk the earth as humans and that ending a healthy animal's life is a moral failure on the part of man. Perhaps the fault lies with the average person's perception of animals. We dispose of our animals so readily because we do not really see them as lifelong companions but as commodities, something owned, like an automobile, and easily replaced. We lack empathy, notes Craig Bestrup, author of *Disposable Animals: Ending the Tragedy of Throwaway Pets*, which is why we can destroy without feeling. Bestrup asks, "What is it like to live in a cage in a strange place, surrounded by anxious animals and unfamiliar people, approached and repeatedly stepped away from by strangers, and perhaps aware that death lies just around the corner?" Animal shelters, well-meaning as they are, may add to the tragedy by making it so easy for people to dispose of their pets. Bestrup asserts that we must end the mass killing of animals and that the need for the macabre practice of euthanasia will end once people become more responsible caretakers. This commitment involves seeing animals as our companions rather than our possessions, recognizing the value of an animal's life, taking charge of its reproduction, and realizing that adopting an animal is a lifetime commitment.[14]

Finding Alternatives. If you absolutely must give up your pet, take the time to find it a good home. Seek out people you know who truly love and want an animal, or find someone through word of mouth. Ask everyone you know—friends, family members, and co-workers, and put up a sign in your veterinarian's office. Be sure to screen applicants, visiting their homes, if possible, and ask for references, as there are lots of unsavory people out there who abuse animals.

If your pet is a purebred, contact a breed rescue group. These groups are composed of volunteers who are fans of a specific breed. Whenever they hear of a dog from a certain breed about to lose its home or its life they will place the animal in foster care until a permanent placement can be found. Breed rescue lists can be found through the ASPCA and the American Kennel Club Association, and on the Internet. Contacting a breed rescue group is also a great way to adopt a purebred. Not only will you be providing an animal with a desperately needed home, but you will spend just a fraction of the cost charged by a breeder.

Other options are small rescue groups and local shelters that are non-animal-control facilities. If your animal is accepted, it will remain there until it gets adopted (barring any severe behavior or serious and irreversible health problems). The ASPCA in New York—not to be confused with independently run SPCA's around the country—is one such organization. Founded over 135 years ago, and long thought of as the dog catchers of New York City, the institution ended its policy of destroying animals in 1995. At that time, the ASPCA reconsidered their mission as a humane organization and shifted its focus to education. The ASPCA spays or neuters all animals before releasing them for adoption and teaches people about why this is so important. It also advocates adopting from a pound rather than buying from pet stores for ethical and practical reasons. Other small non-animal- control facilities include

Bide-a-Wee in New York and the Humane Society of New York.

Finally, it is wise to plan ahead for your companion animal in the event you become injured or die. Talk to a family member or friend who might be willing to take your animal into his or her home, or contact a non-animal-control shelter. "Remember, there are options," states Angeli, "but you have to be your animal's voice and your animal's advocate because you're all they have."

NOTES

1. *Journal of the American Veterinary Medical Association*, 207:4, Aug. 15, 1995, p.421.

2. "Are we vaccinating too much?" *Journal of the American Veterinary Medical Association*, 207:4, Aug.15, 1995.

3. Pitcairn, Richard H., D.V.M., Ph.D., "A new look at the vaccine question," *Proceedings of the 1993 American Holistic Veterinary Medical Association Annual Conference*, p.22.

4. Moskowitz, Richard M.D., "The case against immunization," *The Journal of the American Institute of Homeopathy*, March 1983, 76, p.7.

5. Richard Moskowitz, M.D., ibid.

6. Gary Null interview with Jean Dodds, V.M.D., 3/10/00.

7. Gary Null interview with Dr. Charles Loops, 4/13/00.

8. Gary Null interview with Richard Palmquist, V.M.D., 3/14/00.

9. Gary Null interview with Lester Morris, V.M.D., 7/13/00.

10. "The Vaccination Question," *Love of Animals*, January 1999, p.3.

11. Gary Null interview with Janette Grainger, 3/14/00.

12. Gary Null interview with Dr. Robert Goldstein, 3/23/00.

13. Gary Null interview with Valerie Angeli, 9/10/00.

14. Brestrup, Craig, *Disposable Animals: Ending the Tragedy of Throwaway Pets*, Camino Bay Books, 1997.

CHAPTER 10

Pets and People

I t's great to grow up with a pet. Everyone who has done so knows the unique value of the relationship between animal and human. Growing up with a pet allows a child to see the world as full of animal energy and love, and as an adult, that person will understand, without thinking, that animals are a vital part of our life and world. Dogs are our companions and best friends—which is so much easier to understand when one isn't any taller than the family's German shepherd or Irish setter; and cats are... well, at least we can say they are our superiors and role models. Underneath, though, we know that they really love us too; otherwise, why would they let us feed and take care of them?

Humans have wavered in their view of animals through the ages. In ancient times, many cultures revered animals, most notably Egypt, which deified cows, serpents, fish, and, most of all, cats. So sacred was the feline that anyone bringing harm to the cat, even accidentally, risked being put to death. At the end of its glorified life, the animal's body was carefully wrapped and masked, and placed alongside mummified pharaohs and other noble beings in preparation for the next life. The tides turned dramatically for cats in 13th-century Europe, just when their function as mouse killers was needed most to ward off the plague. During the Inquisition, when "witches" and other heretics were burned en masse, cats were also tortured and killed by the hysterical masses, who thought cats to be yet another manifestation of the devil himself. Fortunately, the madness stopped before the species became extinct, although in the so-called Age of Reason, another less than ideal view of animals developed—the belief that animals were merely mechanisms, and, as such, incapable of feeling and emotion. Charles Darwin, who studied animal populations with scientific detachment, was one who initially adhered to this philosophy. But his thinking about animals and humans was turned around when he witnessed a vivisection of a live, unanaesthetized dog. The dog, with its paws nailed to the operating table, licked the hand of its vivisectionist, and in that gesture Darwin saw the capacity of dogs to love, forgive, and communicate with humans. At this moment, Darwin recognized what the animal truly was—not an exalted god, not a robotic machine, but a sentient being.

A Bond Like No Other. People who do not grow up with animals, but acquire them in adulthood, have their eyes opened, and frequently their hearts softened, by the experience of bonding with a pet. It's never too late to make friends with an animal, as shown by the success of pet therapy in nursing homes and other assisted-living situations. It's been demonstrated again and again that if you go into a nursing home and give the residents any animal companion, from a goldfish to a golden retriever, their spirits lift and their physical conditions improve. Animals bring with them the gift of living in the moment; they're capable of enjoying to the fullest every second of life. Domesticated animals give this gift to people by demonstration, and frequently people give back through the rescue movements that exist now for almost every breed of dog and cat.

Our animal companions are here to love us. This is true of all pets, not just cats and dogs. Pet owners have meaningful relationships with house-trained pigs, rabbits, and ferrets, guinea pigs bought or adopted or brought home from a child's school, snakes that owners "wear" around their necks, fish, and birds that talk or fly around the house. A bond can be established between almost any animal and its human companion or caretaker. By loving us unconditionally, they show us how to love better and more freely. This is their first lesson for us. But according to Dr. Stephen Sinatra, there are several other lessons that our pets or companion animals teach us:

They teach us to appreciate life itself and its smallest pleasures, including our own bodies. Animals are always in tune with their bodies.

They teach us how to relax. Dogs and cats are masters of relaxation and sensual pleasure. Cat and other animal stretches are frequently imitated in yoga classes. If you're tired but not relaxed, look at your cat and get a lesson in loosening up.

They teach us how to be silent, as we observe them not needing constant noise or conversation, but rather listening to the smallest sounds, quietly lounging in our presence, content simply in our company.

They teach us how to reduce stress, not only by relaxing and stretching, but also by prioritizing what's important and what can be let go of. Cats, in particular, know how and when to usefully tune out a situation that is too noisy or stressful. Cats know innately how to detach.

And of course a cat never suffers from low self-esteem, so at the end of a day or a night out a cat never worries about what anyone else thought of him. To thine own self be true—this is a lesson that people seem to need to learn over and over again, and animals can help teach it.

Finally, the animals in our lives teach us how to play—spontaneously, that is, and just for fun—not in an organized, competitive way. This, of course, reduces stress... and so the lessons go on and on.

Animals know things—possess specific knowledge that is beyond our grasp—as well. This is why it is essential to respect all wildlife, not just the animals we share our homes with. Butterflies and geese know when to fly south and how to get where they're going without a map. Squirrels bury their collected nuts in the late fall and can remember for months or even years the exact locations of their different stashes. Perhaps we can learn things from these species. Also, let's remember that such "non-pets" as squirrels, feral cats and dogs, and even pigeons, can have ongoing, loving relationships with those who feed them in parks, on the street, and in alleys. All of these are examples from everyday life of the profound interconnectedness of people and animals on our planet.

PETS AND CHILDREN

Many people think of their pets as children, especially if they have no children of their own. Certainly, similarities exist. Companion animals, like children, depend on others for care and attention, and offer unconditional love in return. But if a child enters the family, the differences between the species become obvious, and the child-substitute risks a loss of status. A parent may begin to worry about the germs that the child will come in contact with as a result of playing with the animal. As a rule of thumb, if you keep your dog or cat clean and well groomed, and maintain its good health through regular veterinary checkups, there shouldn't be a problem. Another concern is the possibility of animal jealousy of the new arrival in your family. This should not be a problem either, though, if you develop a savvy strategy to introduce the baby to your pet.

Doggie, Meet Baby. When your baby is on the way, you have many months to prepare for the exciting event. Be sure to use this time to help your pet get ready for the new arrival too. Animals are sensitive and will notice your change in routine, so do your best to help your pal feel included. For instance, you could allow your pet to follow you into the nursery while you play a tape of a baby crying. The more you include your animal in the preparations, the more accepting it is likely to feel when the baby arrives home.

If you have a dog, you may also need to review basic obedience commands, such as "sit," "down," or "stay," so that in your child's presence the animal will be calm and well behaved. If your animal exhibits any behavior problems, now is the time to resolve these issues, as you will have far less time and patience to deal with them later. If your dog won't learn from you—perhaps the animal is undisciplined, wild around people, fearful of new situations or strangers, or aggressive—check with your holistic veterinarian to make sure there is no physical illness at the core of your animal's problem. Then once your animal's overall health is confirmed, seek out the services of an obedience teacher who trains with gentle, not punishing, methods. Flower remedies may be a useful tool here as well.

When you bring your baby home, you may need to isolate your pet from the child for the first few days. Although you are feeling excited, greet your pet calmly, and even though the bulk of your time is now spent with the newborn, be sure to spend quality moments with your animal each day. During this time of separation, you should present your pet with a blanket containing your baby's scent, allowing your pet to explore the new odor and sleep with it.

At the dog's and baby's first meeting, hold your dog on a short leash in a "sit" or "stay" position while another adult, across the room, holds the baby. Each day allow Rover to get a little closer. In a few weeks, your dog should be alright off its leash, but you should remain cautious, never leaving your infant unsupervised in the presence of an animal. Be especially wary if the animal exhibits fear or aggression around people. If for any reason you feel your dog might harm your baby, as an extra precaution keep a muzzle on your pet during training. Whenever you are uncertain of your dog's trustworthiness, err on the side of your child's safety. Hire babysitters that are experienced with pets, instructing them to keep the two apart.

Dogs will sometimes eat soiled diapers. This seemingly strange behavior is meant to protect new offspring from predators that detect their prey's odors. To prevent this from happening, get a pet-proof hamper. Cats and dogs may also urinate or defecate on baby blankets, baby clothes, or a newborn's crib. These territorial markings help relieve anxiety by covering the baby's scent with their own. Rather than adding to your animal's stress during this time of adjustment through scolding, prevent access to its targets and spend more time with your pet.

Take Care With Toddlers. When your baby gets a little older, new problems could arise as he or she learns to crawl, and then walk. Some dogs fear small children and run from them, but others, those with strong hunting instincts, might attack because they do not recognize these moving creatures as the same babies that were, until recently, being carried about. Be sure to keep your dog in a "sit" or "stay" position while the baby moves, and reward good behavior with verbal and physical expressions of praise. Cats are less likely to accidentally hurt a child because their prey is normally far smaller.

A more likely scenario involves protecting your animal from your toddler or young child. Children do not understand that they can inflict pain upon animals by biting, stepping, jumping, kicking, squeezing, hitting, or pulling body parts. A child may toss a light pet, scream in its ear, chase it, or give it no peace. Monitor children's interactions with animals, and teach them how to respect pets by talking to them and demonstrating proper handling techniques. Children must learn that pets are living beings that feel pain. Supervise child/animal interactions, intervening whenever necessary to demonstrate acceptable behavior, and praising appropriate actions. Show children which parts of a pet's body can be touched and how to gently pet them. Teach them not to disturb an animal that is sleeping, resting, eating, playing with a favorite toy, or chewing on a bone. Getting your child to role-play, pretending to be a dog or cat, can be helpful. After all is said and done, if your child still doesn't exhibit self-control around the family pet, keep the animal isolated until your child exhibits maturity. Remember, every animal, no matter how tolerant, has its limits. It is unfair to allow any animal to be harassed or abused.

By the time your child is a little older, and the family pet is a faithful companion, your child might make the generalization that all animals are trustworthy. Teach your child to be cautious around other animals and continue keeping an eye on your child at all times, even around a friend's trusted pet, as attempting to show affection to another animal could prove dangerous if the animal becomes scared or just doesn't take to your child.

Pets Can Build Character. Having pets in a household is a wonderful way to teach children responsibility, provided that the tasks assigned are age-appropriate. You shouldn't expect a young child to be the animal's primary caregiver—he or she doesn't yet have the mental or physical capability for such a big responsibility—but your child can certainly contribute in small ways. You may want to keep a chart of specific pet-related tasks to be accomplished for the week that you and your child can check off when completed. An easy way to do this is to use a piece of poster board or paper and list the days of the week horizontally and the chores to be accomplished vertically. After each task is completed, place a check or sticker in the appropriate grid. This is not only a wonderful way to teach children how to do routine tasks, but a lesson in organization.

To help your child remember, keep the chart in a highly visible place. You may want to structure pet chores around daily rituals. An example would be feeding the dog at dinnertime. If the child forgets to fill Fido's bowl, simply remind him that just as he is hungry for his dinner, so is the dog.

The experience of owning a pet can also help your child to love and appreciate animals. Most children develop intense bonds with their companion animals, which helps build the foundation for a healthy, loving relationship between the species. Parents can add to their children's awareness by including them in family discussions about the pet at a level geared to their understanding. For example, children can be included in discussions about taking the dog to the veterinarian, why the animal is, or is not, receiving vaccinations, the pet's nutrition, and any health or behavior problems that the animal may be experiencing. Discussing your animal's needs will help your child see the pet as a living, feeling being.

CAN OUR PETS MAKE US SICK?

Our companion animals love us dearly, and we, in return, want to display our affection to them. We express those feelings through petting and sometimes kissing our pets, and we accept a lick from a dog or cat as a sign of genuine affection. In general, no one should withhold affection from a beloved animal for fear of germs any more than they would stop kissing people because it is unsanitary. There are, however, certain people who need to be more cautious than others. Go ahead and kiss your animal, but don't let your child do it because youngsters are more susceptible to what are called zoonotic diseases, advises Paula Cooper, author of *The 277 Secrets Your Dog Wants You To Know* and *277 Secrets Your Cat Wants You To Know*. Also, Cooper points out that if your child and your German shepherd kiss each other regularly, your child might see another German shepherd and, not fully understanding that this is someone else's, want to kiss that dog, an act that can prove dangerous. In addition to children, the elderly and individuals with poorly functioning immune systems should probably not get on kissing terms with Fluffy or Fang.

Actually, animal diseases are spread mostly through biting and scratching. Because a cat's teeth are long and thin, their bites may inject bacteria deep under the skin, and so cat bites are potentially harmful if left untreated. Dog bites may look worse, but their damage is generally on the surface and less severe. Cat scratches can be the cause of cat scratch disease (bartonellosis) when their thin, sharp claws inject bacteria under the skin. Whenever an animal bites or scratches you, clean the wound thoroughly, and, if you suspect infection, see your physician.

Probably the most serious and well-known zoonotic disease is rabies, a virus that attacks the brain and is generally fatal. The disease is transmitted whenever a wild or domesticated animal infected with the virus bites a human or another animal. In addition to pets, possible carriers include bats, skunks, foxes, coyotes, and raccoons. Fear of this dreaded disease has prompted most states to enact strict rabies vaccination requirements for dogs and cats. You must therefore vaccinate your animal for rabies, remembering not to over-vaccinate—according to homeopathic philosophy, that could cause chronic side effects that mimic the disease—but rather checking blood titers periodically to see that the animal is still immune to rabies. When immunity is no longer present, your doctor should once again vaccinate for the condition.

If you or your pet are ever bitten by an animal, and the skin is broken, the incident must be reported to local public health authorities. This is especially important if the animal is not your own, there are injuries to the head or neck, the injury is serious, the attack was unprovoked, or the animal was behaving abnormally. Health officials will want to observe the animal and, if the animal is suspected of having rabies, you may need to be immunized against the disease. The animal could also be destroyed, another reason it is important to immunize your animal against rabies and to keep proof of the vaccination in your records as well as on a tag that is worn on the collar at all times in case the animal gets lost.

Contact with an animal's feces could result in the transmission of intestinal parasites, such as roundworms or tapeworms. To prevent this, check the animal for worms on a regular basis, wash your hands after scooping up after your dog or changing the cat's litter, and wear shoes when outside. In addition, monitor young children when they are playing outside, making sure they do not eat sand or soil, which may contain the eggs of these worms.

Another serious health concern is toxoplasmosis, a parasitic infection shed in cat feces that could result in miscarriage or organ damage to a fetus. A pregnant woman who thinks she is at risk can get a blood test to see whether or not she has the disease. Also at high risk are immune-compromised individuals, such as people with AIDS or cancer. In these people, toxoplasmosis could result in damage to the central nervous system. Pregnant and immune-compromised individuals should not change cat litter and should be careful about handling cats that have not been tested for the parasite. If having someone else change the litter is not an option, these individuals should wear rubber gloves when doing so, and wash both gloves and hands afterwards.

Cats may carry ringworm, a fungal infection that can cause an itchy ring-shaped rash to develop on the skin. Often, animals show no outward sign of the disease. Though ringworm is highly contagious, creams are available to speed recovery and increase comfort during the healing process.

Certain diseases are not truly zoonotic but can be transmitted by pets nonetheless because the pets carry the disease-causing ticks. These tiny creatures, which cause Rocky Mountain spotted fever and Lyme disease, can attach themselves to larger animals and then crawl onto humans who touch them. Ticks being so small—about half the size of a grain of black pepper—are difficult to identify, but anyone living with an animal that goes outdoors should be aware of what the insect looks like and get into the habit of checking the animal's fur. Dogs are more prone to Lyme disease than are cats, which tend to get rid of ticks by licking their fur. Still, cats should be checked around the ears and head for ticks.

Some diseases are shared by animals and humans, but not spread from one species to another. These include leukemia, AIDS (sometimes called feline immunodeficiency disease in cats), hookworm, pinworm, and systemic fungal infections. Animals do not spread colds, flu, or sore throats, with the exception of ferrets, which are susceptible to influenza A and B strains. These viral strains can be passed back and forth between ferrets and humans. Dogs do not give humans bordetella (kennel cough), although this disease is highly contagious to other dogs. Nor do dogs spread heartworm.

Many diseases we get from animals can be prevented with proper care and hygiene. Common-sense practices such as changing cat litter on a regular basis, and scooping up after your dog, are essential to good health. In addition to good grooming and hygiene, regular health check-ups are important. When you first adopt a pet, take the animal to your veterinarian for a thorough examination before the animal comes in contact with family members. The pet's stool and blood should be checked for parasites, and tests should be run to determine antibody levels for diseases. This preventive measure is recommended even if you are given a veterinary history at the time of adoption. Thereafter, your companion animal should be examined by a veterinarian at least yearly. Your vet will advise you about the health-maintenance measures that may be needed, such as a minimal number of immunizations, and regular worming. If you stick to the program you needn't worry too much about being close to your companion animal.

Zoonotic Bird Diseases. Birds can transmit a number of diseases to humans, but you can significantly reduce the chances of this happening by having your bird examined by an avian veterinarian, feeding it a healthy diet, and keeping its living quarters clean.

One of the diseases a bird can carry is salmonella, a condition people we know of in connection with contaminated foods. Birds too can get the disease through ingestion of contaminated food or water. A bird infected with salmonella may exhibit lethargy, loss of appetite, watery droppings, and arthritis. Parrots may become profoundly depressed and die. Birds with salmonella can be treated with antibiotics, although they may remain carriers for life.

Parrot fever, or chlamydiosis, is an airborne bacterial parasite most often contracted from pigeons, turkeys, and ducks, and spread from person to person. Many birds with the condition are asymptomatic, but outward signs of infection could include inflamed eyes, difficulty breathing, and watery droppings. Symptoms in humans are flu-like and can include fever, diarrhea, chills, conjunctivitis, and sore throat.

Avian tuberculosis is an airborne disease usually transmitted via exposure to infected feces. Humans with compromised immune symptoms are at greatest risk. A bird owner infected with tuberculosis could also infect a bird and should therefore avoid contact with the animal while sick. Symptoms of avian tuberculosis in an infect-ed bird are species-specific but generally include weight loss, depression, diarrhea, increased urination, abdominal distention, lameness, and breathing difficulty. Treatment of affected birds is difficult and traditionally includes antibiotics. Infected birds are generally quarantined for up to two years while being tested for the disease every six to twelve weeks.

Of the three main strains of influenza (A, B, and C), only influenza A appears to infect birds. Migratory birds such as water-fowl are believed to be at high risk for carrying influenza A. Symptoms in birds may include depression, appetite loss, coughing and sneezing, and some birds may die suddenly with no apparent symptoms. A companion bird may infect a human, but a more like-ly scenario involves a human infecting a companion bird. A bird owner with clinical signs of influenza should therefore avoid contact with his or her pet.

Allergic alveolitis is a condition that can affect people who are ultra-sensitive to bird feathers, feather-dust, or feces. Initial symp-toms include coughing, breathing difficulty, chills, and fever. If the condition is left untreated, more serious long-term consequences can occur, including progressive breathing difficulty, dry cough, and weight loss. But measures can be taken to prevent any of these problems. Hypersensitive individuals should minimize the amount of dander in their environment by keeping the bird cage clean, bathing their birds frequently, not overcrowding their animals, pro-viding adequate ventilation, and using an air purifier.

TRAVELING WITH YOUR PET

In this highly mobile world, there is often a need or opportunity to travel, and that sometimes means traveling with your pet. Whether it's a short trip to the vet, a long-distance move to another part of the country, or a vacation together, you will want to be well pre-pared to keep your animal safe and happy.

Vacationing together is a great way to bond and, in recent years, it's gotten much easier with thousands of accommodations through-out the country that, for an extra charge, are now welcoming pets. Some, in fact, prefer animals to children! Accommodations range from the extravagant—The Ritz-Carlton will pamper both you and

Fifi—to the economical—if you are budgeting your income, try such motel chains as Motel 6, Best Western, and Comfort Inn. The Appendix lists a number of pet-friendly lodgings throughout the country. You could also get help through the Automobile Club of America or online at such websites as takeyourpet.com or petopia.com.

When contemplating a pet-accompanied journey, your first consideration should be whether or not your animal is in condition to travel at all. Whenever possible, avoid traveling with animals that are very young or old, or that are pregnant, sick, or recovering from an illness or operation. Unless you are taking a short trip to the vet, it's best to leave these animals home. You should also avoid traveling with animals that are aggressive, disobedient, or in any way not socialized.

On the Road Again. Are you are planning on taking a long car trip with Spot? If so, be sure Spot is accustomed to car travel. Before the excursion, take short, frequent, car trips with your pet, increasing the length of the journey little by little. This will help your pet become used to car travel and reduce the likelihood of carsickness.

These frequent shorter trips are an ideal time to get your dog accustomed to a doggie seat belt, and your cat or other small pet acclimated to riding in a carrier. An unrestrained animal in a moving vehicle spells danger. In the event of an accident or sudden stop, the animal could be catapulted through the windshield. Moreover, a loose animal could endanger itself by trying to jump through an open window. In addition, driver and passengers, not to mention other people in the car's path, could be harmed if the animal decides to climb under the gas or break pedal. When traveling by truck or camper, keep the pet near you, not in the back of the pick-up truck or camper.

Solid walls on the carrier provide a sense of security, especially when you add a familiar blanket, a favorite soft towel, and a piece of your unlaundered clothing (your scent has a soothing effect). Fresh water should always be available. Since a water-filled bowl could easily spill its contents in a moving vehicle, placing a few ice cubes into it is a good idea. They melt slowly, providing a constant supply of fresh water. When traveling in a carrier, your pet should never wear a leash. The animal could become tangled in it and even choke.

Keep a leash with you in an easy-to-access place, even if your animal is a cat and doesn't normally use a leash at home. Cats as well as dogs need to stretch their legs, and a harness and leash will keep the animal from running away. Cats sometimes have difficulty adjusting to harnesses and leashes, so you may want to practice ahead of time for short periods.

In addition to a leash, your pet will need its own duffel bag filled with items important to its safety and comfort. You will want to include familiar food and a few gallons of water from home, or distilled drinking water. This is important to prevent your animal's sensitive stomach from reacting to the different bacteria found in unfamiliar water. Also important are a portable water bowl or water bottle, a leash, an extra collar, a first-aid kit (see Chapter 7 for contents), a brush and comb, a lint remover, a blanket and familiar soft toy for the carrier, and a flashlight for walks at night. You should also bring a roll of paper towels, plastic bags, and a pair of rubber gloves to clean up any accidents or sickness. Be sure to bring a litter pan and litter for your cat and a pooper scooper for your dog.

Hopefully your animal won't get lost, but if it does you will want to maximize chances of a quick reunion. Make sure that your pet is wearing a secure collar with tags that show your name and phone number, as well as proof of rabies vaccination. Also, carry a recent photo and description of your pet that includes its name, breed, sex, and age. You could then photocopy the picture and description to post throughout the area. For extra protection, consider micro-chipping. Humane societies, kennels, and shelters across the nation are now scanning found animals to see if they can access identification information in order to reunite animals quickly with their loved ones.

Pack up-to-date veterinary records just in case your animal needs emergency medical treatment or you must board your pet unexpectedly. Many kennels require kennel cough (bordetella) and other vaccines. To avoid over-vaccinating, get your animal's blood titer taken and if levels indicate immunity have your holistic veterinarian write you a letter stating that.

While traveling, you will need to take periodic breaks in order to give your pet the opportunity to eat, drink, exercise, and relieve itself. Schedule a stop every couple of hours. To lessen your chances of losing your pet, never let your animal roam; always walk it on a leash.

HEAT ALERT! Animals are very sensitive to heat, so you should drive with air conditioning in the summer, or during the coolest hours of the day—before 10 a.m. and after 4 p.m. Take care in the winter, too, as sunlight intensifies through the windows. To prevent tragedy, don't leave an animal unattended in a car, especially when the weather is hot. Whether the windows are open or closed, the car can become unbearable in a very short time, and the animal can die a terrible death from heatstroke in just minutes. Any season, even winter, poses dangers, as sunlight intensifies through windows.

Flying With Fido. If you will be traveling by air with your pet, be sure to let the airline know when you're making reservations. They will advise you on their particular guidelines. Some airlines keep animals with the cargo, while others allow them to remain with their owners provided the kennel fits securely beneath the seat. You will need to find out where and how to claim your pet if it is checked into the cargo hold. Also, check the temperatures at your takeoff airport, your destination airport, and any connecting airports. Animals may not be accepted if temperatures are extreme—below 40 degrees or above 80 degrees can be dangerous. If it's at all possible, fly nonstop.

It is important to purchase an airline-approved kennel. These crates, which are approved by the Department of Agriculture, withstand in-flight jostling. The kennel should also be labeled "Live Animal" in large letters on the top and sides. Should your flight be delayed or canceled, this message will aid airline personnel in finding your pet and taking it out of the heat or cold. Your name, address, phone number, and destination should also be clearly and securely attached to the top of the kennel. These measures should be taken even if your pet is going to be traveling with you in the cabin, just in case the airline suddenly decides not to allow you to carry the pet on board.

Here are some important tips for flying with a pet:

Exercise your pet before placing it in the kennel and do not feed the pet six to eight hours before the trip.

Do not sedate your pet. The drug will impair your animal's ability to adjust to the speed and vertical movement of the jet, which can result in an injury.

Place soft bedding in the kennel to absorb any accidents.

Keep a leash in your carry-on bag, not in the kennel. The leash could fall out of the kennel, or, worse, strangle your pet.

If you will be flying for more than 12 hours, put food in a zip-closing plastic bag and leave it in the kennel with feeding instructions for airline personnel.

Do not lock the kennel door; just keep it securely closed. Otherwise, if you and your pet should become separated, or if there is an emergency, airline personnel will not be able to open the kennel.

Lodging Logistics. Before checking into your hotel or other accommodation, be sure the arrangements are mutually beneficial. Some hotels, motels, inns, and lodges have restrictions on the size of the pet. Kennels are usually required. Some places have designated areas for dog walking, but many do not. You will also want to inquire as to what type of room you will have. If possible, get a room with an outside door or one on a lower level near an exit. If you make a request in advance, some pet-friendly hotels will have your brand of pet food waiting for you when you arrive. The cost will be added to your bill, but this may be better than having to carry along a 10-pound bag of food. You should ask for a recommendation of a nearby veterinarian should your pet become ill during your stay. If you will be traveling with an exotic animal, be sure to get the name of a veterinarian familiar with that species.

Consider a Sitter. We should mention here that there may also be times you will want to travel alone, and that, in those instances, there is no need to place the animal in a stress-provoking kennel or cattery. If trustworthy friends or relatives are unwilling or unable to help you out, consider contacting a pet-sitting service. These agencies can recommend responsible caretakers to attend to your pets in your own home. Some of their employees are even qualified to

NATURAL PET CARE

administer medication to animals. Look for a licensed and bonded sitter who is accredited by the National Association of Pet Sitters (NAPPS). You can reach that organization by calling (800) 296-PETS.

HOW ANIMALS HELP PEOPLE

A sailor swept overboard is miraculously pushed to shore by a compassionate sea mammal. Dolphins are legendary for saving the lives of drowning people fortunate enough to be in their paths. More recently, these magnificent animals have been recognized for their ability to help autistic and other disabled children, an effect scientists attribute to their calming sonar vibrations. Truly we are on the threshold of understanding how humans can heal with the aid of the animal kingdom, although we already do utilize animals' help to some degree. Everyone is familiar with the wonderful Seeing Eye dog that, through its intelligence and devoted hard work, brings independence to a blind person. Less known, but also of great value, are the specially trained dogs that assist paralyzed people by helping with chores such as shopping, doing laundry, and even banking by ATM! Other dogs have been trained to help people with epilepsy; they remind them, with the aid of timers, to take their medication; they help them recover from seizures, a task that includes standing at rigid attention to provide physical support for the person to use in standing up; and they fetch the phone when necessary. Then there are pet "therapists." These animals, usually dogs and cats, periodically visit the most despairing populations—the terminally ill, the mentally and emotionally disturbed, the elderly living in nursing homes, and prisoners. Their mission: to promote joy. An animal's natural ability to bring a smile to a face has made pet-assisted therapy a valuable new branch of the health care profession.

Seeing Eye Dogs. Before The Seeing Eye organization was founded in 1929, dogs were generally bred for show. But Dorothy Harrison Eustis, a wealthy Philadelphian who was breeding German shepherds in Switzerland, did not feel that producing animals for this purpose made use of their best qualities. With the help of her staff, Eustis designed a training program where the alertness, stamina, and sense of responsibility of German shepherds could be brought out through work as patrol dogs, army dogs, and Red Cross dogs. Then, while visiting a school in Germany, Eustis realized the full potential of her beloved German shepherds. The dogs she observed were being trained to serve as guides to blind veterans of World War I. Eustis was so impressed with what she saw that she wrote an article about it for the *Saturday Evening Post* (November 1927). When Morris Frank of Nashville, Tennessee, had the story read to him—Frank had been blinded in two separate accidents, each affecting one eye—he was moved to write to Mrs. Eustis, "… Thousands of blind persons, like me, abhor being dependent on others. Help me and I will help them. Train me and I will bring back my dog and show people here how a blind man can be absolutely on his own."

In those days, blind people were considered invalids. They were either institutionalized or completely dependent upon others. Simple things like getting a haircut, shopping for groceries, or holding down a job were beyond a blind person's reach. Eustis responded to Frank's letter, stating that if he could get to Europe, she would train a dog for him. These goals were accomplished, and upon his return to the United States, Frank spent a year touring the country, explaining to people what a dog could do for a sightless or sight-impaired individual. In this way Frank and Buddy, his dog, changed sighted people's perceptions of the blind.

Morris Frank and Dorothy Eustis opened The Seeing Eye school in Nashville, Tennessee, in 1929. (The school was later moved to New Jersey, as Nashville's temperatures were too high to train dogs year-round.) The first class had only two people, but by the end of one year, 17 men and women were enrolled and rewarded with the gift of greater independence. Initially the dogs were imported from Germany, but as the need grew, they were bred in New Jersey.

Today's Seeing Eye is supported only by philanthropic donations. A blind or sight-impaired person need only pay a first-time fee of $150 (a price established in 1934 that was not changed with inflation), and $50 for subsequent use. This token fee gives a blind person a sense of contributing toward his or her own independence, rather than taking a handout. This low fee is quite remarkable when you consider that the cost of breeding, training, and placing a guide dog into service for one person is approximately $45,000. The difference in cost is made up by donations from individuals, foundations, and corporations.

Seeing Eye dogs come from a fine stock. After litters are born, careful records are kept of the animals' temperament, hip condition, size, intelligence, and various other factors that would enable a dog to enter the program or preclude it from participating. Candidates must work particularly well with humans and enjoy being able to please their owner. Generally, Labrador retrievers and golden retrievers are used today because of their trainability, ease of care, and moderate size. These breeds are big enough to pull on a harness to guide someone, but small enough to fit comfortably under chairs in restaurants or desks at work. Also, their coats require little maintenance outside of normal cleaning. Dogs with long hair or dogs with very curly hair, such as poodles, often require the care of a professional groomer, making the cost of owning the dog a factor.

Puppies are raised in volunteer homes. This is preferable to kennels where the dogs don't form strong early bonds with humans, which are so crucial for future bonding experiences. Volunteer families receive the puppy at about seven weeks of age and agree to raise it according to specific guidelines. The family teaches the dog basic obedience commands and manners, and exposes the puppy to the many kinds of situations it may encounter in its work as a guide dog (such as bus travel, city streets, restaurants, and stores). The family is compensated for all veterinary costs, and they receive a quarterly stipend for food. But money is not the main incentive; families raise these puppies out of the goodness of their heart. It is essential to the success of the program that the puppies' first experience be in a loving environment.

Young dogs remain with the host family for a year to a year-and-a-half. At that point, the animals are returned to The Seeing Eye for formal training. The first month back is spent in a kennel where the dogs receive a thorough physical examination. Veterinarians make sure the general health of the dogs is good. Dogs with health problems—a chronic skin allergy, for instance—are taken out of the program, so that a future owner will not be responsible for expensive veterinary bills.

Once a dog is deemed fit to enter the program, it is assigned to an instructor to thoroughly train for its future work. After lessons in basic obedience and manners, the dogs begin harness training where they learn to pull with just the appropriate amount of force. It is this tugging that allows a dog to guide a blind person. The dogs must become accustomed to the harness and learn that wearing it means paying attention to their surroundings. The dogs are taught to take their work seriously.

During the period of training, instructors reinforce desired behaviors—sitting at a curb, stopping at the foot of stairs, halting at a street curb—through praise, while undesirable behaviors—sniffing food in a restaurant, being overly friendly to strangers—earn a reprimand. Initially, a reprimand consists of a verbal correction. Should the behavior remain unchanged for a longer period of time, a trainer might try a leash correction—a small tug on the leash to refocus the dog to attend to its job.

Once the dogs are accustomed to the harness and understand where to stop, they are introduced to more sophisticated concepts. The animals learn clearance; they are taught to think in terms of the height and width of their human companion in order to provide clearance around obstacles and under low-hanging objects, such as signs and awnings. Next is traffic work. Dogs do not naturally understand that moving cars are dangerous, so their instructors may play-act a scene, running into a car and slapping the door to make a loud noise. That gets the dog's attention and teaches the animal that a car is to be respected, but not feared. Dogs learn to check for traffic in a simulated environment before they are exposed to the real world. A dog will learn to stop at red lights and to halt ahead of time any time a car heads toward the path of its person. If the dog comes across a hole in the sidewalk or a barrier, it will learn to safely lead its person around the obstacle.

Instruction is given in small increments so that the dog can master each step before progressing to the next. Periodic evaluations are given throughout the process to be sure that the animal is performing at a satisfactory level. Halfway through the training the instructor will blindfold himself and, accompanied by a supervisor, take the dog out to practice what was learned. The supervisor watches to make sure there are no serious concerns with the dog's progress that might keep the animal from becoming a successful guide dog. If, for example, the dog is too timid in traffic, or too bold, or too friendly with strangers, the supervisor may recommend that the dog not continue with the balance of training.

Generally, guide dogs complete their training and are placed with a person at two-and-a-half years of age. Their average working life is seven to ten years. Some schools for guide dogs retire the animals at a predetermined cutoff age, whether or not their health is declining. But if the dogs are from The Seeing Eye organization, the retirement date is left to the owner's discretion. Usually, once a dog begins to slow down or develop arthritis, the owner decides to retire the dog. The retired dog may stay with its owner, along with a new guide dog, or it can be placed in a new home, with a family member, perhaps, or some person in the community. If the owner does not keep it or find it a home, a third option is to return the dog to The Seeing Eye for the school to place. The organization has a long list of homes for puppies that don't graduate from the program, and the retired dogs are worked into that list.

A working animal's colorful backpack alerts people to the fact that concentration on an owner's safety is a top priority. So these animals should not be petted, talked to, fed, or otherwise distracted; that might put the owner in jeopardy. Trying to direct a blind person, either by pulling on his or her arm or on the dog's harness, is analogous to pulling on the steering wheel of a car while someone else is driving. If a blind person appears lost, it's okay to ask if assistance is needed (one should not assume that the dog automatically knows how to take the blind person to and from places). The guide dog leads the blind person, but only in response to commands from its master such as forward, right, or left (orientation and mobility skills are taught to people before they are given the dog). While guide dog and master are walking, the blind person is concentrating on the sounds of parallel traffic and other sounds to give him his location. Distracting a dog or its master could cause the person to lose orientation and become lost.

Protected under the Americans with Disabilities Act of 1992, these wonderful dogs are given full access to public places. The animals are granted this special privilege because they are highly trained, vital to a blind or seeing-impaired person's independence, and behave properly in any environment.

Pet-Assisted Therapy. Nowhere is the significance of the human/animal bond more apparent than in the cases of people touched by animal-assisted therapy (AAT). Simply put, AAT is the presence of animals in clinical environments. Accompanied by human volunteers, animals visit nursing homes, psychiatric hospitals, drug rehabilitation facilities, children's hospitals, schools for children with special needs, or any institution where people are confined for treatment. While there, the animals spend time with the residents individually or in groups. It's an opportunity for people living in limited, confined situations to have a visit with a friendly, loving animal that doesn't care what the person looks like, smells like, or sounds like. Although cats and dogs are most commonly used in AAT, birds, guinea pigs, hamsters, ferrets, and other "exotics" have been known to make visits too.

While AAT has been gaining in popularity for the past 25 years or so, it was actually used as early as 1792, in a Quaker-run asylum. During World War II the American Red Cross sponsored a program at the Army Air Force Convalescent Center in Pawling, New York, in which dogs, horses, and farm animals were used as a diversion from the strain of daily physical therapy for recovering servicemen. Nonetheless, AAT has become established and widely used as a form of therapy only in the past couple of decades. Why? Like many holistic medical practices, AAT was at first rejected by many conventional facilities and therapists as too "far out there" and nonscientific. But studies have confirmed what the pioneers of AAT—and many a pet-owner—have known all along—that having loving, accepting, nonjudgmental animals around makes a person feel better. Just as our society's awareness of the human/animal bond and the sanctitiy of all animal life has deepened, so too has the realization that animals can help those in physical, emotional, or spiritual pain. Florence Nightingale once said that pets are wonderful companions for the sick. Studies have long shown that animal owners have a greater chance than non-pet-owners of surviving a year or longer following a heart attack. Now, studies have confirmed that patients who receive AAT experience quantifiable physiological benefits, including lower blood pressure, improved muscular movement, and an overall improvement in feelings of well-being.

People living in nursing homes are often profoundly lonely, sometimes spending long periods without a single visitor from outside the facility. In the 1970s, volunteers began to realize that nursing home residents could use some extra visitation of the four-legged variety. The benefits of animal visits are immediately visible in the reactions of residents, who may smile, reach out to the animals, and talk in ways that they ordinarily don't, or aren't encouraged to. Renee Lamm Esordi, a photographer and dog owner who has collected photos of AAT in her book *You Have a Visitor*, observed how the visits spark conversations between volunteers and residents, who frequently begin to reminisce about pets they owned in the past. These stores seem to get some reticent people going, and often residents will go from there into talking about where they used to live, what kind of work they did, and other subjects. The animals become a great aid to socialization in this way. By taking along different kinds of animals, volunteers can usually match a resident's personality with that of a pet—many people, for example, don't feel comfortable with the friendliness of large dogs, but love the warmth and companionship of a cat sitting in their lap, ready to listen to every word and enjoy every stroke.

Originally AAT was intended only for adult-care facilities; a reason for this was that liability insurance was a concern. Nowadays, however, volunteer organizations carry their own insurance, and most organizations check out a volunteer animal first to make sure it has the right personality for this kind of work. Animal-assisted therapy is now commonly practiced in facilities for children. In children's hospitals, dogs must remain on leashes, but they are allowed to jump on patients' beds. For children who may be facing a lifetime of institutionalization, or who may never be able to own a pet, these visits open up a whole range of positive emotional and physical experience. For depressed patients of any age, animal visits can be a real asset; the animals frequently help them to come out of themselves through physical touch and play. For people, especially children, with severe physical limitations, rubbing the animals can increase the patient's range of motion, another tangible benefit of AAT.

For anyone who would like to become involved with the wonderful volunteer work, there are plenty of opportunities. Please note, though: You should not simply show up at a nursing home with Fido for an unannounced visit! What you should do is contact any local SPCA or animal organization to find out who does AAT in your area and how you can get involved. As we've mentioned, your pet will probably have to undergo an evaluation for proper personality and behavior before it can participate. Because the visits can be extremely emotionally draining for the human volunteers, you may want to limit how often you do them. One side benefit of volunteering, Esordi points out, is that it's quality time for you and your pet to spend together. DeltaSociety.org is a good website to check out for more information.

PAWS. Pets Are Wonderful Support is a different type of volunteer organization for animal-lovers. In this case, instead of bringing animals to institutionalized patients, human volunteers come into the homes of HIV/AIDS patients to care for the patients' pets when they are unable to. A PAWS volunteer will bring food, clean bowls, change food and water, clean litter boxes, walk dogs, and just generally spend time with pets whose owners are too ill to do these things themselves. A bonus for volunteers in this program is the formation of friendships with the human patients, who often appreciate beyond words what the volunteer is doing for them. For an HIV or AIDS patient who is still able to live at home but unable to keep up with the demands of pet ownership, the prospect of having to give up a pet is devastating. Now more than ever, these patients need the love and companionship of their pets. By volunteering for this organization you can help a pet and its owner at the same time. If you're interested in volunteering, call a local humane society to get information, or simply call phone information to see if there's a PAWS listing in your area. The organization exists in many large cities across the U.S., including Los Angeles, Philadelphia, and New York, but there are not chapters in every city. Perhaps you could even start one!

SAYING GOODBYE

Eventually, of course, our pets have to die. Almost always, we outlive our pets, and that loss can be one of the worst of our own lives. Dr. Donna Raditic is another holistic vet who is concerned with what animals have to teach us, and she believes that our pets show us two things—how to live, and how to die. Raditic says that one of the unexpected joys of being a vet, as opposed to a "people doctor," is seeing the entire life cycle of a pet, from babyhood into old age and death. Raditic believes that each pet comes into our lives to teach us something specific, and if we are lucky in that relationship, the pet lives long enough to complete the lesson, and then moves on.

For animals, death is not a disease or a disaster, but another natural process. It's only humans who have medicalized death and made it something to fear. So when a pet owner is facing the choice of whether to euthanize a suffering animal, Raditic and other practitioners are able to look at the situation with empathy for the animal, which does not fear death and may need to move on. It's the owner who is left with grief, and there are many support groups available for people suffering over the loss of a pet. These can be a safe haven for the person who is reluctant to speak to colleagues or friends about this grief, fearing ridicule from someone who has never experienced the human/pet bond and cannot understand it. As for the process of euthanasia itself, it is not painful for the animal, and many animal technicians report feeling the animal's peacefulness at being allowed to pass on. It is for the bereaved owner, counsels Dr. Raditic, to reflect on the lesson that animal taught you, and honor your pet's eternal memory by living what you have learned.

CHAPTER 11

People on Pets

In the last chapter we looked at different aspects of human/animal interaction. One thing I've noticed about people who live with pets is that they always seem to have stories about them. Like doting parents of little children, pet people can go on and on about their charges. But like parents, they have willing listeners in others who are sharing the same problems and joys.

I love to listen to stories about animals told by their human friends. They illustrate the delightful individuality of every creature. As all pet people know, you could have five cats, and every single one will have as distinct a personality as five of your colleagues at work. But unlike your colleagues at work, animals are generally uninhibited about going after what they want when they want it, as well as letting you know what they don't like when they don't like it, which is one of the reasons that pet stories can get pretty wild.

The following special section consists of people's experiences with their own animals, told in their own words. The men and women who related the following stories to me kindly gave permission for me to share them with you. Some of the stories have been shortened because of space considerations (yes, pet people do have a lot to say!) but they all describe experiences that I can relate to, and I think you will be able to also. Some of them are about building animal health and healing sick animals. You may get some helpful ideas and inspiration from them. More are about the companionship, sense of peace, and just plain fun that come from living with pets. From these you may get, as I did, a reinforcement of your own feeling that a life with animals is an enriched life. Enjoy!

IRENE "I wonder why it took me so long to get one."

I was thinking about getting a cat, but not totally sure about whether I was more committed to my furniture than to an animal. I was afraid it might claw my carpet, furniture, and a valuable painting given to me by my father. Still, I was semi-prepared for one, my boyfriend having given me a pet food dish and litter box. A few days later I walked up the stairs to find a black and white cat exploring the apartment. My boyfriend said she followed him home. I put up signs to see if anyone would claim her, and since no one did I happily kept her.

Now I'm a true cat lover and wonder why it took me so long to get one. Cassie is a loyal friend who follows me from room to room and rests near my feet or sleeps at the edge of the bed. I can see why people say that having a pet is calming and a good antidote for loneliness. Recently I've been reading about TTouch and trying the circular massages on Cassie. This simple technique seems to really relax her.

SONDRA "I understand that we do not own anyone."

I do not call my dog and cats pets. They are my nonhuman children, my family, my companions. They mean responsibility, curtailing travel, settling for a less luxurious home, sharing my income, scratches, and packages of litter on my closet floor. My dog sleeping near me on the grass means sharing a lovely place with someone I love. It gives me inner peace knowing that she enjoys being in that space with me. She is part Border collie and should, by nature, be outdoors most of the time. I am delighted I can give that brief time to her.

Because I have always had animals in my life I can feel and speak without words. I can love them without parameters and let go when they pass over. I understand that we (all living beings) do not own anyone. We share them awhile but must allow them to go back as others must do with me. This is normal, and universal, and the pain at their passing is a tribute to the souls I mothered for a while.

My pets are unique. My intelligent dog understands human language. She found my glasses and remembers people by name. She herds the cats and breaks up their fights. My cat, Wolfgang, "plays" piano. Simon looks in mirrors, turns around, and examines the objects he viewed. Maurice puts his paw in someone's food bowl, pulls it away with his paw, sometimes out of the room. Of animals past, Me Too sang as my son conducted him with a baton. Linda said "bye-bye" in a high-pitched voice while waving a front paw. Gina ran to me whenever I wondered where she was or thought about her.

ELIZABETH "My cats 'walk on water.'"

I have two young cats, one five months old and one five weeks old. They are the most precious creatures that walk the face of the planet. They walk on water in my eyes, and when I grow up I want to be just like them.

I can watch them all night long. I've learned how much meaning and pleasure they can add to life. I've learned what incredible values they have, that they love unconditionally. They accept everyone for who and what they are, whether they are black or white, rich or poor, fat or skinny. They have purity.

My pets are my best friends. They run to me the moment I come home. They sit on the side of the tub while I shower. They even jump in the shower at times. They continually hug and groom us. They eat and sleep with us. Whatever room we are in, they are in. I cannot look or watch them without smiling. They are proof of perfection.

MARIE-CHRISTINE Another amazing cat

When my pet, a cat named Velvet, is outdoors, I sometimes worry about her. When I do she reads my thoughts and appears at the doorstep. It's amazing! What I have gained from owning a cat is a sense of bonding with nature.

EMILY "...the best hello there is."

My dog is my best friend. She loves me no matter what. I got her when she was seven-weeks old and five pounds. She gives me tons of affection and the best hello there is.

When I brought her home she had been treated badly. She had been neglected and under-loved. I'd pick her up, and she'd wrap those tiny little paws around my neck. She melted my heart. As I started my business and worked very hard she was always great to come home to.

What a great sense of humor she has, wagging her tail so hard that her whole back end wiggles. She sees people in the street and decides to flirt with her Mae West wiggle. I have to stop to say hello. My dog has helped me to realize the enormity of unconditional love.

BOB Three pets, three personalities

It's interesting to see how my three pets show me they like me in completely different ways. Pawford, a yellow Labrador retriever, goes completely crazy, wagging his tail like some sort of engine that's permanently on, and licking me as if I were a delicious ice cream cone. He can knock a person over in his enthusiasm. One cat, Chestnut, will jump up and settle near me, wherever I am, asking to be petted. The other cat, Blackie, the most reclusive and demure of the three—maybe because she was "previously owned"—*lets* me pet her, and that's about it. Plus she lets me know when "time's up" in no uncertain terms!

The three animals never seemed to relate to each other all that much, or so we thought. But then we went away on vacation, leaving them with caretakers who were in and out of the house, but away for more of the time than we would have been. When we came back the pets seemed to have banded together out of necessity; they were now "hanging out" with each other much more. They had actually become friends.

ANONYMOUS The pigeon of the house, and other flying friends

Percy, a pigeon that is my best buddy, arrived four years ago and continues to amaze me each day. He was raised by a lady who, after a couple of months, decided she could not provide him with the care she felt he needed. I was contacted by a vet to see if I could get him "strong on the wing" and released. As soon as I saw his face I knew he was going to be a permanent resident. This was a sweet and special bird.

His diet had been restricted to "human food," which did not include seeds, fruit, or vegetables. Our first order of business was to introduce seeds to his diet. I spent the next two weeks "pecking" at the seeds with my index finger to show him what to do with them. I finally got my nose to the ground to really get the point across. Sometimes you have to go that extra mile to get these "kids" to eat. Finally, as if the switch was activated, he began to peck at the seeds. He never progressed past a seed diet despite my attempts, but he has done well, and he maintains his weight, as well as his overall health.

Percy is the pigeon of the house. He is *very* neat and has his own room. He has become my nurse whenever I have a new bird to care for, and he watches my every move as if to make certain I am careful with him. I could fill many chapters with the adventures and stories of Percy, but that is for another time.

Della is a very small female pigeon. She was raised by the same lady that found Percy, but this time she kept the bird for one year. Again, the vet called to see if I could help, but this was going to be a long process. Della had been fed a very poor diet (lots of love, but the lady's resources were minimal). She had 30 percent of her feathers missing or in very poor condition. Her spirit was good, but her diet was insufficient for good health. She had very few head or neck feathers, patches were missing on her chest, and the wing feathers had stress lines. All of this indicated a poor diet. She was not thin, but very ragged. I took her to see my vet, and we agreed that nutrition was first-priority. She was given a thorough physical exam that included tests.

The first step was to get her diet changed gradually, but from what? No information about what she had been eating was provided. I tried numerous tactics to get her to eat during the transition. As with Percy, I got my nose down to the dish to simulate a beak, and finally she got the idea. In the weeks that followed, she learned to eat a variety of seeds and grains; whole wheat bread as a snack; dark, leafy greens; and, occasionally, a bit of fruit. She would not take nuts or fruit on a regular basis.

There were times that I would just look at her in that condition and get tears in my eyes, but she seemed happy. When I took her back to my vet, two months later, no one could believe it was the same bird. Her old feathers had been replaced by new and shiny plumage, her excess weight dropped, and she looked radiant. Della became a member of my bird family and continues to thrive.

Last September, the vet called to see if I could foster a young pigeon a client had found sitting in her yard. This youngster was approximately 18 days old. He still had gold natal down mixed with his juvenile plumage and was unable to fly. He could try to stand up, but not completely. This concerned me, as he was not standing up on his toes as he should. He was started on baby bird formula and placed in a nice, warm basket with a heating pad. Little Pigeon went back and forth to work with me for the next week.

A few days after he arrived, he became very fluffed and looked like he felt terrible. He was unusually warm to the touch, and his knee was very swollen. The vet felt we needed to take x-rays to get a good look at the knee and allow her to drain some fluid for evaluation. It was necessary to anesthetize him for the procedure. When we looked at the films, we saw five different fractures involving both wings and legs. It wasn't from a fall, as far as we could tell, as there was no bruising or other trauma apparent. She consulted another doctor and they came to the conclusion that he had a severe calcium deficiency.

He was very sore after this procedure, but now we had a plan to help put him back together. He was given liquid calcium and avian vitamins and was kept on a hand-feeding formula in addition to seeds. We started to see improvement after three weeks. The staff at the hospital could not believe the difference in this baby.

His left leg remains crooked; he waddles like a duck, but he is very fast and grew into a large, happy, beautiful pigeon. In December, he noticed Della and the two fell in love and are a bonded pair. They are welcome members of the bird family and give me much inspiration to learn more about how I can help the others I will encounter.

MAXINE Herbal help for cats

I have two cats. They're usually very healthy, but last summer my oldest cat became very ill. My apartment was extremely hot last summer. She became limp; she wouldn't move; she just lay there. I became afraid, so I took her to the vet, and he gave her antibiotics. After she got well I continued to give her vitamin C, echinacea, and goldenseal, and she got better. If she sneezes I'll continue to give her the combination of herbs and vitamins and the next day she'll be all right.

CARRIE A cat named Kramer

Kramer, my cat, helps my life so much. He grounds me when I'm running around and feeling stressed. I place him on my lap, we cuddle for a while, and I instantly calm down. I talk and he listens. He listens well and looks me right in the eye when he does.

A memorable experience is the day Kramer was adopted. My whole family went to a rescue shelter organization called Cat Crossings in Los Angeles to find a cat. We wanted a short-haired female. But when we saw Kramer, a long-haired male, sitting in a cage, looking very regal, handsome, and self-confident, we thought, this is the one for us. The woman who brought in Kramer was still there. She was a writer for the *Seinfeld* television show. We loved the show, Kramer winked, and we took it as a good omen. That day, he became a part of our family. And true to his name he skids and slides into the room to make his entrance.

Kramer is graceful and talented. He will bring us things we ask for, and he can jump enormous heights. I gain something every day from my experience with Kramer. I've learned about relaxation just by watching him sleep and stretch. That is the ultimate in relaxation.

NELLIE Two great dogs

I have owned two dogs. They are unconditionally accepting, totally loving, and wonderful, quiet company.

One of my dogs protected me against a possible attacker in the street. The other allowed me to touch him while he was ailing. I felt his sweet, wonderful energy, which made me feel more peaceful. I was able to help him through the crisis he was going through at the time. Owning my dogs has made me more generous, humble, and loving.

SHERRY Herbal relief

My cat seemed to have some sort of infection involving his eyes. I put a few drops of goldenseal into his food for a few days, and he got better.

VIVIAN "I just love my cat Angel...."

...When we first got him he jumped on the stove and stuck his face in a pot of spaghetti sauce (fortunately it was cooled!) He got some of the red sauce on his nose and looked so cute.

Cats love to lie around and be with people. Angel loves to get into my daughter's room to rest and sleep on her bed. When the door is closed he cries to get in.

I know from having a cat that I'm capable of loving one. Before Angel, I didn't believe I could love an animal.

MARK Sheepdog a great friend

Vinca is very open and loves to be rubbed and brushed. She is a source of great unconditional love and a great friend.

Vinca is a unique breed, a sheepdog. She is always friendly to people she greets. Vinca always barks at trucks. They get her agitated and angry. Vinca is also very sensitive and makes a great guard dog for the house. She will respond to any unusual sound by being alert and barking.

Vinca is always straightforward and honest about asking for whatever she needs. She does this by using body language. For example, if she wants to go outside for a walk, to eat, or just be loved by having her head and back rubbed, she will let me know. She likes being massaged.

KAREN "My cats have become my children, my friends, my family."

My cats, eight-year old Heather and one-and-a-half-year-old Amanda, teach me love, comfort, sweetness, softness, magic, and a connection to nature. We have many memorable experiences. We play string games together. I bathe my cats and then wrap them in a big, soft towel, holding them like a mother would hold her child. That's a real bonding experience. I dance with Heather, letting her experience the world upside-down.

Heather is very perceptive and knows me well. She comforts me when I am feeling less than optimal. She is a bit hostile to others who come to my home. Amanda is very affectionate and is learning to trust again. She was abandoned at an early age by a previous owner and used to play very rough. Amanda loves to lick me for long periods of time (very hygienic!)

My cats have become my children, my friends, my family. They have taught me peace, relaxation, and how to communicate without words. Their eyes speak volumes. They are wiser than I. They operate out of intuition and instinct.

HARRY "I take care of them, and, in turn, they offer me friendship."

Castor and Pollux, my two conure parrots, bring nature and company into my home. Their large vocal repertoire sounds like relaxing background noise. Their intelligence made it possible for a two-way friendship to develop.

What do I mean to my conures? They chose to live with me because when I put their cage in the backyard and opened it, they stayed close by and returned to it. I take care of them, and, in turn, they offer me friendship. I clean my home (more than I used to) and their cage. I'm generally more relaxed from having two Conures.

ROBERT Dogs can teach us

Scampers, a chowchow belonging to my roommate, has a loving, sweet personality. Formerly an abandoned pet that had been abused, she has responded wonderfully to love and care. It's hard to imagine that she entered the house vicious and growling. The guy who brought her in from a chow rescue organization communicated that this behavior was unacceptable, and she is now loving and protective.

I constantly wonder about my relationship with Scampers and what she is teaching me about relationships with other people. I have kept people distant so as to not get hurt. I constantly contemplate the idea of opening up.

JUNE An affectionate snake—and more—

Goliath, my four-year-old ball python, has been with me since he was a baby. He's healthy and loving and means the world to me. People wonder how a snake could be caring, but he is incredibly affectionate. If I would give him to you to hold and start to walk into another room, he would keep turning his head until he found me—snakes don't have peripheral vision. They only see straight ahead. He trusts that I will feed him, keep him warm, and give him a clean home. An emotional bond is as important to me as physical health; the love has to be there.

NATURAL PET CARE

Goliath likes being around people. Sunday is his outing day with me. We'll either go to the flea market or to the park. He likes to stay around my arm, or even better, wrap himself around my pocketbook so that no one puts their hand in there. I normally don't put him around my neck; that would look like I was showing him off. He rides in the car with me, wrapping himself partially around the door handle and looking out the window as I drive. He curls up on my lap and sits with me for long periods. Whenever I take him out I bring a pouch for him to crawl into if he's hot or tired. And I always bring a water bottle to cool him down. If we don't go anywhere, he'll go out on my sunny terrace. There's also a tree in my bedroom for him to climb.

Goliath eats homebred mice or rats (bought at the pet store), about four or five a week. He only eats when hungry and does not torture his prey the way a cat would. If he is not hungry, he will leave his prey alone. Once a week I give him a vitamin rub. It helps him to shed. On the bottom of his tank I put ground calcium that gets absorbed by his skin into his body. Snakes need calcium to avoid a calcium deficiency, which can cause bumps on their skin and a crooked shape. A lot of snakes get skin ulcerations and mouth sores. He doesn't get any of that. He's in dynamic shape.

Goliath never gets sick, but about two years ago he got a teeny boil on his stomach after going into the water. What I did was place a hot compress on him every day for about five days. I also put peroxide on him. It burst, I wiped away the residue, and he never got a boil again. Snakes are very prone to boils, so I'm really proud of the fact that he had only one little one, and that was a couple of years ago. Snakes are also prone to mites. I wash his cage every week, but once a month, everything in it goes into my tub, and it's total washdown. I clean his stuff with an all-natural product called Oxyclean. Then I examine him for mites, putting the light on in the middle of the night to see them. He's never ever had a mite.

I have to be careful to keep the temperature warm enough. I buy him special bulbs that simulate daylight, which are pretty expensive. I give him 12 hours of light in the cage and 12 hours of night because it wouldn't be healthy to leave the lights on all the time. He has a little cave in there that I bought him. Also, when he sheds, he scrapes on his bed of all-natural wood—it's like a tree trunk—and the skin comes off more easily. I have to be careful to keep that clean. He also has a heat rack in there, but I don't want him to get burnt, so I always wrap a small towel around it. He goes on it when he needs to, but his skin doesn't hit it.

I have a lot of other pets, too. Molly and Chester are two white rats. They are excellent pets and great with children. Molly and Chester were supposed to be Goliath's dinner around three years ago. I had taken them out of the cage, but he wasn't hungry. Then I put them out the next day, and he wasn't hungry again. I did that about three times. By that time I was getting attached to the mice, so I made them my pets. I went out and got them a huge cage. Now they're on a total health food diet. I give them fresh vegetables every day. They eat nuts, fruits, sunflower seeds, peanuts, and whatever is the remainder of my food. Whatever organic items I eat they get as snacks. They also love to eat natural alfalfa. Every day I give them natural vitamins, a drop in their water and a drop in their food. I also wash them once a week—could you believe it? Otherwise, rodents develop a pungent aroma. I wash their cage once a week also; I clean it with Orange Glow or Oxyclean. All my cleaning products are 100-percent natural. I play with the rodents. They know their names, and they come running to me. On Sundays, when Goliath comes in, they go out on the terrace and they play.

I have five cats as well, of assorted ages. The baby is about two. All the cats eat a low-residue diet. It's easy on the stomach and has a very low ash content. The food sold in the supermarket has a high ash content, which causes a painful condition called cystitis, especially in the boys. The girls can get it also, but it usually affects the boys. I began this diet when my cat Freedom started vomiting. My veterinarian gave her a drug that she took for about a year to help stop the vomiting. Then I went to a different veterinarian who suggested that I start giving her a low-residue diet. With that she was able to get off the medicine. It's been over a year now that she's not needed any medication. In addition to the low-residue diet, I also give my cats some of what I eat, especially the vegetables.

Freedom is also diabetic. Because of the low-residue food with the low ash content, her diabetes is totally under control with food alone. Freedom also has arthritis in the hind legs. So every day I give her half a capsule of powdered glucosamine mixed into her food. We both take it. You should see her now. Before the glucosamine she was practically dragging her hind legs. It was getting hard for her even to climb on my lap. Now she can climb onto the kitchen counter and jump off. That's amazing for a 16-year-old.

My cats also take garlic and brewer's yeast. As a result they all have beautiful, shiny coats. They love the flavor, and it repels fleas. Everybody gets combed once a week to prevent hairballs. Once a month they get their ears swabbed down with lukewarm water. They're not too crazy about that, but I do that so they don't get mites in their ears. Also, when cats catch cold they get a runny eye. That has happened. I don't really get anything fancy. A few times a day I'll wipe down the eyes with warm water and sterile cotton balls. Then I just wipe the eye again to dry it. I've had to do that a number of times.

With cats, you have to be careful of what plants you keep around. I can't buy poinsettias, for instance, or the cats will eat them, and they're poisonous. I do have a nice garden on my terrace, though. To get rid of fruit flies and other insects on my plants I use something that's 100-percent natural so as not to hurt my animals or plants. The stuff I use for the gnats is called Orange Guard. The label says, "Kills on contact. May be used around food, humans, and pets." The active ingredient, orange peel, seems to do something to kill little bugs without harming my animals or myself.

I have one other very exotic animal, a sugar glider. A sugar glider is about the size of a hamster. It's got hands, enormous eyes, and a little face. When you let it out it makes itself into the shape of a box and it flies like a flying squirrel. His diet is 100-percent vegetarian. He's always eaten nuts, vegetables, and fruit. He gets calcium drops once a week that I mix into his food.

I have a huge fish tank, also, with Discus, a huge cichlid, and angelfish. My Siamese fighting fish are in a separate bowl. Otherwise they'd fight and eat the other fish. My son takes care of the tank, making sure the pH and temperature are just right. He has little bushes growing in there. They eat a lot of that. He has algae in there and banana plants. They seem to like that.

Then we have frogs, and they eat crickets. My son set up a little aquarium for them with water in one part and rocks on the other side. When they want to be wet they can go into the water, and when they want to dry off they can go onto the rocks. He has a special light for them, too, that simulates sunlight. My apartment is super-sunny, by the way, and that's good for my animals.

I used to have a green iguana. He wasn't a desert iguana; he was a tropical iguana. He had to be sprayed down twice a day with water so he wouldn't dry out. Once a week I would put him in the bathtub so his skin wouldn't dry out. He would swim for about half an hour. The iguana was 100-percent vegetarian—that's how they eat in the wild—and would only eat vegetables. He was here for quite a while, but he took a lot of care. I had to run home to him so much. Going on vacation was impossible because a lot of people would be there to take care of the cats, but wouldn't want to deal with a reptile. With Goliath when I go on vacation I make sure he eats extra mice and if I leave him extra water there's no problem. But the iguana had to be sprayed with water twice a day, which was becoming a real problem. Also, his nails were getting really long, and he had gotten very big. I had to handle him with work gloves so as not to get scratched. He didn't scratch me on purpose, but whenever I went to pick him up I'd get scratched all over. Truthfully, it got to be too much for me and I gave him to a veterinary student. He's in a really good home.

All my pets get along with each other. In fact, my Siamese, Cocoa, cleans everybody, and they love it. She washes them all with her tongue. I guess that's the mother instinct because she's the only cat who has ever had kittens. Because they're loved, they're very happy animals that live long lives. My pets get really old. Gregory, my oldest, is 20. My other cat, Meow—I found her in an empty lot—lived to be almost 17. When she died, she was under the table, curled up in a little circle. The hard part is losing an animal you love. It doesn't matter how many you have; you miss the one you don't have.

I volunteer at an animal shelter once a week, and get my cats from an animal shelter. I've been an avid animal lover my whole life. As a teacher, I always kept animals in the classroom. I taught the second graders how to wash out the cage and how to give vitamins. I would do the same thing in the classroom that I did at home.

My son is all grown up and my pets are now my babies. I am an avid animal lover and take excellent care of them. My cats have never been boarded when I was on vacation. I had people come in and take care of them. My animals are very healthy and happy. They mean the world to me.

RITA "When no one was there for me, they were."

My nine cats are my loving companions who always provide me with emotional support. They are psychic, sometimes finding things that I am looking for and either brining them to me or locating them and alerting me. They communicate their feelings to me and are a reminder that the human form is not the only form of intelligence. One of my cats, Salviera, gets upset if I cry and comforts me, licking my tears and putting her paw on my hand in a reassuring manner. Another, Spot, has feline immune deficiency syndrome and is still healthy. I'm sure it's because of the bonding, energy, and time spent together in companionship. They are each different. Some act like they are my children, some act like they are my friends. Scott, the FIDS cat, acts like he is the father of all the others and is my partner in watching over and caring for them.

My cats mean responsibility as well. I don't take long vacations because I worry about how the separation will affect them. They have kept me going in times when I felt I might give up. When no one was there for me, they were. When others are around they seem happy to see me exchanging pleasantries and visits with them. I love them for the wonderful souls they are.

I could write a book about each one of my pets, how they were rescued, why no one would adopt them, and why I could not part with them. Christopher, for example, was found in a garbage can with three siblings, just a day or two old. They, unfortunately, died, but he fought to live with a rat tooth hole in his rump that abscessed and burst before I noticed it. (That rat probably put the hole in the plastic bag that allowed him to breathe.)

I have gained so much from my experience with animals, more than space permits me to tell. Animals are not indifferent, selfish creatures, contrary to a recent "study" I heard about. To know that, one must live with them, and make a commitment to one's pets.

BARBARA "My pet ferret gives me joy...."

...Most of the time she is fearless. I love her boldness and wish I had half her willingness to try new things. Her curiosity brings a smile to my soul, and her innocence and playfulness warm my heart. She's my buddy.

Having a ferret has taught me to love unconditionally, to be more caring, patient, and compassionate. We have a mutual respect for one another. I now have a sense of belonging to something other than the human race. Having a ferret is a responsibility, but it's nice to be needed. She depends on me for her health and well-being. I'm sure all ferrets are playful, but she's just so much fun!

MASON "My dog is a beautiful creature..."

...white with black spots and a great dog physique. He has the most independent mind of any dog I know. My dog is a full and valuable presence in my life. He is a jogging partner and a being to give love to and get love from. He is social. I have met many people through him, and some are now good friends. He has helped me to understand what it means to take care of something, which I sometimes resent but know is an invaluable thing to have learned. Although I sometimes wish I didn't have him around to deal with, I also can't imagine life without him.

TINA "My pet is my friend...."

...She is always happy to see me. It makes me feel good. I feel responsible for her. She counts on my company and affection.

Pets need to be free, to be themselves. I've had many cats in my life. Each one has his or her own personality. This one is very patient, but when she's mad she shows it.

ANONYMOUS Diet makes a difference for a jay

A young scrub jay was raised for six weeks by a vet tech from a local hospital. Jay was hand-fed with baby-bird-feeding formula, but weaned off a bit too soon and given human food in its place. The human food consisted of dry cereal, some cooked vegetables, cooked chicken, cooked hamburger meat, salami, cheese, bologna, and various other not-so-healthy choices.

I was contacted to take a look at this bird, as the surrogate mother was worried about it, describing it as "deformed." The deformity was a bad case of poorly developed feathers; they were all turned outward, making it look like he "went poof." His weight was very low, and his keel bone extremely palpable. This bird had noticeable energy, but could not get enough lift to fly properly. He ran and hopped everywhere, but his feathers weren't able to provide him much service for flying.

I took him home to "fine-tune" him and immediately started him on mealworms, wax worms (good protein and calories), fresh fruits, and lightly steamed green vegetables to ease the transition to healthy foods. He would attack his food voraciously and look at me for more healthy goodies. His weight almost doubled in the first week. I added more raw vegetables to his diet, which he always enjoyed along with cooked millet, quinoa, and oats.

After five weeks, Jay was fully feathered with new feathers, his weight was good, and his flying ability much improved. Overall, he responded ideally to the improvement in his diet, proving that proper diet makes the difference. He was released to a veterinarian friend of mine who assisted me with his recovery. Jay is getting acclimated to the outside world again and learning to hunt and enjoy the life he was intended to live.

ROSARIA Kangaroo-like cat

I have three cats—Eloise, Lola, and Stranger. They are my children. I love them, and they love me unconditionally. Each one has a unique personality, needs, and quirkiness. Eloise sits up like a kangaroo and has a passion for my slippers. Lola carries on with her stuffed mouse as if it were her child. And stranger is fascinated with my bathtub.

TERRY "By having cats I have learned to understand people better."

My cat reminds me of myself. Her traits are different aspects of mine. I can tell my mood by how my cat reacts to me. My pet helps me to relax and get comfortable. She always finds new ways to do things she wants and is a great source of entertainment.

By having cats I have learned to watch and understand people better, especially subtle personality aspects (facial expressions, sounds, habits). I can look at my cat and know what she is thinking. I can listen to her sounds and how what they mean. By dealing with people's cats I have learned that you usually pick the cat that best relates to you.

My cat is unique in that she always seems to be doing something new. Her facial expressions change, she makes different sounds, and she likes to hide in different places. She knows whom to trust and whom not to trust. She doesn't come out when there are people I don't trust.

LUCILLE Rabbits have special needs

My house rabbit was a member of the family with complete rights. We gave her a lot of attention. She shared our hours at home whether it was good times or not. She was unique in that she actually enjoyed listening to Pavarotti.

Three years ago, my beloved rabbit passed on. I have since realized that I formed a strong attachment to her. I carry around an excessive amount of guilt over the care of this pet and her passing. Most important, I discovered that rabbits need the care of veterinarians who specialize in their particular physiology. Our vet was homeopathic but knew nothing about her needs and problems. She could have been saved if we had the right veterinarian.

WALTER The healing power of human warmth

Eight years ago, in October, there was an unusual snowstorm. While I was away, my cat got pneumonia from being outside for six hours. He had a cough and couldn't smell his food. He wouldn't eat for a week. I called the vet, but refused to give him antibiotics. For two weeks my cat slept on me, lying directly on my chest. I gave him my warmth and positive energy, and he gradually got better.

HELEN "I have a cat who is a natural healer."

I used natural foods to treat my cat after she was diagnosed with a kidney disease at the age of 12 and given just two to three months to live. Heather's food consisted mostly of two recipes. One was raw meat, rice, and adzuki beans. The other was cooked liver, rice, and eggs. I was also giving her glandular supplements, but she wouldn't accept those for a while. As a treat, I would give her cooked beets and mix the beet juice into her food—she loved it! A book I used for recipes and a lot of information was Dr. Pitcairn's *Complete Guide to Natural Health for Dogs and Cats*. She lived to be 16!

Heather was with me through many stages of life—from college to marriage. We had a very strong bond and still do. We shared many memorable experiences, so many, in fact, that I could write a book about it and have often though about doing so. Two days before Heather died I told her I loved her and gave her permission to go. She was waiting for that permission. The energy of our bond is still there.

Now I have a cat named Hally who is an intuitive, natural healer. Once I woke up at 4 a.m. with a horrible earache. I wondered how I would feel when I went to work at 7 a.m. I somehow went back to sleep. Halley positioned herself on my pillow against my left ear. I woke up at 6:30 a.m. without an earache. She has stretched herself over my stomach and cured my menstrual cramps. And she has spent days sitting against my husband's knee after his knee surgery to help with his recovery. It goes on and on....

PEARL The Clark Gable of the dog world

My foxhound Buster came into our lives when he was just 12 weeks old. The man who owned him was very cruel and ignorant. He got Buster specifically for hunting, but he was just a puppy. Because he couldn't hunt, Buster's owner wanted to give him to an animal shelter where he probably would have been destroyed. He kept Buster in a dark basement, and the dog was full of worms. My husband, who shared an office with this man, asked for Buster. The man wanted $65, so my husband paid him. He not only saved Buster's life, but he brought home a wonderful companion animal that has been a joy to us both.

Buster is highly intelligent. He won't allow us to argue. If we have any harsh words he will jump right in the middle. He goes to sleep at 11 every night, and if we don't come to bed he starts barking at us. He keeps us laughing and has made our relationship much better. We both love Buster, and he's an integral part of the family. We have our own boat, and Buster has his own life jacket and his own towel. Buster is incredible, and we both love him very much.

Now at nine, Buster is starting to develop a faint white film over his eyes, the beginning of cataracts. My veterinarian said there wasn't anything I could do to help him. He did recommend vitamins—vitamin E, and essential fatty acids—even though he didn't believe these would correct his conditions. Another problem I was having was with Buster's shedding. Since he was a young pup,

GARY NULL

268

Buster has been shedding a lot all year round. The veterinarian thought that shedding was normal for this type of dog, but I suspected that he was deficient in some nutrient.

I tried lots of formulas designed to stop shedding, but he wouldn't take any. Whenever I would put vitamins into his food he would refuse to eat. Buster is very choosy; if something doesn't smell right to him he won't eat it. Every six months, I would also give Buster a pill to prevent heartworms. Heartworm pills are known to shorten an animal's life, and Buster was showing symptoms of early aging. His youthful look started to disappear and was now replaced by an aged look.

I found out about the Earth Animal company and started using their herbal vision formula for his eyes. The ingredients are eyebright, chamomile, gingko, goldenseal, bayberry with flower essence, nasturtium, and Shasta daisy. A side benefit of the vision formula is emotional balance. I put seven drops into his water every day.

I also started to add their multivitamin in treat form, Daily Health Nuggets, to his food. Those were the first vitamins he would accept. His ability to discriminate between artificial and natural smells amazes me. He is very sensitive and picks up on everything. The Daily Health Nuggets are a complete vitamin/mineral formula that is designed to boost the immune system.

Within a week, Buster's shedding was cut in half. I believe the essential fatty acids in the Daily Health Nuggets are what made a difference. He is looking better and is not as nervous as he once was.

For the past few years I've been feeding Buster a diet of rice, organic free-range chicken, and organic meat, not raw meat as some experts recommend. Buster likes his meats cooked, and I believe this is healthier. Raw store-bought meats have the potential for transmitting pathogens; they're not fresh like just-killed prey in the wild. I also add vegetables and acidophilus to Buster's food. I buy Buster water from the Fiji islands. The water tastes pure and it has an alkaline pH.

In place of the pill to prevent heartworms, I give him an herbal powder from Earth Animal made up of human-food-grade ingredients—brewer's yeast, garlic, B vitamins, minerals, and special nutrients that work together synergistically. It's supposed to do the same as the heartworm pill without the damaging effects. I just started the regimen, so it's a little early to tell how well it will work.

Because of Buster's good looks and beautiful personality, I was approached by filmmakers to see if he could be in a movie. (The movie is named *The Passenger* and it will be aired on cable TV on the Sundance Channel.) We spent three 15-hour days of intensive filming, and he was fantastic. Buster made friends with everyone on the set, and although he never acted before he was absolutely superb. Our neighbors now call him the Clark Gable of the dog world.

Buster is lovable, highly intelligent, and so magnetic that people cross the street to ask me if they can pet him. (And some don't even ask.) Many children gather around him when I walk Buster past their school. He goes to each and every one, standing on his hind legs, never leaving out a child. I'm moved by his sensitivity. I don't know where or how he learned to do this and the other numerous things he does that express such feeling and love. My husband brought Buster home in December of '91, right after my breast cancer surgery. I really believe my most loyal and very best friend is keeping me alive.

SANDRA Detoxing a cat

Thirteen years ago, I was advised to euthanize my eight-year-old cat Gina by at least six veterinarians because she was having kidney and cardiac failure. I would not kill her. I couldn't quite place it, but I just felt something was blocking her. Because she had a very foul odor, I thought this cat should be detoxed. This is before I ever detoxed myself, but I must have read about it somewhere. She wouldn't eat, so I had to learn how to give her fluids at home, which I did several times a day. And I used plain aloe without a flavor. I also used bentonite clay and some type of very mild fiber for a while. After a week, she started to clean out. Then I started to give her this substance in a tube—I don't remember the name—but it stimulates appetite in animals. I put some on her paw, and she couldn't stand it, so she licked it off. Little by little, I was able to introduce foods to her. I found a wonderful book called *Ten Essential Herbs*, and I slowly gave her herbs and baby food.

As she started to clean out I was able to give her fluids twice a day and eventually she didn't need extra fluids at all. She lost a lot of weight. She had been a fat cat, and she was very, very thin and weak at this point. After I detoxed her I started to introduce nutrients. I read the labels of veterinary nutrients and then went into a health food store and tried to get the natural products and break them down to a small proportion of the amount that they would use for humans. I made my own little recipes, gave that to her, gave her the baby food, and slowly started to give her other foods.

About three weeks later, I brought her back to the veterinarian and her tests were much better. Her kidneys were practically normal. When I brought her back a third time for a follow-up test she was normal. This was miraculous.

In addition to that, I used visualization. When she was very, very sick and I wouldn't let her be euthanized, she only wanted to sleep on the floor in the closet, which a lot of animals do, and which I like to do. I like to creep in a little hole when I don't feel good. I put a blanket on the closet floor, and I was lying next to her. There was no light on in the closet, but there was a little bit of light coming from the bathroom. When I looked at her, I saw a flat band of gray outlining her body. I sat in the lotus position and looked at the gray band. In my mind, I made that gray band lighter and lighter, lighter and lighter. I started to breathe deeply and rhythmically. I saw something happening that I didn't really understand, but I let it happen. I let the band get lighter and lighter, lighter and lighter, until it was silvery, almost effervescent. I just looked at her body and visualized her body absorbing it. I was able to do this in the evenings when we went to sleep. On some days I did it twice in a day. I don't know if it was imagination, but I'm telling you this cat was a dead cat when I brought her into the vet's office, and she started to walk the day after this happened. Before that I had been carrying her. She wasn't walking anymore.

So something happened. Eventually she didn't want to sleep in the closet anymore, but in bed. I didn't see the gray band anymore and she was healthy. This was a miraculous healing. This eight-year-old cat lived to be 18. On the day of her passing she waited 12 hours for me to come home. I knew she was going to die that day. When I left in the morning for work I said, "You wait for mommy. Don't go until I come back." When I came back she put her arms up. I picked her up, and she passed over. It was a very close relationship that I had with her. She passed over very nicely, very quietly and gently.

ALAN A cat full of energy

My first cat lived for 19 years despite being a street cat rescued when she was six weeks old. Our current cat is one-and-a-half years old. We took the cat in at six weeks. At that time she had diarrhea and extremely pale-colored stools. She was lethargic. Now she has dark-colored, solid stools, and is regular and full of fun and energy.

I use nutritional yeast, fish (either canned mackerel or sardines, both packed in water), kelp, and organic old-fashioned rolled oats to feed our cat. We also give our cat natural digestive enzymes with almost every meal. We only use organic, all-natural wood pellets as cat litter in her box, and we clean it on a regular basis. We also give our cat vitamins and natural liver de-fattening agents from time to time.

BARBARA Restored health in cats

My cats were becoming constipated, so I purchased psyllium husk from the health food store. The veterinarian said to give them laxatives. If that didn't work he thought I might need surgery on the colon of one cat. Thank God the psyllium husk fiber worked.

ELIZABETH Energy healing

I've been trained in energy healing science and have a private practice as a healer. In my practice I work with people, but I will work the energy field of my own children and animals. Working on people or pets in your own family is not recommended. I just do it because I love them, and I can't keep my hands off them.

I can see the energy field in most cases. But my primary method of high sense perception is kinesthetic. Sometimes I can see where the lines of energy are broken in the body, and I work to repair them.

There are different causes of an imbalance. For instance, my dog has a sensitivity in her hindquarters because before I got her, when she was a pup, they clipped her tail. This is just a sore spot with her. The other problem that I've had with her is that when we go away she tends to excessively lick the hair off her body (poodles have hair, not fur). Not coincidentally, she's chosen to lick it off from the hindquarters. Another problem that I've had with her is excessive barking. So I've worked with that energetically.

When they've gotten sick what I've done with them is use energy healing as a complement to the veterinary care that I've given them. I've found that the recovery time is much faster. For instance, my cat recently became very ill. She lost a lot of fluids in her body, and we didn't know whether she had kidney trouble or not. I took her to the vet, who gave her some medication, prednisone, which I hated giving to her. But 16 years earlier I had a cat that had the same symptoms, and I remembered that prednisone was wonderful. Yet there comes a time when the animal gets anxious on it. So I didn't use it for the full course. I just did it enough to help her turn the corner, and then I used energy work. She's great now. She had tests, and she's doing beautifully. She's back to normal.

When I do energy work my clients need to be still. Curiously, my animals will sit still much more readily than my children. I have to work on my children when they're asleep because that's about the only time they'll let me into their fields. But the animals will always let me in.

I feed them a diet called Eukanuba, a healthy diet for pets. Sometimes I sprinkle Green Stuff into their food.

VICTORIA A wonderful wheaten

I have a wheaten terrier, and they have a tendency to get overexcited and charge into other dogs. Before training sessions, I give him Rescue Remedy and lark, and I also take Rescue Remedy myself because it's a little overwhelming. The lark is for nervousness and lack of confidence. It's also for people who think they're going to fail a test. My dog wasn't taking a test; he was going for training. And sometimes he would just get a little undone. And me—during the class people are so intent watching one another I found that if I took Rescue Remedy or lark myself I would be calmer, and as a result my dog would be. So that's also why I did it.

My dog is a year-and-a-half old, and he's never gotten sick. I feed him a raw foods diet based on Pitcairn's diet in *Natural Foods for Dogs and Cats*. My husband gets a kick out of it when he says, "Is that for us or the dog?" At times, I will have him fast for a day and then have him go back on track the next day.

I give my family a lot of raw food, and it just didn't seem right to give him dried food all the time. So that's why I figured I had to research it, and that's what I did. I found out about dried foods, how they go against the dog's natural tendencies and how many diseases are associated with them. And when I started talking to people who had animals in other countries, they would say that you had to feed your dog and take responsibility for it and prepare its food. The more I learned, the more it made sense to me. Feeding dried food only is like feeding your child dry cereal every day.

It's not all that time-consuming to prepare your dog's food because you can make all the food up at one time, freeze it in little sections, and then defrost one bag at a time. And then, if I'm in a pinch, I'll mix it in with the dry food. It's a little bit of work, but I'm not that put off by it. I also give him raw marrowbones. I'll go to the butcher, get the big marrowbone, and let him eat that, especially if I'm having company, to give him something to do. But my friends' first response to me is, "Oh, you have to be careful with that." They're alarmed and can't believe that I do give him marrowbones or raw carrots and stuff like that. But my family's fine with it.

In the book, Dr. Pitcairn has a formula that he calls healthy powder. In that healthy powder is yeast, lecithin, kelp, bone meal, and vitamin C. Then I also take Gary Null's Green Stuff, and I put that in the dog's food, especially if he's not eating vegetables.

One time he was limping, and I knew he had jumped off the porch and hurt himself. I gave him some arnica and he seemed to be fine after a short time.

After he was groomed, he wouldn't let anyone touch him on the back legs. They must have been overly aggressive towards him. I met a woman who did Tellington Touch with animals. She showed me how to do it. And by doing that with him, he's much calmer. He goes in to be groomed a lot easier now. If I'm at a place, and he seems to be nervous, I'll start doing that with him. Or even when people come over. Any time I feel that he's looking a little stressed I do it—or even if I'm just sitting with him.

I've done a lot for my dog, and people will say, "How do you know it's working?" The only thing I can really say is that I've had him groomed at different places and different groomers have all commented to me on what a nice looking dog he is, and what a nice coat he has. Anyone who knows the wheaten dog will have the same comment, "He's not your typical wheaten." He's just a nice dog. He doesn't have any behavior problems. I would like to think that through all this combined effort the dog has come into his own.

PATRICIA "My cat Ripple is a blessing and a gift...."

...She is a window to another realm of existence—the noncerebral zone. I love to just sit and watch her, even when that's all *she* is doing—sitting and watching. She is a beautiful little spirit that brings me immeasurable joy. She is truly her own soul. She prefers to keep to herself, especially if there is more than one human around and most especially if it is not one of her inner circle of human friends. However, without fail, whenever I have been sick or depressed she always comes and jumps on me, lays on my stomach, my back, my lap. She sleeps there, right on me, but only at those times. It must be her sensitivity and awareness of energy.

There are no words to describe the feeling I get from lying with my cat—my face on her warm, fuzzy belly. I really don't like it when people say that cats are stupid, mean, or evil. I hear this more frequently than I care to remember. Ripple is a very emotional spirit. She is loving, but she is shy. When there are people around that she doesn't know very well she prefers to keep to herself. But when her favorite people are here she comes out, bumps your legs, is very talkative, lies on her back, and begs for belly-tickling.

Here is something unique and peculiar about Ripple. She makes this funny bird sound, a deep-throated warble that none of the other cats I've had ever made.

TOM Responsibility strengthens a bond

Our two cats provide a topic of conversation and amusement for my wife and me. When my wife was away once for two-and-a-half weeks, I was solely responsible for them, and I developed a greater affection for my animals and a stronger bond. Many animals seem to have a need for humans, and humans a need for them.

LUANNE
"Hearing pets tell you 'I love you' in perfect English is a rush."

I have two beautiful parrots, an African gray and a yellow-naped Amazon. I use full-spectrum lights in the area where my birds' cages are. They eat only organic seeds and nut mixes, filtered water, and treats of Gary's Green Stuff, Red Stuff, and Muscle powder. I keep a clean environment for them. I clean their cages and toys regularly and clean the floors around their cages with alcohol. I keep an air purifier on for two hours a day. I believe that their friendly disposition and robust health are a result of these habits.

I also bond with the birds daily, playing catch with the empty vitamin containers that double as their toys. I use cuddling and touch therapies with them. To say the least, hearing your pets tell you "I love you" in perfect English is a rush.

As a holistic R.N., I understand that real results come from an integrated approach to health. I apply this to me as well as my birds. They are a source of joy and unconditional love.

CHERI Curing a cat

I had a cat that got sick. There seemed to be something wrong with her, and it was getting progressively worse. The cat had a cold in her eye. It was partially closed, and it didn't seem to be getting any better.

Since I don't like taking a lot of drugs—I used to take goldenseal and chlorophyll and all kinds of natural supplements—I figured the cat should be able to take these types of things too and that they would probably be healthful. I knew goldenseal was good for infections. I figured I'd just mix some up in her food and see what transpired. So that's what I did. I took 500 mg of goldenseal out of the capsule, and I mixed it up in her food so she wouldn't be able to tell it was there. I just fed it to her for about three days.

I started to see a difference, so I just continued on. And I know it wasn't a long period of time. It wasn't more than a week that I gave it to the cat, and it seemed like the infection went away and she was back to normal.

JOAN "My passion and purpose in life is to take care of birds..."

...whether they are ill, injured, orphaned, or simply bewildered. I live with a family of birds that includes past charges that could not be released back to the wild, and a family of domesticated Australian zebra finches. This is the story of one tiny zebra finch named Fluffy and the impact she recently made upon my life.

Zebra finches are naturally vigorous, fast-paced little birds with infinite energy. Fluffy's plumage is a striking light silver color with contrasting cream-colored feathers on her chest. She has a distinct orange beak and legs that add further contrast to her overall length of three inches.

Early in April 1999 I noticed that Fluffy was not feeling like her normal energized self. She had grown quiet and reclusive and was no longer socializing with the rest of the flock during their usual daily routine. I picked up the little bird that seemed suddenly very fragile and vulnerable. I performed a basic physical exam to check for obvious causes of her condition. I noticed that her left eye appeared swollen and some of the feathers had fallen away from her cheek and upper neck area and she had experienced weight loss. It was time to schedule a visit to see Dr. Gloria, her veterinarian, for further evaluation.

Fluffy was placed in the avian hospital cage, which is a clear plastic box measuring 14 by 20 by 10 inches, comfortably equipped with a heating pad, a perch, a tube-style bamboo nest, food, and water. The trip we would take to the vet hospital that day was the beginning of an intensive journey of discovery and healing.

As we arrived at the veterinary hospital, Jennifer [the assistant] greeted us. She always has a wonderful smile and comforting words of encouragement for any patient I bring to see the doctor. We were escorted to the examination room, which must seem disconcerting to a little bird like Fluffy with the high ceilings and shiny medical devices. I spoke quietly to Fluffy, assuring her that all was well and we needed help to determine what was causing her discomfort.

Dr. Gloria carefully examined Fluffy and determined there was an eye infection; we would treat the problem with oral antibiotics and eye ointment. A simple-enough solution, or so I thought. The medication would prove to help at first, then the symptoms would recur. We had to administer several additional treatments during the course of the summer, each time fighting the problem, but never really eradicating it altogether. In September, things began to go terribly wrong with Fluffy. Her right eye had atrophied into the eye socket, 75 percent of her feathers were missing, and the left foot and leg had become swollen.

Something had invaded her body and was spreading. Was it cancer? I kept thinking that I took such good care of my birds, and now something was killing her, and we could not determine exactly what it was. With all of the medical technology and treatment available to humans, this one-ounce bird could not be easily diagnosed because of the lack of diagnostic tools for someone her size. We were running out of time and options and were forced to return to the hospital.

The infection had spread and settled into the joint and bone of her left leg. Dr. Gloria came into the examination room looking deeply concerned about the options available for treatment. The prognosis didn't look good for Fluffy. The further use of antibiotics could eventually kill her, and it was no longer proving useful. The decision was before us to either put her to sleep and end the misery or amputate the leg. Surgery could kill her because of her weakened condition.

We went home to ponder the next course of action. As we entered the house all of the zebra finches greeted her with their beeps and chirping, but she barely had the strength to answer them. I dropped myself onto the couch in an emotionally drained state while Percy, my companion pigeon, stood at my shoulder consoling and counseling me. This evening he looked particularly wise with his combination of charcoal gray feathers highlighted by green iridescent neck feathers. The birds and I act as a family unit; decisions affect all of us. Percy and I studied each other's face. He has been with me for three years and had seen other sick birds pull through and had never seen me give up. Fluffy then started to beep a very strained call to me. It was chilling as I listened to the cry in her voice telling me that she wanted to live and we had to keep trying. The next couple of weeks we would be preparing her for surgery by building up her strength and weight.

October 27th was a beautiful autumn day but time to go to the hospital for the surgery. I was feeling enormous guilt, wondering if I was sentencing her to certain death as soon as the anesthesia was administered. Jennifer greeted us in the usual manner, but I saw the concern in her face as she checked us into the exam room for Fluffy's pre-op exam.

Dr. Gloria lovingly placed Fluffy on the scale to weigh her and examine her leg before we went to surgery. I would be with Fluffy during the procedure. She was ready; I could tell by her appearance and demeanor. I, on the other hand, was feeling the grip of uncertainty the morning held for us, but knew we were doing the right thing for her.

It was time. I carried Fluffy in her hospital cage down the hallway to the surgery room. I had been in there before during procedures and observed other surgeries, but this one was chilling me to the bone. "Concentrate—this isn't about your fears; it is about Fluffy and her survival," I told myself.

Dr. Gloria and Nurse Peggy prepared the instruments and operating table as I held Fluffy and comforted her. Time was starting to move slowly at this point. Dr. Gloria looked at me and said, "We are ready." I gave Fluffy a kiss and gave her to Dr. Gloria. A small makeshift mask was devised to fit over her tiny face; now the combination of oxygen and isoflurane gas began to billow into her air sacs. I kept telling her to breathe deeply and we all breathed with her. Slowly her little eyes began to close and her body became limp. The anesthetic was taking her into a deep slumber and no doubt provoked some very strange dreams. I wanted her to quickly go to sleep so we could do the surgery and see if she would wake up.

She was positioned on her back, and the surgery began. We could tell she was breathing by the pulsation in her legs from the beating of her heart. Dr. Gloria worked quickly to amputate the leg and tie off the excision site to prevent bleeding. Her small hands swiftly moved with precision as her dark eyes darted effortlessly from the small patient beneath her hands to the gauges on the tanks of gas and oxygen, balancing all of the components to keep her patient alive.

Finally the surgery was done and it was time to bring her back to consciousness. Oxygen began replacing the gas that had dropped her so near death. Dr. Gloria and I waited and watched as her chest heaved up and down as she breathed in the oxygen. The entire hospital had become very quiet. Her continued breathing indicated she was still with us. An eyelid opened to welcome the world. "Come on Fluffy, fight your way out," I said to her. She slowly came out of the deep sleep; she had survived the surgery.

After she stabilized, I took her home. Once again, as soon as we walked through the back door, all of the birds chirped and cooed to welcome her home. "Beep!" she cried out to them. She announced her arrival to the flock. I placed her in my bedroom to rest quietly and recover from the anesthesia. Now we waited during this critical 24 hours to see what would happen. One day merged into the next few days, then into 10 days after surgery and a remarkably recovering patient.

Early one evening I was working in another room when I heard all of the birds chirping excitedly. I went into the living room to see what was happening, but nothing appeared wrong in the aviary. I stopped a moment to check on Fluffy as I had habitually done since the surgery. Her left wing had a dark red stain all over it. I wasn't too alarmed at first, thinking she had scraped her wing while trying to maneuver it like a crutch. I picked her up and turned her over to check further and was horrified to see blood rushing from the surgical site. She had been very active that day, and the clot must have fallen off the wound.

Bleeding bird in hand, and pigeon sitting on my shoulder to supervise me, I applied direct pressure to stop the flow of blood. Fluffy has only about 4 cc's of blood in her body, which is the equivalent of 3/4 teaspoon. Each time I looked to see if it stopped it started again when she moved. This was more than my expertise could handle. I hurriedly called Dr. Gloria at her home for assistance. She instructed me to use direct pressure again, but I was unable to stop the bleeding for very long. The bird's life was draining right out of her into my hands. Dr. Gloria advised us to meet her at the hospital.

Fluffy had come so far and had been improving; now she was facing another fight to stay alive. I wrapped the stump as tightly as I could, placed her in a warm blanket, and proceeded to the hospital. It was dark at 6:45 p.m. and silent as we arrived at the hospital. I didn't know if she was still alive as I carried her into the surgery room. Dr. Gloria and I didn't say anything as I removed the blanket from her. "She is still alive!" we exclaimed. This little bird was continuing to battle for life, despite the fact that she had practically bled to death. A clotting agent was applied to the surgical site, and we waited that long wait once again to watch her stabilize. She was clinging on to any spark of life left in her. The spark ignited and the flame grew more intense. We went home to recover.

This fight was proving to be the worst for her. Now she had the added burden of blood loss, which made her weaker, as well as the pain from the amputation, the possibility of infection, and the loss of her tail feathers that assisted in her balance. A bird so small does not have the benefit of a pain reliever available without the threat of serious side effects. She became noticeably weaker the next few days. She would lie on her side, trying to stay off the stump that must have been excruciatingly painful. I consulted with a physician who had undergone amputation of a leg as a young man to gain perspective on what she was enduring. He assured me it was very painful and just the touch of the bandage hurt. As I sat and watched her I felt absolutely helpless. I could not take away the pain.

The following Tuesday she returned to the hospital for a checkup. I wasn't sure what her doctor would say about her progress since she was still so weak. Was it time to end her misery and let her go? Dr. Gloria carefully held her as she examined the stump and suddenly noticed feathers starting to grow at the base of her tail. This was a sign that her body was regenerating! After all these months and times of being near death she was coming back; she was winning! The growth of her tail was measured daily and provided us with a measurement of recovery.

Today she is a healthy, feathered bird that is sitting near me as I write this. She has inspired me to go forward with my education in avian studies to do whatever I can to help other birds like her. I now have a clear idea of how I must continue my education. She taught me to find options when faced with formidable obstacles, explore possibilities, and realize I am capable of much more than I ever imagined. Thank you, Fluffy.

HOLISTICALLY ORIENTED VETERINARIANS

Following is a list of doctors of veterinary medicine, organized by state and listed alphabetically by city. Some are more conventional than others, but they all incorporate principles of holistic healing into their practices to some degree.

Most of the veterinarians listed here work with dogs and cats only. However, a few of them work with exotic animals, horses, and other species.

ALABAMA

Twila G. Floyd, DVM
Nature's Oasis
448 Day Lily St.
Auburn, AL 36832
Ph: 334-826-6624,826-NOAH

S. Allen Price, DVM
Vespridge Veterinary Clinic
1444 Montgomery Hwy
Birmingham, AL 35216
Ph: 205-822-0210

ALASKA

Jeanne Olson, DVM
1890 Hollowell Road
North Pole, AK 99705
Ph: 907-488-2906
corvi@mosquitonet.com

ARIZONA

S. Anne Smith, VMD
29834 North Cave Creek Road
Suite 118
Cave Creek, AZ 85331
Ph: 619-225-2121

Judith A. Stolz, DVM
2682 North El Dorado Drive
Chandler, AZ 85224
Ph: 480-899-1624
Fax: 480-917-5981
homeopvet@aol.com

Karen Ivin, DVM
2021 East Amber Lane
Gilbert, AZ 85296
Ph: 480-497-6362
Fax: 480 497 3908
zooowner@earthlink.net

Norman Ward, DVM
Hoistic Animal Center of Arizona
6990 East Shea Blvd., Suite 120
Scottsdale, AZ 85254
Ph: 480-609-1147
Fax : 480-609-1012

Deborah C. Mallu, DVM, CVA
215 Disney Lane
Sedona, AZ 86336
Ph: 520-282-5651
Fax: 520 282 3586
2suns@sedona.net

ARKANSAS

Pat Bradley, DVM
Ph: 501-329-7727
Telephone consultation practice

CALIFORNIA

Beth Wildermann, DVM
17333 Bear Creek Road
Boulder Creek, CA 95006
Ph: 408-354-1576

Monica A. Laflin, DVM
2159 San Elijo Ave.
Cardiff, CA 92007
Ph: 760-436-3215
Fax: 760-436-4126

Tom Boekbinder, DVM
Holistic Veterinary Clinic
26135 Carmel Rancho Blvd.
Carmel, CA 93923
Ph: 831-620-0115
Fax: 831-620-0116

Adrienne Moore, DVM
Southland Veterinary Care
2762 South Mission Road
Fallbrook, CA 92028
Ph: 760-723-6633

Linda K. Johnson, DVM
Commonwealth Animal Hospital
1941 West Common Wealth Ave
Fullerton, CA 92833

Ph: 714-525-2355
Fax: 714-525-7646

Don E. Lundholm, DVM
Adams Pet Clinic
10130 Adams Ave.
Huntington Beach, CA 92646
Ph: 714-964-1605
Fax: 714-965-0765

Richard Palmquist, DVM
721 Centinela Ave.
Inglewood, CA 90302
Ph: 310-673-1910
Fax: 310-673-8089

David A. Gordon, DVM
22421 El Toro Rd.
Lake Forest, CA 92630
Ph: 949-770-1808
Fax: 949-770-8984
arroyopet@aol.com

Manjit S. Nagi, DVM
2335 "F" Street
Livingston, CA 95334
Ph: 209-394-8556

Donna K. Fernandez, DVM
2047 Palosverdes Drive North
Lomita, CA 90717
Ph: 310-530-3833
Large animals only

Jennifer S. Burke, DVM
VCA Rossmoor El Dorado
10832 Los Alamitos Blvd.
Los Alamitos, CA 90720
Ph: 562-598-8621
Fax: 562-598-9561

Marc Bittan, DVM
11673 National Blvd
Los Angeles, CA 90064
Ph: 310-231-4415
www.theholisticvet.com

Douglas Coward, DVM
Animal and Bird Clinic
24961 Chrisanta Drive
Mission Viejo, CA 92691
Ph: 949-768-3651
Fax: 949-768-1333

Thomas Van Cise, D.V.M.
1560 Hamner Ave.
Norco, CA 92860
Ph: 909-737-1242

Henry Pasternak, DVM
Highlands Veterinary Hospital
526 Pacific Palisades Drive
Palisades, CA 90272
Ph: 310-454-2917
Fax: 310-454-3412
puppydoc@aol.com

Megan Bamford, DVM
2121 East Foothill Blvd.
Pasadena, CA 91107
Ph: 818-947-8258

J. Lauren De Rock, DVM
16311 Gustafson Ave
Patterson, CA 95363
Ph: 209-664-1764
Fax: 209-892-7702
drderock@evansinet.com
www.equineacupuncture.com
Equine only

Dirk B. Yelinek, DVM
200 S. Catalina Ave. No 208
Redondo Beach, CA 90277
Ph: 310-374-4399

Jacqueline McAndrew, DVM
South San Diego Veterinary
Hospital
2910 Coronado Ave.
San Diego, CA 92154
Ph: 619-423-7123
Fax: 619-423-5477

Dean D. Beyerinck
Irving Street Veterinary Hospital
1434 Irving Street
San Francisco, CA 94122
Ph: 415-664-0191
Fax: 415-664-6708
www.irvingsvet.com

Jeffrey N. Bryan
Irving Street Veterinary Hospital
1434 Irving Street
San Francisco, CA 94122
Ph: 415-664-0191
Fax: 415-664-6708
www.irvingsvet.com

Kelly E. Jensen
Irving Street Veterinary Hospital
1434 Irving Street
San Francisco, CA 94122
Ph: 415-664-0191
Fax: 415-664-6708
www.irvingsvet.com

Claire Mollard
Irving Street Veterinary Hospital
1434 Irving Street
San Francisco, CA 94122
Ph: 415-664-0191
Fax: 415-664-6708
www.irvingsvet.com

David W. Penney, DVM
Irving Street Veterinary Hospital
1434 Irving Street
San Francisco, CA 94122
Ph: 415-664-0191
Fax: 415-664-6708
www.irvingsvet.com
www.drdavepenney.com

Cheryl Schwartz, DVM
San Francisco Vet Specialists
3619 California St.
San Francisco, CA 94118
Ph: 415-387-6844
Fax: 415-387-6799

Pamela Bouchard, DVM
Tendercare Veterinary Hospital
1569 Fourth St.
San Rafael, CA 94901
Ph: 415-454-4994
Fax: 415-491-1196

Stanley Goldfarb, DVM
Home Vet
450 4th St.
San Rafael, CA 94901
Ph: 415-459-2195
Fax: 415-456-3687

Douglas Lemire, VMD
Mobile Alternative Veterinary Care
P.O. Box 40521
Santa Barbara, CA 93140
Ph: 805-565-3985
Fax: 805-565-3985
dr.douglasvet@home.com

Greg Ugarte, DVM
P.O. Box 42003
Santa Barbara, CA 93140
Equine

Carolyn Araiza, DVM
Pager: 408-231-4034
House calls in the Santa Clara,
Sunnydale and San Jose area

Darren Hawks, DVM, DACVIM
Veterinary Alternatives
2585 Soquel Drive
Santa Cruz, CA 95065
Ph: 831-475-5400
www.jps.net/dhawks

Linda Wells, DVM
Santa Cruz Veterinary Hospital
2585 Soquel Drive
Santa Cruz, CA 95065
Ph: 831-475-5400

Roger W. Valentine, DVM
Rahnie Valentine
Pet Allergy Center, Inc.
1637 16th Street
Santa Monica, CA 90404
Fax: 310-392-7369
petallctr@aol.com
Offers training for vets in NAET

Stephanie Chaumers, DVM
Holistic Animal Care
4918A Sonoma Highway
Santa Rosa, CA 95409
Ph: 707-538-4643

Jack M. Long, VMD
Forestville Veterinary Hospital
5033 Gravenstein Hwy No.
Sebastopol, CA 95472
Ph: 707-823-7312
Fax: 707-823-9247
info@forestvillevet.com

Neal K. Weiner, DVM
15290 Hwy 299W
Shasta, CA 96087
Ph: 530-242-0911
Fax: 530-242-0195
www.thenaturalpetcarecompany.net
emailpcn-lac@webtv.net

Dean R. Bader, DVM
Shingle Springs Veterinary
Corporation
4211 Sunset Lane Suite 101
Shingle Springs, CA 95682
Ph: 530-677-0390
Fax: 530-677-0613

Kerry J. Ridgway, DVM
1420 Grove St.
Sonoma, CA 95476
Ph: 707-935-1825
Fax: 707-935-1988
optionsvet@aol.com
www.horserehab.com
Equine only

Linda C. Boggie, DVM
Village Veterinary Hospital
3125 W. Benjamin Holt
Stockton, CA 95219
Ph: 209-951-5180

John B. Limehouse, DVM
Priscilla Taylor-Limehouse, DVM
Limehouse Veterinary Clinic of
Holistic Medicine
10742 Riverside Drive
Toluca Lake, CA 91602
Ph: 818-761-0719

COLORADO

Jean Hofve, DVM
jhofve@earthlink.net

Holly S. Foster, DVM
7805 W. 62nd. Ave.
Arvada, CO 80004
Ph: 303-456-4136

David Fong, DVM
P.O. Box 440410
Aurora, CO 80044
Ph: 303-693-9314

Douglas E. Amy, DVM
Gunbarrel Veterinary Clinic
4636 North 55th St.
Boulder, CO 80301
Ph: 303-530-2500
Fax: 303-530-2885

David H. Jaggar, MRCVS, DC
5139 Sugar Loaf Road
Boulder, CO 80302-9217
Ph: 303-449-7936
Fax: 303-449-8312
djaggar@aol.com

Robert J. Silver, DVM
Boulder's Natural Animal
685A South Broadway
Boulder, CO 80305
Ph: 303-494-7877

www.naturaldvm.com
www.bouldersnaturalanimal.com

H.C. Gurney, Jr. DVM
Aspen Park Veterinary Hospital
26497 Conifer Road
P.O. Box 222
Conifor, CO 80433
Ph: 303-674-0280
Fax: 303 838 4244

James Gaynor,, DVM
Critter Veterinary Care
2633 S. College Ave.
Ft. Collins, CO 80525
Ph: 970-226-4620
Fax: 970-226-4675
cvc@verinet.com

Marla Schwent, DVM
Critter Veterinary Care
2633 S. College Ave.
Ft. Collins, CO 80525
Ph: 970-226-4620
Fax: 970-226-4675
cvc@verinet.com

Steve Scibelli, DVM
Critter Veterinary Care
2633 S. College Ave.
Ft. Collins, CO 80525
Ph: 970-226-4620
Fax: 970-226-4675
cvc@verinet.com

Ron Carsten, DVM
Birchtree Animal Hospital
1602 Grand Ave.
Glenwood Springs, CO 81601
Ph: 970-945-0125

Rhonda L. Rodman, DVM,
CVA, CVC, CVH
7910 W. 20th Avenue
Lakewood, CO 80215
Ph: 303-202-0420

Bettye Hooley, DVM
Morningstar Veterinary Clinic
717 N. Cascade
Montrose, CO 81401
Ph: 970-249-8022

Betty Jo Black, DVM
7125 W. 27th Ave.
Wheat Ridge, CO 80215
Ph: 303-239-9917
HolisticVet@netscape.net

CONNECTICUT

Neil C. Wolff, DVM
Blue Cross Animal Hospital
530 E. Putnam Ave.
Greenwich, CT 06830
Ph: 203-869-7755

Gregory C. Azzolin, DVM
Northford Veterinary Clinic
1411 Middletown Ave.
Northford, CT 06472
Ph: 203-484-0736
Fax: 203-484-7966
northfordvet@juno.com

Allen M. Schoen, DVM
15 Sunset Terrace
Sherman, CT 06784
Ph: 860-354-2287
Fax: 860-350-3482
www.drchoen.com

Alan M. Busek DVM
The Pet Hospital of Stratford
1185 Linden Ave.
Stratford, CT 06615
Ph: 203-381-9488
Fax: 203-375-0503

Jeff Feinman, VMD, CVA
49 White Birch Road
Weston, CT 06883
Ph: 203-222-7979
Fax: 203-227-3231
www.homevet.com
drjeff@homevet.com

Robert Goldstein, DVM
Earth Animal Veterinary Practice
606 Post Road East
Westport, CT 06880
Ph: 203-222-0260

Teaches veterinarians how to do
BNA; for BNA training info:
1-800-670-0830, or bnaweb.com
rgoldstein@earthanimal.com
sgoldstein@earthanimal.com

DELAWARE

Shelley R. Epstein, VMD
Wilmington Animal Hospital
828 Philadelphia Pike
Wilmington, DE 19809
Ph: 302-762-2694
Fax: 302-762-1620

FLORIDA

Jeff Saunders, DVM
Saunders Veterinary Clinic
2801 U.S. Hwy 27 S.
Avon Park, FL 33825
Ph: 863-453-5700
Fax: 863-453-2549

Anthony Krawitz, DVM
5030 Champion Blvd. Suite G11
Calusa Animal Hospital
Boca Raton, FL 33496
Ph: 561-241-7177
Fax: 561-241-5029
calusaah@bellsouth.net

Beth Brown, DVM
Braden River Animal Hospital
5012 State Road 64 East
Bradenton, FL 34208
Ph: 941-745-1513
Fax: 941-746-0515
brhvet@mindspring.com
bbrowmdvm@mindspring.com

Peggy Fleming, DVM
Florida Equine Acupuncture
Center
21412 Field of Dreams Ln.
Dade City, FL 33523
Ph: 352-583-2400
Fax: 352-583-4007
Large animals only

Gregory Todd, DVM
1355 Pinehurst Rd.
Dunedin, FL 34698
Ph: 727-733-9351

Ronald A. Johnson, DVM, PhD
Mobile practice
680 Tennis Club Drive
Fort Lauderdale, FL 33311
Ph: 954-731-2000
Boca Raton: 954-426-0620
Palm Beach: 561-833-8777
Del Ray Beach: 561-740-3339

Iris Ramirez, DVM
Affectionately Pets House Calls
Ft. Myers, FL
Ph: 941-454-7387

Gerald J. Johnson, DVM
Quality Care Animal Hospital
7970 Miramar Parkway
Hollywood, FL 33023
Ph: 954-964-5557
Fax: 954-964-5558
gjohn3183@AOL.com
www.herbalvetmed.com

Robert H. Foley, DVM
VCA Upper Keys Animal Hospital
Upper Keys Veterinary Clinic
87108 Overseas Highway
Islamorada, FL 33036
Ph: 305-852-3665
Fax: 305-852-9646

P. C. Hightman, DVM
Brentwood Animal Hospital
4605 Brentwood Ave.
Jacksonville, FL 32206
Ph: 904-354-0547
Fax: 904-358-7566
hightmanap@aol.com
www.hightman.ap.net

Alyce Sims, DVM
Manadarin Veterinary Clinic
11587 San Jose
Jacksonville, FL 32223
Ph: 904-268-8880

John C. Haromy, DVM
Haromy Veterinary Clinic
3631 Hwy 60 E
Lake Wales, FL 33853
Ph: 863-676-5922
Fax: 863-676-7342

Betsy Coville, DVM
Alternative Animal Care
510 Stratfield Dr.
Lutz, FL 33549
Ph: 813-949-1818

Joseph Demers, DVM
Holistic Animal Clinic
496 N. Harbor City Blvd.
Melbourne, FL 32935
Ph: 407-752-0140
Fax: 407-752-0150
jdemers@prodigy

Robert Ferran, DVM
8271 South Dixie Hwy.
Miami, FL 33143
Ph: 305-662-4202
Fax: 305-662-7973

Diane M. Borreson, DVM
9633 Conservation Dr.
New Port Richey, FL 34655
Ph: 727-376-8984
Fax: 727-376-8984

Jan Bellows, DVM
Pet Healthcare Center
9111 Taft St.
Pembroke Pines, FL 33024
Ph: 954-432-1111
Fax: 954-431-8550

Anita S. Holt, VMD
Charlotte Animal Clinic
1825 Tamiami Trail Unit A-2
Port Charlotte, FL 33948
Ph: 941-624-4004
Fax: 941-624-4007
petassist@earthlink.net

Laura Earle, DVM
Coastal Animal Hospital Wellness
Center
545 Gus Hipp Blvd.
Rockledge, FL 32955
Ph: 407-632-3800
Fax: 407-632-2366

Lisa R. Edwards, DVM
Coastal Animal Hospital Wellness
Center
545 Gus Hipp Blvd.
Rockledge, FL 32955
Ph: 407-632-3800
Fax: 407-632-2366

Robin L. Cannizzaro, DVM
Holisic Veterinary Care
326 49 Avenue North
St. Petersburg, FL 33703
Ph: 727-528-0298
Fax: 727-525-7005

Robert Katz, DVM
Stuart Animal Hospital
3003 S. Federal Hwy.
Stuart, FL 34994
Ph: 561-287-2242
Fax: 561-287-0089

Gerald A. Wessner, VMD
Holistic Veterinary Clinic
14402 S. Hwy 475
Summerfield, FL 34491
Ph: 352-245-2025
Fax: 352-245-3360
holisiticvet@earthlink.com
www.holisticveterinaryclinic.com

Russell Swift, DVM
7154 N. University Drive #86
Tamarac, FL 33321
Ph: 561-391-5615
Fax: 954-720-0978
petsfriend@zim.com

Anne Lampru, DVM
Animal Alternatives/Holistic
Health Care
Tampa, FL
Ph: 813-265-2411
Fax: 813-962-4477

Michael J. Herman, DVM
1795 10th Avenue
Vero Beach, FL 32960
Ph: 561-562-0666

Constance DiNatale, DVM
Veterinary Acupuncture &
Complementary Therapy, Inc.
742 Clay St.
Winter Park, FL 32789
Ph: 407-644-0080
Fax: 407-644-0046

GEORGIA

Deneen C. Fasano, DVM
Noahs Arch Mobile Veterinary
Service
5410 Bridge Pointe Dr.
Alpharetta, GA 30005
Ph: 770-752-7237
Fax: 770-754-4133
veggievet@aol.com
Mobile Practice

Julia L. Partin, DVM
Hickory Flat Animal Hospital
2939 E. Cherokee Dr.
Canton, GA 30115
Ph: 770-345-2816
Fax: 770-704-0365

Taffy Shields Rhyne, DVM
Oak Mountain Animal Hospital
1155 Stripling Chapel Rd.
Carrollton, GA 30116
Ph: 770-834-1000

Howard L. Rand, DVM
2000 Bill Murdock Road
Marietta, GA 30062
Ph: 770-973-4133
Fax: 770 565 7684

Susan Wynn, DVM
Greater Atlanta Veterinary Group
1080 N. Cobb Parkway
Marietta, GA 30062
Ph: 770-424-6303
Fax: 770-426-4257
swynn@emory.edu

Bill Connolly, DVM
Gwinette Animal Hospital
2184 McGee Rd.
Snellville, GA 30078
Ph: 770-972-0447
Fax: 770-978-0542

Michelle Tilghman, DVM
Loving Touch Animal Center
1975 Glenn Club Drive
Stone Mountain, GA 30087
Ph: 770-498-5956
Fax: 770-498-3458
Ltac99@aol.com

Charlene R. Kickbush, DVM
Art Of Healing
2231 Hog Mtn. Rd.
Watkinsville, GA 30677
Ph: 706-769-1533
Fax: 706-769-2042

Allison B. Earls, DVM
Allatoona Animal Hospital
6733 Bells Ferry Road
Woodstock, GA 30189
Ph: 678-445-1111
Fax: 678-445-6200

HAWAII

Ihor Basko, DVM
P. O. Box 159
Kapaa, HI 96746
Ph: 808-828-1330
Fax: 808-822-2829

Robin M. Woodley, DVM
Kapa'au, HI 96755
Ph: 808-889-0430
rwoodley@interpac.net

Suellen J. Kotake, DVM
All Pets Clinic Waipahu, Inc.
94-366 Pupupani St.
Waipahu, HI 96797
Ph: 808-671-7424
Fax: 808-676-2391

IDAHO

Debra J. Mack, DVM
A Natural Choice
3660 Flint Dr.
Eagle, ID 83616-4534
Ph: 208-939-4800
Fax: 208-939-7304

Ronald L. Hamm, DVM
2337 Lago Liberty Rd.
Grace, ID 83241
Ph: 208-427-6233

ILLINOIS

Kathleen M. Von Ruff, DVM
VCA Aroma Park
3302 Old Waldron Road
Aroma Park, Illinois 60910
Ph: 815-937-9314

Julie A. Mayer, DVM
Portage Park Animal Hospital and Dental Clinic
5419 W. Irving Park Rd.
Chicago, IL 60641
Ph: 773-725-0260
Fax: 773-725-1830

Judith Rae Swanson, DVM
1465 W. Catalpa Ave.
Chicago, IL 60640-1255
Ph: 773-561-4526

Pamela Ann Craig, DVM
Animas Veterinary Clinic
320 East Neville
Grayslake, IL 60030
Ph: 847-223-5593
Fax: 847-223-4748

Annie Logan, DVM
17513 Streit Rd.
Harvard, IL 60033
Ph: 815-943-3101

Sharon L. Willoughby, DVM
Animal Chiropractic Center
623 Main Street
Hillsdale, IL 61257
Ph: 309-658-2920
Fax: 309-658-2622
www.animalchiro.com

Robert Williams, DVM
13835 N. State Hwy. One
Marshall, IL 62441
Ph: 217-826-5621
Fax: 217-826-6067

Herbert W. Preiser, DVM
Animal Natural Health Annex
2975 North Milwaukee Avenue
Northbrook, IL 60062
Ph: 847-827-5200
Fax: 847-827-7176

Karen Shaw Becker, DVM
Natural Pet Animal Hospital
17236 South Harlem
Tinley Park, IL 60477
Ph: 708-342-1111
Fax: 708-342-1608

Ellen M. Paul, DVM
Lipton Animal Hospital
908 East Maine
Urbana, IL 61802
Ph: 217-344-1017
Fax: 217-344-0654

INDIANA

William J. Hathaway, DVM
Trail Creek Animal Hospital
3025 E. Michigan Blvd.
Michigan City, IN 46360
Ph: 219-879-8241

Mark P. Haverkos, DVM
Village Veterinary Clinic
22163 Main St. Box 119
Oldenburg, IN 47036
Ph: 812-934-2410

ulie A. Anderson, DVM
Rockville Animal Clinic
P.O. Box 150 US 41 North
Rockville, IN 47872
Ph: 765-569-3210
Fax: 765-569-0837

Suzanne D. Michel-Quintero, DVM
Quintessential Health
615 Hillcrest Road
W. Lafayette, IN 47906-2349
Ph/Fax: 765-463-9520

IOWA

Fred Mulch, DVM
Whitehaven Veterinary Clinic
5725 Brady St.
Davenport, IA 52906
Ph: 319-386-9680
Fax: 319-386-9681

Marilyn Lowe, DVM
Crawford County Veterinary Clinic
720 Broadway
Denison, IA 51442
Ph: 712-263-6089

KANSAS

Larry Snyder, DVM
Box 4135
Topeka, KS 66604
Ph: 785-233-3185
Fax: 785-233-5807

KENTUCKY

Kirk A. Weber, DVM
6008 Taylor Mill Rd.
Latonia Lakes, KY 41015
Ph: 606-356-2145
Fax: 606-356-2156

Virginia E. Garrison, DVM
4750 Hartland Pkwy #147
Lexington, KY 40515
Ph: 606-971-0947
Fax: 606-971-0947

Elizabeth Boswell, DVM
5607 Oxford Ct. #862
Louisville, KY 40291
Ph: 502-499-9663

Joy Dunn, DVM
RR #3 Box 236A
Mt. Vernon, KY 40456
Ph: 606-256-5360

LOUISIANA

David Murphy Lowdermilk, DVM
2220 Landau Lane
Bossier City, LA 71111
Ph/Fax: 318-742-9997
Equine

Elizabeth A. Ford-Jones, DVM
PO Box 11120
Jefferson, LA 70181-1120

Ph:504-734-7946
Mobile house calls

Mary Finley, DVM
Leonville, LA
Ph: 337-879-2020

Lowell K. Roger, DVM
539 Bonnabel Blvd.
Metairie, LA 70005
Ph: 504-832-5113
Fax: 504-832-5115
Equine

Casey Lestrade, DVM
P.O. Box 339
#4 Westbank Expressway
Westwego, LA 70094
Ph: 504-436-7911

MAINE

Judith K. Herman, DVM
95 Northern Ave.
Augusta, ME 04330
Ph: 207-623-1177
Fax: 207-626-5799
hermandvm@aol.com

Donald McLean, DVM
965 Crockett Ridge Rd.
Norway, ME 04268
Ph: 207-743-8346
holvet@megalink.net

MARYLAND

Gary Brooks, DVM
VCA Academy Animal Hospital
5915 Belair Rd.
Baltimore, MD 21206
Ph: 410-483-5162
Fax: 410-483-4331
www.vcai.com

Monique Maniet, DVM
Veterinary Holistic Care
4820 Moorland Lane
Bethesda, MD 20814

Ph: 301-656-2882
Fax: 301-656-5033

Scott B. Sanderson, DVM
East Columbia Animal Hospital
6490 Dobbin Rd.
Columbia, MD 21045
Ph: 410-992-7087
Fax: 410-992-0463

Nancy Ruth, DVM
2151 Defense Highway Suite 1
Crofton, MD 21114
Ph: 410-721-7387
Fax: 410-721-7385

Francine K. Rattner, VMD
South Arrundel Veterinary
Hospital
85 West Central Avenue
Edgewater, MD 21037
Ph: 410-956-2932
Fax: 410-956-3755
savet@annap.infi.net

Linda Gray, DVM
1200 W. Old Liberty Rd.
Eldersburg, MD 21784
Ph: 410-795-6106

John A. Eagling, DVM
11843 Ocean Gateway
Ocean City, MD 21842
Ph: 410-213-1170
Fax: 410-213-2128

Grace L. Calabrese, DVM
P.O. Box 245
Phoenix, MD 21131-0245
Ph: 410-557-6040

Cindy Dahle, VMD
Bay Area Veterinary Hospital
150 Kent Landing
Stevensville, MD 21666
Ph: 410-643-7888
Fax: 410-604-0081

MASSACHUSETTS

Ellen R. Crighton, DVM
130 Centre Street
Danvers, MA 01923
Ph: 978-739-4556
Large and small animals

Donna M. Raditic, D.V.M.
440 Stockbridge Road
Great Barrington, MA
Ph: 413-528-5577

Bud Allen, M.S., DVM
Family Vet Center
99 Main St.
Haydenville, MA 01039
Ph: 413-268-8387
Fax: 413-268-3899

Brian Corwin, DVM
Dog and Cat Housecalls
96 Inverness Lane
Longmeadow, MA 01106
Ph: 413-565-5104;
1-888-567-3840
brianvet@aol.com

Dorsie R. Kovacs, DVM
Monson Small Animal Clinic
125 Palmer Rd.
Monson, MA 01057
Ph: 413-267-5141
Fax: 413-267-4963

Rosemary L. Burdon, DVM
Carlee Memorial Animal Hospital
21 Crooked Lane
Nantucket, MA 02554
Ph: 508-228-1491
Fax: 508-325-5547
www.mspca.org

Stuart R. Hodder, DVM
Bliss Pond Veterinary Services
43 Smith Hanson Rd.
North Brookfield, MA 01535
Ph: 508-867-6898

Regina M. Downey, DVM
Coastal Animal Clinic
91 Bridge Road
Salisbury, MA 01952
Ph: 978-463-3309
Fax: 978-463-6930
www.coastalanimalclinic.baweb.com

Mark E. Broady, DVM
3 Mohawk Trail
Shelburne Falls, MA 01370
Ph: 413-625-9517

Jeffrey Levy, DVM
Natural Veterinary Care
71 Ashfield Road
Williamsburg, MA 01096
Ph: 413-268-3000
www.homeovet.net

MICHIGAN

Jeanne L. Romanik, DVM
Silverwood Veterinary Center
6994 Dutton SE
Caledonia, MI 49316
Ph: 616-554-9556
Only acupuncture and chiropractic
for small animals and horses

Charline S. Wilson, DVM
9964 Cherry Valley Suite 4
Caledonia, MI 49316
Ph: 616-891-7737

Harold D. Sheridan, DVM
West Michigan Veterinary Service
16025 68th Ave.
Coopersville, MI 49404
Ph: 616-837-8151
Fax: 616 837 7853

Susan G. McFall, DVM
Davison Veterinary Hospital
1510 Cummings Rd.
Davison, MI 48423
Ph: 810-653-4108
Fax: 810-653-4109

Lynne Friday, DVM
Lexington Veterinary Clinic
5346 Main St.
Lexington, MI 48450
Ph: 810-359-8828
Fax: 810-359-5046

Elizabeth Routson, DVM
Parkway Veterinary Clinic
41395 Wilcox Rd.
Plymouth, MI 48170
Ph: 734-453-2577

John M. Simon, DVM
Woodside Animal Clinic
27452 Woodward Avenue
Royal Oak, MI 48067
Ph: 248-545-6630
Fax: 248-545-7979

Grace Chang, DVM
Southfield Veterinary Office
24130 W. 10 Mile Road
Southfield, MI 48034-3038
Ph: 248-356-0822
Fax: 248-356-0826

Anne S. Rice, DVM
P.O. Box 373
Williamston, MI 48895
Ph/Fax: 517-655-3479

Sharon G. Yaskulski, DVM
Carr's Veterinary Clinic
P.O. Box 980304
Yasilanti, MI 48198
Ph: 734-482-8171

MINNESOTA

Dan Hartsell, DVM
6282 County Road 8 NW
Alexandria, MN 56308
Ph: 320-762-8076
Fax: 320-762-5027

Roger DeHaan, DVM
Holistic Veterinary Services
33667 Peace River Ranch Road
Frazee, MN 56544
Ph/Fax: 218-846-9112

Heather L. Evans, DVM
All Creatures Acupuncture
P.O. Box 50084
Minneapolis, MN 55405-0084
Ph: 612-243-0260

Glenn Nielsen, DVM
Waite Park Veterinary Hospital
and Holistic Health Center
37 2nd Ave. S.
Waite Park, MN 56387
Ph: 320-253-1061
Fax: 320-529-0125

MISSOURI

Ann Broeder, DVM
Animal Healthy Healing
2615 S. Big Bend Blvd
St. Louis, MO 63143
Ph: 314-781-1738

Christine J. Crosley, DVM
Animal Healthy Healing
2615 S. Big Bend Blvd
St. Louis, MO 63143
Ph: 314-781-1738

Robert Schaeffer, Jr., DVM
St. Louis Hills Veterinary Clinic
7001 Hampton Avenue
St. Louis, MO 63109
Ph: 314-353-3444
Fax: 314-353-1245

MONTANA

John K. Harshman, DVM
P.O. Box 371
Chinook, MT 59523
Ph: 406-357-2936
Fax 406-357-3367

Sara Stephens, DVM
Alpine Veterinary Service
500 South 5th West
Missoula, MT 59801
Ph: 406-728-4605

NEBRASKA

Diane Simmons, DVM
8625 1/2 Q St.
Ralston, NE 68127
Ph: 402-593-6556
Fax: 402-593-8810

NEVADA

Nancy Brandt, DVM
6160 W. Oquendo Rd.
Las Vegas, NV 89118
Ph: 702-598-5130
Fax: 702-658-1800

Linda Steelman, DVM
Bonanza Cat Hospital
7550 West Lake Mead Blvd. Ste 1
Las Vegas, NV 89128
Ph: 702-438-7000
Fax- 702-838-8512

Joanne Stefanatos, DVM
Animal Kingdom Veterinary
Hospital
1325 Vegas Valley Drive
Las Vegas, NV 89109
Ph: 702-735-7184
Fax: 702-735-8139
jstefanato@aol.com

J. Alan White, DVM
P.O. Box 1565
Minden, NV 89423
Ph: 775-782-8735
Equine

NEW HAMPSHIRE

George Tarkleson, DVM
Colebrook Veterinary Clinic
123 Main St.
Colebrook, NH 03576

Ph: 603-237-8871
Fax: 603-237-8248

Rosemary Manziano, DVM
Coltsneck Animal Clinic
85 Rt. 34 South
Coltsneck, NJ 07722
Ph: 732-780-4211
Fax: 732-294-4699

Charles T. Schenck, DVM
VCA Edgebrook Animal Hospital
777 Helmetta Blvd.
East Brunswick, NJ 08816
Ph: 732-257-8882
Fax: 732-254-2303

Robert W. Mueller, DVM
Fair Chance Farm
261 Randolph Rd.
Freehold, NJ 07728
Ph: 732-780-2202
Fax: 732-780-5159
rnmueller@exit109.com
Chiropractic care only

Kenneth D. Fischer, DVM
Hillsdale Animal Hospital
201 Broadway
Hillsdale, NJ 07642
Ph: 201-358-6520
Fax: 201-358-8332

Karin L. Johanson, DVM
Three Rivers Veterinary Services
Housecalls
28 Kitchell Road
Madison, NJ 07960
Ph: 973-292-3889
Fax: 973-292-3913

Mark D. Newkirk, DVM
Margate Animal Hospital
9200 Ventnor Ave.
Margate, NJ 08402
Ph: 609-823-3031
Fax: 609-822-9152

Gloria B. Weintrub, VMD
Countryside Veterinarian Hospital
190 Rt. 70
Medford, NJ 08055
Ph: 609-953-3502
Fax: 609-953-5329

Gerald Buchoff, DVM
North Bergen Animal Hospital
9018 Kennedy Blvd.
North Bergen, NJ 07047
Ph: 201-868-3753
Fax: 201-868-0453
drbuchoff@aol.com

Lori Walker-Wilson, DVM
Veterinary House Calls
9 Main Street
Sparta, NJ 07871
Ph: 973-729-7121
Fax: 973-726-0459

Michael Dym, VMD
28 B Holly Cove
Mt. Laurel, NJ 08054
Ph: 856-235-2524
Fax: 856-722-9240

Mona Ann Boudreaux, DVM
A Time to Heal
1925 Juan Tabo Suite E
Albuquerque, NM 87112
Ph: 505-450-4325

Annet L. Sheffield, DVM
2705 Juan Tabo NE, B-1
Albuquerque, NM 87112
Ph: 505-292-3666
Fax: 505-332-8187

Don Hamilton, DVM
P.O. Box 67
Ocate, NM 87734
Ph: 505-666-2091

B. Dee Blanco, DVM
Los Animales
P.O. Box 5865
Santa Fe, NM 87502-5865
Ph: 505-986-3434

Robert Norman Schwyzer, DVM
Santa Fe Equine
P.O. Box 2677
Santa Fe, NM 87501
Ph: 505-988-7999
Equine only

NEW YORK

George Glanzberg, VMD
64 White Creek Road
No. Bennington, VT 05257
(Near Albany, NY)
Ph: 802-442-8714
Fax: 802-447-2326

Christing Ochrymowych, DVM
Knoll's End Animal Hospital
106-7 Hartwell Rd.
Berkshire, NY 13736
Ph: 607-657-8555
Fax: 607-657-2803
info@knollsend.com

James M. Okrepki, DVM
Knoll's End Animal Hospital
106-7 Hartwell Rd.
Berkshire, NY 13736
Ph: 607-657-8555
Fax: 607-657-2803

Douglas Kappstatter, DVM
144 7th St.
Bethpage, NY 11714
Ph: 516-932-3089

Barbara Eisner-Leiman,
DVM, CVA
233 Berry Street
Brooklyn, NY 11211
Ph: 718-387-0541
and

163 Woodhollow Lane
New Rochelle, NY 10804

Sarah Ober, DVM
Candor Animal Care
2 Mill Street
Candor, NY 13743
Ph: 607-659-4220
Fax: 607-659 3346

Cynthia Lankenau, DVM
Holistic Center for Veterinary Care
9002 Sunset Drive
Colden, NY 14033
Ph: 716-941-9477

Wayne K. Herr, DVM
Suburban South Animal Hospital
1230 French Rd.
Depew, NY 14043
Ph: 716-668-0503
Fax: 716-668-0943

Noelle M. DeMasi, DVM
Petmend Animal Hospital
1999 Palmer Ave.
Larchmont, NY 10538
Ph: 914-834-9000
Fax: 914-834-9253

Steven M. Schultz, DVM
Countryside Veterinary Clinic
5860 South Transit Road
Lockport, NY 14094
Ph: 716-434-2838
Fax: 716-434-2921

Paul K. Johnson, DVM
The Animal Health Center
488 East Main St.
Middletown, NY 10940
Ph: 914-343-9888
Fax: 914-342-5006

Anne M. Apple, DVM
Apple Veterinary Care
P.O. Box 98
New Baltimore, NY 12124
Ph: 518-756-6600

Beatrice Ehrsam, DVM
New Paltz Animal Hospital
230 Main Street
New Paltz, NY 12561
Ph: 845-255-5055

Steven Kasanofsky, DVM
Riverside Animal Hospital
250 W 100th Street
New York, NY 10025
www.holisticvets.com

Phillip Raclyn, DVM
Riverside Veterinary Group
219 W 79th St.
New York, NY 10024
Ph: 212-787-1993
Fax: 212-787-1397

Peter L. Brown, DVM
Keuka Lake Veterinarian Clinic
112 W. Lake Road
Penn Yan, NY 14527
Ph: 315-536-2771

Marilyn I. Schmidt, DVM
The Equine Clinic at Oaken Croft
880 Bridge St.
Ravena, NY 12143
Ph: 518-767-2906
Fax: 518-767-3503

Burton D. Miller, DVM
Riverhead Animal Hospital
1182 W. Main St.
Riverhead, NY 11901
Ph: 516-727-2009
Fax: 516-727-7540

Michele A. Yasson, DVM
Holistic Veterinary Services
1101 Rt. 32
Rosendale, NY 12472
Ph: 845-658-3923
Fax: 845-658-3884
and

Heart of Chelsea Animal Hospital
257 West 18th Street
New York, NY 10011

Ronald A. Scharf, DVM
Animal Hospital of Noskayuna
2764 Troy Rd.
Schenectedy, NY 12309
Ph: 518-785-9731
Fax: 518-785-9741

Christine E. N. Aiken, D.V.M.
Smith Ridge Veterinary Center
400 Smith Ridge Road
South Salem, NY 10590
Ph: 914-533-6066
Fax: 914-533-6405

Martin Goldstein, DVM
Director, Smith Ridge Veterinary
Center of South Salem, New York
400 Smith Ridge Road
South Salem, NY 10590
Ph: 914-533-6066

Cliff N. Conarck, D.V.M.
810 Middle Country Rd.
St. James, NY 11780
Ph: 631-265-1438

John F. Sangiorgio, DVM
The Veterinary Emergency Center
1293 Clove Road
Staten Island, NY 10301
Ph: 718-720-4211
Fax: 718-720-4212

Patrick Tersigni, VMD
Equipower
1807 Hemmer Rd.
Wayland, NY 14572
Ph: 716-728-5562
Small and large animals

Craig H. Russell, DVM
Westport Animal Hospital
PO Box 396 Pleasant St.
Westport, NY 12993

Ph: 518-962-8228
Fax: 518-962-8308

Marc A. Franz, DVM
Woodbury Animal Hospital
145 Woodbury Road
Woodbury, NY 11797
Ph: 516-367-7100
Fax: 516-367-7119

Andrea Jacobson, DVM
30 Woodybrook Lane
Croton-on-Hudson, NY 10520
Ph: 914-271-2227
Fax: 914-271-7922
Feline only

NORTH CAROLINA

Laurel M. Davis, DVM
Asheville Veterinary House Calls
3 Webb Cove Rd.
Asheville, NC 28804
Ph: 828-254-2221
Fax: 828-254-2227

Margaret Federhart, DVM
Whispering Waters Veterinary
Clinic
122 Astor Cook Rd.
Blowing Rock, NC 28605
Ph: 828-295-9181
Fax: 828-295-9112

Kim V. Hombs, DVM
Atrium Animal Hospital
6520 McMahon Drive
Charlotte, NC 28226
Ph: 704-542-2000
Fax: 704-543-8455

James E. Schacht, DVM
Idlewild Animal Hospital
6400 E. Independence Blvd.
Charlotte, NC 28212
Ph: 704-535-6688
Fax: 704 535 6669
idlewild@charlotte.infi.net

Dana L. Lehr, VMD
Academy Pet Hospital
200 Owen Drive
Fayetteville, NC 2830
Ph: 910-484-7153
Fax: 910-484-0527

Ann M. Davis, DVM
Greensboro Veterinary Hospital
3741 High Point Rd.
Greensboro, NC 27407
Ph: 336-299-5431
Fax: 336-299-5441

Charles E. Loops, D.V.M.
38 Waddell Hollow Road
Pittsboro, NC 27312
Ph: 919-542-0442
Fax: 919-542-0535
Available for phone consultations

Gale Gilbert Bowman, DVM
Bowman Animal Hospital
P.O. Box 68099
Raleigh, NC 27613
Ph: 919-847-6216
Fax: 919-870-5605

OHIO

Robert E. Neubauer, DVM
Mount Healthy Animal Hospital
9199 Pippin Rd.
Cincinnati, OH 45251
Ph: 513-931-9127
Fax: 513-931-9137

Cathy A. Petrasky, DVM
Acupuncture and Veterinary
Services
house call practice
Cincinnati / Dayton area
Ph/Fax: 513-934-2992

Donn W. Griffith, DVM
Animal Medical and Emergency
Hospital
3859 W. Dublin-Granville Rd.
Dublin, OH 43017

Ph: 614-889-2556
Fax: 614-889-8184

Robert Gaston, DVM
Cincinnati Southwest Veterinary
Care
9970 Harrison Ave.
Harrison, OH 45030
Ph: 513-367-4111
Fax: 513-367-4145
www.vetwellness.com

Ronald L. McNutt, DVM
Lima Animal Hospital
2909 Elida Road
Lima, OH 45805
Ph: 419-331-1456
Fax: 419 331 5598

Pamela Fisher, DVM
Viking Community Animal
Hospital
434 N Main Street
North Canton, OH 44720
Ph: 330-494-7387
Fax: 330-494-8179

Gail E. Counts, DVM
Shawnee Animal Clinic
101 Bierly Rd.
Portsmouth, OH 45662
Ph: 740-353-5758
Fax: 740-353-5438
www.petdoctorohio.com
www.petmall.com

Karen Spracklen, DVM
12318 Midway Road
South Solon, OH 43153
Ph: 937-462-8600
Fax: 937-462-8093
Equine

Sandra M. Snell, DVM
Sycamore Animal Hospital
1277 State Hwy 67 N.
Sycamore, OH 44882

Ph: 419-927-2548
Fax: 419-927-9034

David A. Drake, DVM
Countryside Animal Hospital
5510 Monroe St.
Sylvania, OH 43560
Ph: 419-882-7688
Fax: 419-882-8844

C. Scott Hosket, DVM
Hosket Veterinary Service
4450 Rt. 68 North
Yellow Springs, OH 45387
Ph: 937-767-7422
Fax: 937-767-1701

OKLAHOMA

Nita McNeill, DVM
Mustang Animal Clinic
130 E. Hwy 152
Mustang, OK 73064
Ph: 405-376-4556
Fax: 405-376-2831

Rebecca Coleman, DVM
All Pets Veterinary Hospital
6909 East 6th Street
Stillwater, OK 74074
Ph: 405-624-8622

George A. Carley, DVM
Hunters Glen Veterinary Hospital
9150 South Braden
Tulsa, OK 74137
Ph: 918-493-3332
Fax: 918-493-7401
www.huntersglenvet.com

OREGON

Donna M Starita, DVM
A Country Way
P.O. Box 485
Boring, OR 97009
Ph: 503-663-7277

R.H. Anderson, DVM
Polk Veterinary Clinic
1590 E. Ellendale
Dallas, OR 97338
Ph: 503-623-8318
Fax: 503-623-1109

Doreen Hock, DVM
252 W. 7th Ave.
Eugene, OR 97401
Ph: 541-345-1608

Chuck Hawkins, DVM
Dogwood Pet Hospital
1440 E. Powell
Gresham, OR 97030
Ph: 503-667-9457
Fax: 503-669-1659
www.dogwoodpet.com

Brian Reister, DVM
East Lane Veterinary Hospital
42755 McKenzie Hwy.
Leaburg, OR 97489
Ph: 541-896-0044
Fax: 541-896-9882

Albert J. Simpson, DVM
Berry Hill Veterinary Hospital
19073 South Beaver Creek Rd.
Oregon City, OR 97045
Ph: 503-650-1667
Fax: 503 650 8689
www.berryhillvet.com

Lisa M. Hoberg, DVM
3067 NE Oregon St.
Portland, OR 97232
Ph: 503-239-5670

Jeffrey Judkins, DVM
The Whole Pet Veterinary Clinic
1431 SE 23rd
Portland, OR 97214
Ph: 503-233-2332
Fax: 503-233-7246
wholepet@spiritone.com

Bob Ulbrich, VMD
The Whole Pet Veterinary Clinic
1431 SE 23rd
Portland, OR 97214
Ph: 503-233-2332
Fax: 503-233-7246
wholepet@spiritone.com

PENNSYLVANIA

James L. Bianco, VMD
Ardmore Animal Hospital
24 East Athens Avenue
Ardmore, PA 19003
Ph: 610-642-1160
Fax: 610-896-8790
www.ardmore-ah.com

John C. Harthorn, DVM
2176 Brush Run Rd.
Avella, PA 15312
Ph: 724-345-3350
Fax: 724-345-3706

Douglas E. Knueven, DVM
Beaver Animal Clinic
357 State Street
Beaver, PA 15009
Ph: 724-774-8047
Fax: 724-774-5774
www.beaveranimalclinic.com

Jay N. Leeb, VMD
Bensalem Veterinary Hospital
3462 Bristol Pike
Bensalem, PA 19020
Ph: 215-297-0750/215-638-1595
Fax: 215-638-1693

Susan Beal, DVM
Big Run Healing Arts
Box 550
Big Run, PA 15716
Ph: 814-427-5004
Fax: 814-427-5929

Glen Dupree, DVM
Big Run Healing Arts
Box 19
Big Run, PA 15715
Ph: 814-427-5004
Fax: 814-427-5929

Linda T. Stern, DVM
Avian and Feline Hospital
3300 Hartzdale Drive
Camp Hill, PA 17011
Ph: 717-730-3755

Elizabeth E. Burke, DVM
Thoreau Veterinary Hospital
929 Northampton St.
Easton, PA 18042
Ph: 610-559-0728
Fax: 610-559-0367

Cynthia Maro, DVM
Ellwood Animal Hospital
728 Lawrence Ave.
Ellwood City, PA 16117
Ph: 724-758-8882
Fax: 724-758-2740

Sheldon L. Gerstenfeld, VMD
Chestnut Hill Veterinary Hospital
and Bird Clinic
903 Bethlehem Pike
Erdenhelm, PA 19038
Ph: 215-836-2950

Louise I. Morin, VMD
Delaware Valley Animal Hospital
266 Lincoln Highway
Fairless Hills, PA 19030
Ph: 215-946-1111
Fax: 215-946-7757

Rose M. DiLeva, VMD
Animal Wellness Center and
Mobile Veterinary Services
20 Park Lane
Glen Mills, PA 19342
Ph: 610-558-1616
Fax: 610-558-9190

Christine Makoski, DVM
Landenburg Veterinary Clinic
1611 New London Rd.
Landenberg, PA 19350
Ph: 610-255-5372
cmakowski@dplus.net

Linda S. Bachin, VMD
3268 Barley Lane
Lansdale, PA 19446
Ph: 610-222-0500
Avian

Lee Simpson, DVM
Healing Options for Animals
250 Greenwich Street
Kutztown, PA 19530
Ph: 610-683-9303

Susan Yatsky, VMD
New Britain Animal Clinic
341 W. Butler Avenue
New Britain, PA 18901
Ph: 215-340-0345

Michael S. Tierney, VMD
Keystone Veterinary Hospital
428 Brownsburg Rd.
Upper Makefield
Newtown, PA 18940
Ph: 215-598-3951
Fax: 215-598-3746

C. Edgar Sheaffer, VMD
Park Veterinary Clinic
47 N. Railroad St.
P.O. Box 353
Palmyra, PA 17078-0353
Ph: 717-838-9563
Fax: 717-838-0377

Sally Myton, VMD
999 Killarney Drive
Pittsburgh, PA 15234
Ph: 412-884-2434
Fax: 412-884-5222

Jeanne F. Wordley, VMD
Old Marple Veterinary Hospital
820 West Springfield Road
Springfield, PA 19064
Ph: 610-328-1300

Don M. Heinert, DVM
Natural Animal Veterinary Clinic
42 Waterford Street
Union City, PA 16438
Ph: 814-438-3800

Judith M. Shoemaker, D.V.M.
P.O. Box 130
West Grove, PA 19390
Ph: 610-998-0526

Devea K. Khalsa, V.M.D.
Animal Healing Center
1724 Yardley-Langhorne Rd.
Yardley, PA 19067-5517
Ph: 215-493-0621
Fax: 215-493-1944

RHODE ISLAND

Elizabeth Hassinger, DVM (formerly Dr. Campbell)
Wolfrock Animal Health Center
710 South County Trail
Exeter, RI 02822
Ph: 401-294-0102
Fax: 401-294-8178

SOUTH CAROLINA

Rosemarie Asterino, DVM
Clinton Animal Hospital
P.O. Box 483
Clinton, SC 29325
Ph: 864-833-2487

Jeanne R. Fowler, DVM
All About Pets Incorporated
409 Old Buncombe Rd.
Travelers Rest, SC 29690
Ph: 864-834-7334
Fax: 864-834-1003

TENNESSEE

Rai Kaur Khalsa, VMD
Fountain City Animal Hospital
5630 N. Broadway
Knoxville, TN 37918
Ph: 865-688-0776

Sandra Priest, DVM
Four Winds Holistic Animal Services
600 Bennington Circle
Knoxville, TN 37909
Ph: 865-690-3863
www.homeearthlink.net/~four-winds

Terry G. Brockman, DVM
Richland Animal Clinic
6043 Charlotte Avenue
Nashville, TN 37209
Ph: 615-356-6534
Fax: 615-353-0868

TEXAS

Joseph A. Kincaid, DVM
Anthony Animal Clinic
901 Franklin St.
P.O. Box 2696
Anthony, TX 79821
Ph: 915-886-4558
Fax: 915-886-2556

Nancy A. Bozeman, DVM
The Animal Doctor
5721 SW Green Oaks Blvd.
Arlington, TX 76017
Ph: 817-572-2400
Fax: 817-572-2026

Jerry B. Dittrich, DVM
Animal Healthcare
1115 W. Mayfield Rd.
Arlington, TX 76015
Ph: 817-467-6688
Fax: 817-467-1509

Susan D. Eakle, DVM
Griffith Small Animal Hospital
3407 Northland Dr.
Austin, TX 78731
Ph: 512-453-5828
Fax: 572-453-5889

William Falconer, DVM
Austin, TX
Ph: 512-288-5400

Kathryn Van Winkle, DVM
Barton Creek Animal Clinic
4201 Westbank Drive
Austin, TX 78746
Ph: 512-327-8300

Charles Vandermause, DVM
Crystal Mountain Animal Hospital
8947 Bee Caves Rd. #206
Austin, TX 78746
Ph: 512-263-2900

Madalyn Ward, DVM
Bear Creek Animal Clinic
11608 fm 1826
Austin, TX 78737
Ph: 512-288-0428
Fax: 512-288-1117
www.holistichorsekeeping.com
Equine

Denise Easterling, DVM
Easterling Veterinary Clinic
P.O. Box 248
942 Hwy. 75N
Centerville, TX 75833
Ph: 903-536-2796
Fax: 903-536-6702

Jackie Cole, DVM
Campeche Cove Animal and Bird
Hospital
3802 Cove View Blvd.
Galveston, TX 77554
Ph: 409-740-0808

S. J. Gravel, DVM
Harmony Path Clinic
185 Old Lytton Springs Road
Rte 2 Box 140
Hwy 183 N.
Lockhart, TX 78644
Ph: 512-398-3719

Thomas L. Granger, DVM
Countryside Veterinary Clinic
380 North LHS Drive
Lumberton, TX 77656
Ph: 409-755-7216

Wendy Elaine Culp Blount, DVM
Companion Animal Medicine
Services
1093 Woodhaven Dr.
Nacogdoches, TX 75961
Ph: 936-569-2038
Fax: 936-568-9991
drblount@vonallmen.net

Shawn P. Messonnier, D.V.M.
2145 West Park Boulevard
Plano, TX 75075
Ph: 972-867-8800
naturalvet@juno.com
www.petcarenaturally.com

Paul R. Bruton, DVM
Animal Healthcare Clinic of
Southlake
1615 E. Southlake Blvd.
Southlake, TX 76092
Ph: 817-481-1382
animalhealthcare@aol.com

Betsy Walker Harrison, DVM
House calls and telephone consultations
100 Park Rd. SO.
Wimberly, TX 78676
Ph: 830-935-2596
Fax: 830-935-2590

Kimberly Henneman, DVM
6300 North Sagewood Drive
Suite H #225
Park City, Utah 84098
Ph: 435-647-0807
Fax: 435-647-2985
vuduvet#1@aol.com

VERMONT

Stephanie Woolwick-Holzman,
VMD
Arlington Animal Hospital
3195 Rt. 7A
Arlington, VT 05250
Ph: 802-375-9491
Fax: 802-375-9337

Patty Pruitt, DVM
Open Air Pet Repair
53 Washington St.
Middlebury, VT 05753
Ph: 802-388-7501

George Glanzberg, VMD
64 White Creek Road
North Bennington, VT 05257
Ph: 802-442-8714
Fax: 802-447-2326

William Conrad Kruesi, D.V.M.
87 E. Clarendon Road, Route 103
North Clarendon, VT 05759-9650
Ph: 802-747-4076
Fax: 802-747-0283
www.crvetcenter.com

VIRGINIA

Robert C. Brown, DVM
Cherrydale Veterinary Clinic
4038 Lee Highway
Arlington, VA 22207
Ph: 703-528-9001
Fax: 703-243-8586
www.cherrydalevet.com

Cheryl A. Caputo, DVM
Pet Health Clinic
840 Roanoke Rd.
P.O. Box 240
Daleville, VA 24083
Ph: 540-992-4550
www.pethealthclinic.com

Anne Garrood, DVM
Great Falls Animal Hospital
10125 Colvin Run Road
Great Falls, VA 22066
Ph: 703-759-2330

Rebecca L.G. Verna, DVM
Bullrun Veterinary Hospital
14840 Washington St.
Haymarket, VA 20169
Ph: 703-754-4146
Fax: 703-754-1843

Constance Pozniak, DVM
Boulevard Veterinary Hospital
6636 Virginia Beach Blvd.
Norfolk, VA 23502
Ph: 757-461-4416
Fax: 757-466-7844

Jordan A. Kocen, DVM
6136 Brandon Ave.
Springfield, VA 22150
Ph: 703-569-0300
www.southpawsvet.com

Linda Joyce Taylor, DVM
Rt. 6 Box 86
Tazewell, VA 24651
Ph: 540-988-7984
Fax: 540-988-8200
Horses and farm animals

Paul D. Rowan, DVM
Owl Creek Veterinary Hospital
587 S. Birdneck Rd.
Virginia Beach, VA 23451
Ph: 757-428-4344
Fax: 757-422-2064

Joyce C. Harman, DVM, MRCVS
P.O. Box 488
Washington, VA 22747-0008
Ph: 540-675-1855
Fax: 540-675-1447

Meryl Lessinger-Bely, VMD
Animal Clinic of Williamsburg
7316 Merrimac Trail
Williamsburg, VA 23185
Ph: 757-253-0812
Fax: 757-253-0908

WASHINGTON

Tevinder Sodhi, DVM
Animal Wellness Center
2115-112th Ave. NE
Bellevue, WA 98006
Ph: 425-455-8900
Fax: 425-455-9946
www.holisticpetcare.com

Michelle C. Schraeder, DVM
Mountain Veterinary Hospital
3413 Mt. Baker Hwy.
Bellingham, WA 98226
Ph: 360-592-5113
Fax: 360-592-3112

Frank W. Bischak, DVM
Bremerton Animal Hospital
613 N. Callow Ave.
Bremerton, WA 98312
Ph: 360-373-7333
Fax: 360-373-7457

Will Rowe, DVM
Creekside Veterinary Service
P.O. Box 409
Chewelah, WA 99109
Ph: 509-935-8936
Fax: 509-935-8271

Jan Richards, DVM
P.O. Box 97
Chimacum, WA 98325
Ph: 360-385-4488
www.allmyrelations.org

Lee J. Herzig, DVM
Four Winds Veterinary Clinic
102 Washington Avenue South
Eatonville, WA 98328
Ph: 360-832-6500
Fax: 360-832-6252

Douglas R. Yearout, DVM
9004 Vernon Rd.
Everett, WA 98205
Ph: 425-334-8171
Fax: 425-334-1136

William J. Burlingame, DVM
Quilceda Veterinary Hospital
1263 State Ave.
Marysville, WA 98270
Ph: 360-659-8482
Fax: 360-658-9414

Patti Schaefer, DVM
Canisport Veterinary
Therapeutic Services
Olympia, WA 98501
Ph: 360-923-5759

Charles W. Coleman, DVM
Coleman Veterinarian Clinic
621 W. Clark St.
Pasco, WA 99301
Ph: 509-545-4931
Fax: 509-545-4451

Michael H. Cable, DVM
Big Valley Veterinary
Services P.S., Inc
25297 Big Valley Rd.
Poulsbo, WA 98370
Ph: 360-697-1650
Fax: 360 697-6974
www.bigvalleypetresort.com

Larry Siegler, DVM
Animal Healing Center
8015 165th. Ave. N.E.
Redmond, WA 98052
Ph: 425-885-5400
Fax: 425-869-2304

Michael W. Lemmon, DVM
Highlands Veterinary Hospital
P.O. Box 2085
Renton, WA 98056
Ph: 425-226-8418

Nancy A. Bauer, DVM
Carkeek Park Veterinary Hospital
9756 Holman Road NW
Seattle, WA 98117
Ph: 206-789-8505
Fax: 206-789-1317

Donna Kelleher, DVM
2536 Alki Ave. SW
Box 143
Seattle, WA 98116
Ph: 206-935-3041

Kerry Fisher, DVM
Animal Pain Management Center
11901 North Division
Spokane, WA 99218
Ph: 509-468-0443
Fax: 509-468-0452

WEST VIRGINIA

Jane Laura Doyle, DVM
Berkeley Springs, WV
Ph: 304-258-5819
animalia@intrepid.net

WISCONSIN

Janet D. Schnell, DVM, AVCA
Dairyland Veterinary Clinic
16244 S. Swedish Hwy.
Dairyland, WI 54830
Ph: 715-244-3881
emailjschnell@win.bright.net

Tom Cameron, DVM
Deforest Veterinary Clinic
416 Mohican Pass
Deforest, WI 53532
Ph: 608-846-3933

Maria H. Glinski, DVM
Silver Spring Animal

Wellness Center
1405 W. Silver Spring Drive
Glendale, WI 53209
Ph: 414-228-7655
Fax: 414-228-1072

Barbara Noeldner, DVM
Madison Cat Clinic
601 N. Sherman
Madison, WI 53704
Ph: 608-249-2822
Fax: 608-249-2775

Andrew Zuckerman, DVM
Small Animal Hospital
2163 N. Farwell Ave.
Milwaukee, WI 53202
Ph: 414-276-0701
Fax: 414-276-7019

Jan Harkins, DVM
Reedsburg Small Animal Clinic
222 N. Walnut St.
Reedsburg, WI 53959
Ph: 608-524-6545

Marta Engel, DVM
Rising Sun Animal
Wellness Center
315 E. Decker St.
Viroqua, WI 54665
Ph: 608-637-2227
Fax: 608-637-2648

Barbara J. Smith, DVM
Waterloo Veterinary Clinic
801 Canal Rd.
Waterloo, WI 53594
Ph: 920-478-3234
Fax: 920-478-4044

WYOMING

Vicki Burton, DVM
Healing Ways Veterinary Care
Mobile Practice
Laramie, WY 82070
Ph: 307-742-2488

OTHER HOLISTIC PRACTITIONERS

ANIMAL COMMUNICATORS

Sharon Callahan
Phone consultations
and flower essences
Ph: 530-926-6424
Fax: 530-926-1245
www.anaflora.com.
Phone consultations

Barbara S. Shor
30884 Kings Valley Drive
Conifer, CO 80433.
Ph: 303-838-3419
barbara@barbarashor.com

"I get into a quiet, centered state, and I tune into the animal. I focus my attention totally on that animal, I call in all of our guidance, and I ask for information that's for the highest good of all concerned."
—Barbara Shor

DOG INSTRUCTORS

Melissa Drake Campbell
Manager of Public Relations
The Seeing Eye, Inc.
P.O. Box 375
Morristown, NJ 07963-0375
Ph: 973-539-4425
Fax: 973-539-0922
www.seeingeye.org

For information on breeding, raising, and training dog guides and instructing qualified blind people in their use.

Alan Finn
Designing Dogs
516 Sibley Ave.
Old Forge, NY 18518

Helps dogs with behavior problems

September Morn
Ph: 360-738-4599
morndogs@aol.com
Teaches gentle dog training methods

Susan Travellin
Woodside Farm Dog and Horse Training
Califon, NJ 07830
Ph: 908-832-9453
smtrave@aol.com

NATURAL BIRD CARE

Alicia McWatters, Ph.D.
Ph: 505-281-5168
holisticparrot@mcwatters.org
www.parrothouse.com/
McWatter.htm

HELP FOR HORSES

Sam Powell Equine Consulting Services, Inc
P.O. Box 892
Hendersonville, TN 37077-0892
Ph: 615-826-2876
www.asksampowell.com

Barry Seedman
Hypnosis Institute
New York City
Ph: 800-494-9766

(Also see Susan Travellin under Dog Teacher and TTEAM)

TTEAM AND T-TOUCH INSTRUCTOR

Debra Potts
18505 NE Bald Peak Road
Newberg, OR 97132.
Ph: 503-538-8637

TTeam and T-Touch Santa Fe
Ph: 800-854-8326

TTeam and T-Touch Canada
Ph: 800-255-2336

"Our intent is to help the being be the very, very best it can be. We're looking at physical, mental, and emotional balance. We're looking at the body being as comfortable as it can be, and we're making sure that the animal's getting clear communication from the person s o that the relationship can be the very best that it can be."
—Debra Potts

HOLISTIC VETERINARY ORGANIZATIONS

AMERICAN HOLISTIC VETERINARY MEDICAL ASSOCIATION
2218 Old Emmorton Road
Bel Air, MD 21015
Ph: 410-569-0795
www.altvetmed.com

INTERNATIONAL VETERINARY ACUPUNCTURE SOCIETY (IVAS)

P.O. Box 271395
Fort Collins, CO 80527-1395
Ph: 970-266-0666
Fax: 970-266-0777
www.ivas.org

AMERICAN ACADEMY OF VETERINARY ACUPUNCTURE
P.O. Box 419
Hygiene, CO 80533-0419
Ph: 303-772-6726
AAVAoffice@aol.com

AMERICAN VETERINARIANS AND CHIROPRACTORS ASSOCIATION (AVCA)
623 Main Street
Hillsdale, IL 61257
Ph: 309-658-2920
Fax: 309-658-2622
AmVetChiro@aol.com

NATIONAL CENTER FOR HOMEOPATHY
801 North Fairfax Street, Ste 306
Alexandria, VA 22314
Ph: 703-548-7790
Ph: 877-624-0613
Fax: 703-548-7792
www.homeopathic.org

INTERNATIONAL FOUNDATION FOR HOMEOPATHY
P.O. Box 7
Edmonds, WA 98020
Ph: 425-776-4147
Fax: 425-776-1499
ifh@nwlink.com

ACADEMY OF VETERINARY HOMEOPATHY (AVH)
751 NE 168th Street
North Miami, FL 33162-2427
Ph: 305-652-5372
Fax: 305-653-7244
webmaster@acadvethom.org

ASSOCIATION OF VETERINARIANS FOR ANIMAL RIGHTS
P.O. Box 208
Davis, CA 95617-0208
Ph: 530-759-8106
Fax: 530-759-8116
AVAR@igc.org
www.AVAR.org

RECOMMENDED READING

COMPANION ANIMALS

*All You Ever Wanted to Know
About Herbs for Pets*
by Greg and Mary Tilford
(Bowtie Press, 1999)

*Cherished Messages and Memories
as Told by an Animal Communicator*
by Lydia Hiby with Bonnie S.
Weintraub (NewSage Press, 1998)

*Disposable Animals: Ending
the Tragedy of Throwaway Pets*
by Craig Brestrup
(Camino Bay Books: 1997)

*Dogs Never Lie About Love:
Reflections on the Emotional World of
Dogs* by Jeffrey Moussaieff Masson
(Random House, 1997)

*Dr. Pitcairn's Complete Guide to
Natural Health for Dogs and Cats* by
Richard H. Pitcairn, DVM, PhD
and Susan H. Pitcairn
(Rodale Press, 1995)

*Foods Pets Die For: Shocking Facts
About Pet Food* by Ann N. Martin
(NewSage Press, 1997)
newsage@teleport.com
www.teleport.com/~newsage

*Home-Prepared Dog and Cat Diets:
The Healthful Alternative*
By Donald R. Strombeck, DVM,
PhD (Iowa State University Press,
1999)

*The Natural Pet Care Series of
Pocket Guides* (Crossing Press)

Supernutrition for Dogs 'n' Cats
By Nina Anderson
& Dr. Howard Peiper
Ph: 888-NATURE1

*277 Secrets Your Dog Wants You
to Know* by Paulette Cooper
(Ten Speed Press, 1998)

*277 Secrets Your Cat Wants You
to Know* by Paulette Cooper
(Ten Speed Press, 1997)

*You Have a Visitor: Observations on
Pet Visitations and Therapy*
by Renee Lamm Esordi
(Blue Lamm Publishing, 2000)
www.youhaveavisitor.com

For the Love of Animals
A holistic monthly publication
that talks about the latest
approaches to disease
prevention and treatment.
Ph: 800-211-6365
Fax: 800-711-2292

EXOTIC ANIMALS

*Almost a Whisper: A Holistic
Approach to Working with Your Horse*
by Sam Powell with Lane Carter
Alpine Productions, Inc.
225 South Madison
Loveland, CO 80537-6514
www.asksampowell.com

*Naturally Healthy Bird: Nutrition,
Feeding, and Natural Healing
Methods for Parrots* by Alicia
McWatters (Safe Goods, 1997)

Training Your Pet Ferret by
Geraldine Buscis (Barrons
Educational Series, 1997)

*277 Secrets Your Snake and Lizard
Want You to Know* by Paulette
Cooper (Ten Speed Press, 1999)

PRODUCTS FOR THE NATURAL PET

AVJ Natural Cat
(health foods, supplements,
unique gifts)
6 South Hanover Street
Pottstown, PA 19464
1-610-326-0177
www.naturalcat.com

Anaflora (flower essences)
P.O. Box 1056
Mt. Shasta, CA 96067
Ph: 530-926-6424
Fax: 530-926-1245
info@anaflora.com
www.anaflora.com.

Animals Apawthecary
(low-alcohol herbal extracts)
P.O. Box 212
Conner, MT 59827
Ph: 406-821-4090
animals@bitterroot.net

Arrowroot Natural Pharmacy
(homeopathic remedies)
83 E. Lancaster Avenue
Paoli, PA 19301
Ph: 610-640-2720

Azmira.com
(holistic products for your pet)
2100 N. Wilmot Road, Suite 109
Tucson, AZ 85712
Ph: 800-497-5665
Fax: 520-886-2638
info@azmira.com

Dr. Ian Dunbar
c/o James and Kenneth Publishers
(behavior books and tapes)
2140 Shattuck Avenue
Suite 2406
Berkley, CA 94706
Ph: 510-658-8588

Earth Animal
(a variety of natural health
care products for your pet)
606 Post Road East
Westport, CT 06880
Ph: 800-622-0260
rgoldstein@earthanimal.com
sgoldstein@earthanimal.com
www.earthanimal.com

Mike Reed
(specially formulated fish foods)
M. Reed Enterprises
P.O. Box 1930
Sutter Creek, CA 95685
Ph: 209-267-1175
mreed@mreed.com
www.mreed.com

Flea Busters
(natural flea products)
6555 NW 9th Avenue
Suite 411-412
Ft. Lauderdale, FL 33309
Ph: 800-353-2786

Frontier Herbs
(organic herbs)
P.O. Box 299
Norway, IA 52318
Ph: 800-669-3275
www.frontiercoop.com

Halo, Purely for Pets
(human-grade quality food for
dogs, cats, birds; whole- food
supplements; natural pet care
products)
3438 East Lake Road
Suite 14-PMB 612
Palm Harbor, FL 34685
Ph: 813-854-2214
www.halopets.com

Kent Homeopathic Associates
(homeopathic remedies)
1386 San Anselmo Avenue
San Anselmo, CA 94960
Ph: 415-457-0678
(sold to veterinarians only)

Luyties Pharmaceutical Company
(homeopathic remedies)
St. Louis, MO 63158-8080
Ph: 800-325-8080

McZand and
Natrabio, Inc. (herbs)
P.O. Box 5312
Santa Monica, CA 90405
Ph: 800-800-0405
www.natrabio.com
(manufactured for people,
but some veterinarians
recommend their products)

Natural Animal
(herbs, organic products)
7000 US 1 North
St. Augustine, FL 32095
Ph: 800-274-7387
www.naturalanimal.com

Natural Animal
Nutrition (supplements)
2109 Emmorton Park Rd.
Suite 113
Edgewood, MD 21040
Ph: 800-548-2899

Natural Life Pet
Products (pet food)
P.O. Box 943
Frontenac, KS 66762
Ph: 800-367-2391
www.fament.com/natlife

Nature's Sunshine (herbs)
P.O. Box 1000
Spanish Fork, UT 84660
Ph: 801-798-9861

Pet Guard, Inc.
(pet food and skin products)
P.O. Box 728
Orange Park, FL 32067-0728
Ph: 800-874-3221

PETicular (safe insect repellants
and other herbal products)
Ph: 619-239-0708

Pets 'n' People, Inc.
(Nature's Miracle Stain and
Odor Remover and other natural
cleaning products)
Ph: 310-544-7125

Premier Pet Products
(Gentle Leader Collars)
406 Branchway Road
Richmond, VA 23236
Ph: 888-640-8840
www.gentleleader.com

Prozyme Products, LTD
(Prozyme)
6444 North Ridgeway Avenue
Lincolnwood, IL 60712
Ph: 800-522-5537

Sojourner Farms (pet food)
One 19th Avenue South
Minneapolis, MN 55454
Ph: 888-867-6567
www.sojos.com

Standard Process Labs
(supplements, glandulars)
Ph: 800-848-5061
www.standardprocess.com

Wachter's
(organic sea products)
360 Shaw Road
South San Francisco, CA 94080
Ph: 800-682-7100
Fax: 650-875-1626
www.wachters.com

Weleda Pharmacy, Inc.
(homeopathic remedies,
herbal products)
841 S. Main Street
Spring Valley, NY
Ph: 914-352-6145

Wysong
(human-grade pet food
and supplements)
1880 North Eastman Road
Midland, MI 48642-7779
Ph: 800-748-0188
www.wysong.net

Whiskers
(holistic pet shop)
New York City
Ph: 800-whiskers

NATURAL CAT LITTERS

As cats may not take to a sudden
switch to a new litter, it's a good
idea to mix a little of the new litter
in with the old, gradually adding
more each time you change the
box, until the new brand has completely replaced the old one.

The World's Best Cat Litter
Earth Animal
606 Post Road East
Westport, CT 06880
Ph: 800-622-0260
www.earthanimal.com

Completely safe for kittens
and cats, even when ingested,
because it is made from
crumbled corn kernels.

Care Fresh
Absorption Corporation
1051 Hilton Avenue
Bellingham, WA 98225
Ph: 800-242-2287

Dust-free, biodegradable,
naturally deodorized, flushable,
paper-based product.

Cat Country Organics
Premium Litter for Cats
M.M.P., Inc.
P.O. Box 778
Lewiston, MT 59457
Ph: 800-752-8864
www.mtnmeadowspet.com

Dust-free, biodegradable,
plant-based, naturally deodorized,
flushable product.

Good Mews
Stutzman Environmental Products
P.O. Box 307
Canby, OR 97013
Ph: 888-877-7665
Fax: 503-266-8776
www.stutzman-environmental.com
goodmews@stutzmzman-
environmental.com

100% recycled, palletized organic
fiber, scented with cedar oil.

Hi-Tor Dust-Free
Cat Litter
Triumph Pet Industries
7 Lake Station Road
Warwick, NY 10990
Ph: 800-331-5144
www.triumphpet.com

Biodegradable, dust-free, naturally
deodorized, recycled newspaper
that has been processed and
formed into pellets. Low-tracking.

SWheat Scoop Litter
Pet Care Systems, Inc.
Ph: 800-794-3287

Recyclable, naturally clumping
litter made from wheat and corn.

PET-FRIENDLY LODGINGS

ALASKA

Ivy Inn B&B
Anchorage
Ph: 907-345-4024
www.ivyinn.net/

Susitna Wilderness B&B
Willow
Ph: 907-733-1941
www.alaska.net/~wildrnes/

ALABAMA

The Mansion B&B
Talladega
Ph: 205-761-9051
www.concentric.net/~Devries/

ARKANSAS

Palaver Place—B & B
DeValls Bluff
Ph: 870-998-7206
www.palaver-place.com

A Cliff Cottage & The Place Next
Door
Eureka Springs
Ph: 501-253-7409/800-799-7409
www.cliffcottage.com/

Harvest House
Eureka Springs
Ph: 501-253-9363/800-293-5665
www.eureka-usa.com/harvest

CALIFORNIA

Eagles Nest B&B
Big Bear Lake
Ph: 909-866-6465/888-866-6465
www.bigbear.com/enbb/

White Horse Estate B&B
Duarte
Ph: 626-568-8172/800-653-8886
www.citycent.com/whitehorse/

A Weaver's Inn
Eureka
Ph: 707-443-8119/800-992-8119
www.humboldt1.com/~weavrinn/
weaversinn/

Rosemary Cottage
Inverness
Ph: 415-663-9338/800-808-9338
www.rosemarybb.com

1859 Historic National Hotel, A
Country Inn-
Jamestown/Yosemite
Ph: 209-984-3446/800-984-3446
www.national-hotel.com/

The Inn At 657
Los Angeles
Ph: 213-741-2200/800-347-7512
www.patsysinn657.com

Blair House Inn
Mendocino
Ph: 707-937-1800/800-699-9296
www.blairhouse.com

Inn At Schoolhouse Creek
Mendocino
Ph: 707-937-5525/800-731-5525
www.schoolhousecreek.com

Mono Hot Springs Resort
Mono Hot Springs
Ph: 209-325-1710
www.monohotsprings.com/

Spruce Grove Cabins & Suites
S. Lake Tahoe
Ph: 530-544-0549/800-777-0914
www.sprucegrovetahoe.com

Sea Horse Resort
San Clemente
Ph: 949-492-1720
www.sanclemente.com/
seahorseresort

Inn at Heavenly
South Lake Tahoe
Ph: 530-544-4244/800-692-2246
www.800mycabin.com

COLORADO

Mark I Guest Suites
Denver
Ph: 303-331-7000
www.marksuites.com

Rochester Hotel
Durango
Ph: 970-385-1920/800-664-1920
www.rochesterhotel.com/

Mountain Meadows Barn, Bed &
Breakfast
Gunnison
Ph: 970-641-9501
www.youngminds.com/mtnmead-
ows/

The Ranch House Bed &
Breakfast
Gunnison
Ph: 970-642-0210
www.ranchhousebnb.com

Ute Meadows B&B
Marble
Ph: 970-963-7088/888-883-6323
www.utemeadows.com/

Los Milagros De San Luis B&B
San Luis
Ph: 719-672-3608/800-983-9580
www.localweb.com/proaccess/Drea
mWeaver/DreamWeaver.htm

The Wyman Hotel & Inn
Silverton
Ph: 970-387-5372/800-609-7845
www.thewyman.com

CONNETICUT

Old Lyme Inn
Old Lyme
Ph: 860-434-2600/800-434-5352
www.oldlymeinn.com/

Cumon Inn B&B
South Windsor
Ph: 860-644-8486
www.i-networld.com/CumonInn/

DISTRICT OF COLUMBIA

Hereford House
District of Columbia
Ph: 202-543-0102
www.bbonline.com/dc/hereford/

FLORIDA

Florida House Inn
Amelia Island
Ph: 904-261-3300/800-258-3301
www.floridahouse.com

Midnight Sea Guesthouse
Fort Lauderdale
Ph: 954-463-4827/800-910-2357
www.midnightsea.com/

Oceanfront Cottages & Vacation
Homes
Idialantic
Ph: 321-725-8474/800-785-8080
www.oceanfrontcottages.com

Curry Mansion
Key West
Ph: 305-294-5349/800-253-3466
CurryMansion.com/curry/index.ht
ml

Douglas House
Key West
Ph: 305-294-5269
www.DouglasHouse.com/

Miami Beach Pool Paradise
Miami Beach
Ph: 305-532-3666
members.aol.com/mbhouse/mbho
use.html

Tropical Shores Beach Resort
Sarasota
Ph: 941-349-3330/800-235-3493
www.tropicalshores.com

Gram s Place B&B Guesthouses &
Music
Tampa
Ph: 813-221-0596
www.grams-inn-tampa.com

GEORGIA

Rees Park Garden Inn
Americus
Ph: 912-931-0122
www.americus.net/~reespark

Moon Valley Resort Bed &
Breakfast
Rabun Gap
Ph: 706-746-2466
www.moonvalleyspgs.com

Joan s B&B On Jones Street
Savannah
Ph: 912-234-3863/800-407-3863
www.bbonline.com/ga/savannah/jo
ans/index.html

Goodbread House
St. Mary's
Ph: 912-882-7490
www2.ganet.org/visitga/tour_web_s
earch.pl?webid=1520&search=det
ail

HAWAII

Hale Maluhia Country Inn
Kailua-Kona
Ph: 808-329-5487/800-559-6627
www.hawaii-bnb.com/halemal.html

Becky's B&B
Naalehu
Ph: 808-929-6960/800-235-1233
www.hawaii-bnb.com/beckt.html

IOWA

Inn the Hunt
Kanawha
Ph: 515-762-3370/888-760-3611
www.netins.net/showcase/innthe-
hunt/

IDAHO

Cricket-On-The-Hearth B&B
Coeur D'Alene
Ph: 208-664-6926
members.aol.com/cricketbed/page
2.htm

ILLINOIS

The Archer House
Marshall
Ph: 217-826-8023
www.ourads.com/archerhouse

Isle Of View
Metropolis
Ph: 618-524-5838
www.bbonline.com/il/isleofview/

KENTUCKY

The Fredrick-Talbott Inn
Fishers
Ph: 317-578-3600/800-566-2337
www.fredtal.com

Sanford House B&B
Covington
Ph: 606-291-9133

B&B at Silver Springs Farm
Lexington
Ph: 606-255-1784/877-255-1784
www.bbsilverspringsfarm.com/

Aleksander House B&B
Louisville
Ph: 502-637-4985
www.bbonline.com/ky/aleksander/

La Casa Amarilla
Stanton
Ph: 606-663-6689
www.lacasaamarilla.com

Rose Hill Inn
Versailles
Ph: 606-873-5957/800-307-0460
www.rosehillinn.com/

LOUISIANA

Loyd Hall Plantation B&B
Cheneyville
Ph: 318-776-5641/800-240-8135
www.louisianatravel.com/
loyd_hall/

Cajun Houseboat Rentals
Morgan City
Ph: 504-385-2738
www.petronet.net/
cajunconnection/

St. Vincent's Guest House
New Orleans
Ph: 504-566-1515
www.prytaniainns.com

2439 Fairfield A Bed & Breakfast
Shreveport
Ph: 318-424-2424

MASSACHUSETTS

Rexhame Shores B&B
Marshfield
Ph: 781-837-1900
www.xensei.com/users/yussi/

MARYLAND

Admiral Fell Inn
Baltimore
Ph: 410-522-7377/800-292-4667
www.admiralfell.com/

Hopkins Inn
Baltimore
Ph: 410-235-8600/800-877-3404

Walnut Ridge B&B
Grantsville
Ph: 301-895-4248/888-41.WAL-
NUT
www.bbonline.com/md/
walnutridge

Waterloo Country Inn
Princess Anne
Ph: 410-651-0883
www.waterloocountryinn.com

MAINE

Belfast Bay Meadows,
A Country Inn by the Sea
Belfast
Ph: 207-338-5715/800-335-2370
www.baymeadowsinn.com/

Camden Harbour Inn
Camden
Ph: 207-236-4200/800-236-4266
www.camdenharbourinn.com

The Manor Inn
Castine
Ph: 207-326-4066/877-
MANORINN
www.manor-inn.com/

The Inn At St. John
Portland
Ph: 207-773-6481/800-636-9127
www.maineguide.com/portland/
stjohn/

MICHIGAN

Willow Brook Inn B&B
Canton
Ph: 734-454-0019/888-454-1919
www.bbonline.com/mi/willow/
index.html

Victorian Gardens B&B
and Gift Shop
Chesaning
Ph: 517-845-2511
members.tripod.com/
VictorianGardens/

MINNESOTA

Thayer's Historic B&B
Annandale
Ph: 320-274-8222/800-944-6595
www.thayers.net

Viking Motel
Duluth
Ph: 218-728-3691/800-345-6912
www.cpinternet.com/~viking

MISSOURI

Rock Eddy Bluff Farm
Dixon
Ph: 573-759-6081/800-335-5921
www.rockeddy.com

MISSISSIPPI

Lofty Oaks Inn
Biloxi
Ph: 228-392-6722/800-280-4361

MONTANA

Sacajawea Inn
Three Forks
Ph: 406-285-6515/800-821-7326
www.avicom.net/sacajawea/

NORTH CAROLINA

A Hill House Bed & Breakfast Inn
Asheville
Ph: 828-232-0345/800-379-0002
www.hillhousebb.com

Dunromin: A Rustic Mountain
Rental Cabin
Asheville
Ph: 828-658-3345/800-457-2740
www.dunromin.com/

The Melrose Inn
Tryon
Ph: 828-859-7014

Mountain Creek B&B
Waynesville
Ph: 828-456-5509/800-557-9766
www.sogospel.com/mcbb

Anderson Guest House
Wilmington
Ph: 910-343-8128/888-265-1216

Augustus T Zevely Inn
Winston-Salem

Ph: 336-748-9299/800-928-9299
www.winston-salem-inn.com

NEW HAMPSHIRE

The Balmoral—A Fine Colonial
Inn
Bethlehem
Ph: 603-869-3169
nettx.com/balmoral/index.html

The Horse and Hound Inn
Franconia
Ph: 603-823-5501/800-450-5501

NEW JERSEY

The Pillars of Planfield B&B
Planfield
Ph: 908-753-0922/888-PILLARS
www.pillars2.com

NEW MEXICO

Angels Ascent B&B
Cedar Crest
Ph: 505-286-1588
www.showemall.com/showemall/
angels/

Hilltop Hacienda B&B
Las Cruces
Ph: 505-382-355
www.zianet.com/hilltop

Meson De Mesilla
Mesilla
Ph: 505-525-9212/800-732-6025

Alexander s Inn B&B
Santa Fe
Ph: 505-986-1431/888-321-5123
www.collectorsguide.com/sf/
l008.html

El Paradero
Santa Fe
Ph: 505-988-1177
www.elparadero.com

Inn Of The Turquoise Bear
Santa Fe
Ph: 505-983-0798/800-396-4104
www.bbonline.com/nm/bluebear/
index.html

The Preston House
Santa Fe
Ph: 505-982-3465/888-877-7622
www.prestonhouse.com/index.html

Adobe and Stars B&B
Taos
Ph: 505-776-2776/800-211-7076
www.taosnet.com/stars/

NEVADA

Crooked House B&B
Virginia City
Ph: 775-847-4447/800-340-6353
www.bbonline.com/nv/
crookedhouse/index.html

NEW YORK

Mansion Hill Inn & Restaurant
Albany
Ph: 518-465-2038/888-299-0455
www.mansionhill.com/

Big Indian Springs B&B
Big Indian
Ph: 914-254-5905

Auberge: The Hedges B&B
Clinton
Ph: 315-853-3031/800-883-5883
members.aol.com/hedgesbb/
hedges.htm

Horse Shoe Inn
Cooperstown
Ph: 518-284-2284

Point Lookout Mountain Inn
East Windham
Ph: 518-734-3381
www.thecatskills.com/_plook.htm

River Run B&B
Fleischmanns
Ph: 914-254-4884
www.bbonline.com/ny/riverrun/
index.html

Serenity Farms
Greene
Ph: 607-656-4659
www.geocities.com/
westhollywood/6173/serenity

Sandy Creek Manor House
Hamhn
Ph: 716-964-7528/800-594-0400
www.sandycreekbnb.com

Gateway Lodge B&B
Highmount
Ph: 914-254-4084

Flicker s Stage & Screen B&B
Hillsdale
Ph: 518-325-6467
www.flickersbandb.com

Hudson City B&B
Hudson
Ph: 518-822-8044
www.hudsoncitybnb.com

Fourpeaks—Adirondack Camps
& Guest Barns
Jay
Ph: 518-946-7313/800-373-8445
www.4peaks.com

OHIO

Ohio River House B&B
Cincinnati (Higginsport)
Ph: 937-375-4395
www.OhioRiverHouse.com

Wagner s 1844 Inn
Sandusky
Ph: 419-626-1726
www.lrbcg.com/wagnersinn

OKLAHOMA

Heritage Manor B&B
Aline
Ph: 580-463-2566/800-295-2563
www.cruising-america.com/
heritagemanor

The Sharpe House
Checotah
Ph: 918-473-2832

The Ranch Of Stillwater
Stillwater
Ph: 405-377-2201
www.magicalchild.org/
theranch.html

OREGON

Ashland Patterson House
Ashland
Ph: 541-482-9171/888-482-9171
www.mind.net/patterson

Sea Quest B&B
Yachats
Ph: 541-547-3782/800-341-4878
www.seaq.com

PENNSYLVANIA

The Queen, A Victorian B&B
Bellfonte
Ph: 814-355-7946
www.bellefonte.com/queen/

Pheasant Field B&B
Carlisle
Ph: 717-258-0717
www.pa.net/pheasant

Golden Pheasant Inn
Erwinna
Ph: 610-294-9595
www.goldenpheasant.com

Aaron Burr House Inn &
Conference Centre
New Hope
Ph: 215-862-2570
www.new-hope-
inn.com/Aaron/index.html

Wedgwood Inns of New Hope,
Bucks County
New Hope
Ph: 215-862-2485
www.new-hope-inn.com

The Inn at Georgian Place
Somerset
Ph: 814-443-1043
www.somersetcounty.com/
theinn/index.html

Spring Valley B&B and Horse
Farm
Spring Creek
Ph: 814-489-3695/800-382-1324
www.springvalleybandb.com/

TENNESSEE

Iron Mountain Inn
Butler
Ph: 423-768-2446/888-781-2399
www.ironmountaininn.com/

Masters Manor Inn
Knoxville
Ph: 423-219-9888/877-866-2667
www.mastersmanor.com

The King's Cottage—
Bed & Breakfast—Inn
Memphis
Ph: 901-722-8686
www.thekingscottage.com

TEXAS

Carrington s Bluff B&B
Austin
Ph: 512-479-0638/800-871-8908
www.bbonline.com/tx/governors/
carrington.html

The Governor's Inn
Austin
Ph: 512-477-0711/800-871-8908
www.bbonline.com/tx/governors/
index.html

Heart Cottage B&B
Clifton
Ph: 254-675-3189

Arbor House Inn & Suites
San Antonio
Ph: 210-472-2005/888-272-6700
www.arborhouse.com/

Painted Lady Inn on Broadway
San Antonio
Ph: 210-220-1092
www.bestinns.net/usa/tx/
paintedlady.html

The Katy House
Smithville
Ph: 512-237-4262
www.katyhouse.com/

UTAH

The Garden Bed & Breakfast Inn
Spring City
Ph: 435-462-9285/877-537-2337
www.bedsandroses.com

VIRGINIA

River s Edge
Christiansburg
Ph: 540-381-4147/888-786-9254
www.river-edge.com

Longdale Inn
Clifton Forge
Ph: 540-862-0892/800-862-0386

The Hummingbird Inn
Goshen
Ph: 540-997-9065/800-397-3214
www.hummingbirdinn.com/

Garden And The Sea Inn
New Church
Ph: 757-824-0672/800-824-0672
www.gardenandseainn.com/

The Owl & The Pussycat
Petersburg
Ph: 804-733-0505/888-733-0505
www.bbonline.com/va/owlcat/index
.html

VIRGIN ISLANDS—US

The Danish Chalet Inn
St. Thomas
Ph: 340-774-5764/800-635-1531
www.vi-danish-chalet-inn.com/

VERMONT

The Pond House at Shattuck Hill
Farm
Brownsville
Ph: 802-484-0011
www.bbonline.com/vt/pondhouse/

The Cortina Inn
Killington
Ph: 802-773-3331/800-451-6108
www.cortinainn.com/

Red Clover Inn
Mendon
Ph: 802-775-2290/800-752-0571
www.redcloverinn.com/

Green Mountain Inn
Stowe
Ph: 802-253-7301
www.greenmountaininn.com

Snow Goose Inn
West Dover
Ph: 802-464-3984/888-604-7964
www.snowgooseinn.com/

WASHINGTON

Monarch Manor Estates
Bainbridge Island
Ph: 206-780-0112
www.monarchmanor.com/

Puget View Guesthouse
Olympia
Ph: 360-413-9474
www.bbonline.com/wa/pugetview/

Harbor Pointe B&B
Whidbey Island
Ph: 360-675-3379/800-668-1110
www.whidbey.net/harborpointe/

Red Apple Inn
Yakima
Ph: 509-248-7150

WISCONSIN

Gypsy Villa Resort
Eagle River
Ph: 715-479-8644/800-232-9714
topwebsite.com/gypsy/

Justin Trails B&B Resort
Sparta
Ph: 608-269-4522/800-488-4521
www.justintrails.com

WEST VIRGINIA

Cacapon B&B
Berkeley Springs
Ph: 304-258-1442/888-629-3309
www.mariasgarden.com/b&b/index
.html

General Lewis Inn
Lewisburg
Ph: 304-645-2600/800-628-4454
www.bbonline.com/wv/gener-
allewis/index.html

Yokum's Vacationland
Seneca Rocks
Ph: 304-567-2351/800-772-8342
www.yokum.com

WYOMING

Double Eagles Nest
Buffalo
Ph: 307-682-8841
www.2eaglesnest.com

A. Drummond's Ranch
Cheyenne
Ph: 307-634-6042
www.cruising-america.com/
drummond.html

Adventures Country B&B
Cheyenne
Ph: 307-632-4087
www.cruising-america.com/
country.html

Porch Swing B&B
Cheyenne
Ph: 307-778-7182
www.cruising-
america.com/porch.html

The Howdy Pardner
Cheyenne
Ph: 307-634-6493
www.cruising-america.com/
howdy.html

Davy Jackson Inn
Jackson
Ph: 307-739-2294/800-584-0532
www.davyjackson.com

Cottage House of Squaw Creek
Lander
Ph: 307-332-5003
www.rmisp.com/cottagehouse/

PET FOOD CONTACT LIST

Voice your concerns by writing
to these organizations:

AAFCO Pet Food Committee
Dr. Rodney Noel—Chair
Office of Indiana State Chemist
Purdue University
1154 Biochemistry Building
West
Lafayette, IN 47907-1154
www.aafco.org

FDA Center for Veterinary
Medicine
David A. Dzanis, DVM, Ph.D.,
DACVN
7500 Standish Place
Rockville, MD 20855
Ph: 301-594-1728
www.cvm.fda.gov/

Pet Food Institute
1200 19th Street NW
Washington DC 20036-2401
Ph: 208-857-1120/208-223-4579

PET FOOD MANUFACTURERS

Advanced Pet Diets
Breeder's Choice Pet Foods
16321 East Arrow Highway
Irwindale, CA 91706
Ph: 800-255-4286

Alpo
Friskies Petcare Company
Glendale, CA 91203
Ph: 800-366-6033

Amway
Amway Corporation
7575 Fulton
Grand Rapids, MI 49335

ANF
Century Pet Care
P.O. Box 326
Dana Point, CA 92629
Ph: 800-722-3261

Anmar
Natura Pet Products
1171 Homestead Road #275
Santa Clara, CA 95050
Ph: 800-532-7261

Avo-Diets
Breeder's Choice Pet Foods
16321 East Arrow Highway
Irwindale, CA 91706
Ph: 800-255-4286

Bil Jac
Kelly Foods Corporation
3457 Medina Road
Medina, OH 44256
Ph: 800-321-1002
www.biljac.com

Blue Seal
Blue Seal Feeds
P.O. Box 8000
Londonderry, NH 03053
Ph: 800-367-2730

Breeder's Choice
Breeder's Choice Pet Foods
16321 East Arrow Highway
Irwindale, CA 91706
Ph: 800-255-4286

California Natural
Natura Pet Products
1171 Homestead Road #275
Santa Clara, CA 95050
Ph: 800-532-7261

Cargill
Cargill, Inc.
P.O. Box 9000
Minneapolis, MN 55440
Ph: 800-328-1189

Cornucopia
Cornucopia Pet Foods, Inc.
229 Wall Street
Huntington, NY 11743
Ph: 516-427-7479

Diamond
Diamond Pet Food Company
P.O. Box 146
Meta, MO 65058
Ph: 800-442-0402

Eagle
Eagle, Inc.
P.O. Box 506
Mishawaka, IN 46546-0506
Ph: 800-255-5959

Eukanuba
The Iams Company
P.O. Box 14597
Dayton, OH 45413
Ph: 800-525-4267

Excel
Pet Products Plus, Inc.
1600 Heritage Landing #112
St. Charles, MO 63303
Ph: 800-592-6687

Flint River Ranch Products
Flint River Ranch
1243 Columbia Avenue, B-6
Riverside, CA 92507
Ph: 909-682-5048

FROMM Family Nutritionals
FROMM Family Foods, Inc.
P.O. Box 365
Mequon, WI 53092
Ph: 800-325-6331

Full Balance
Muenster Milling Company, Inc.
P.O. Box 585
Muenster, TX 76252
Ph: 800-772-7178

Gereen
Gereen Enterprises
6216 Baker Lane
Alvarado, TX 76009
Ph: 800-358-4908

Holistic Gold
Jaydan Diversified, Inc.
1222 Fewster Drive, Unit 7
Mississauga, ONT L4W 1A1
Canada

Iams
The Iams Company
P.O. Box 14597
Dayton, OH 45413
Ph: 800-525-4267

Innova
Natura Pet Products
1171 Homestead Road #275
Santa Clara, CA 95050
Ph: 800-532-7261

Joy
Best Feeds
P.O. Box 246
Oakdale, PA 15071
Ph: 800-245-4125

Joy Demand
Best Feeds
P.O. Box 246
Oakdale, PA 15071
Ph: 800-245-4125

Kasco
Pet Products Plus, Inc.
1600 Heritage Landing, #112
St. Charles, MO 63303
Ph: 800-592-6687

Ken-L Ration
Heinz Pet Products
Box 5700
Newport, KY 41071
Ph: 800-828-9980

Matrix
Natura Pet Products
1171 Homestead Road #275
Santa Clara, CA 95050
Ph: 800-532-7261

Natural Life
Natural Life Pet Products
P.O. Box 943
Frontenac, KS 66763-0943
Ph: 800-367-2391

Nature's Recipe
Nature's Recipe Pet Foods
341 Bonnie Circle
Corona, CA 91720
Ph: 800-843-4008

Neura
Old Mother Hubbard Dog Food
Co., Inc.
P.O. Box 1719
Lowell, MA 01853-1179
Ph: 800-225-0904

Nutro
Nutro, Inc.
445 Wilson Way
City of Industry, CA 91744
Ph: 800-833-5330

Optimum
Optimum Pet Care
3775 Southwestern Blvd.
Orchard Park, NY 14127
Ph: 800-833-9224

Pedigree
Kal Kan Pet Care
P.O. Box 58853
Vernon, CA 90058-0853
Ph: 800-525-5273

Perfect Balance
Muenster Milling Co., Inc.
P.O. Box 585
Muenster, TX 76252
Ph: 800-772-7178

PetCo
9151 Rehco Road
San Diego, CA 92121

PetGuard Premium
PetGuard, Inc.
P.O. Box 728
Orange Park, FL 32067-0728
Ph: 800-874-3221

The Pet Pantry
The Pet Pantry International, Inc.
P.O. Box 5148
Stateline, NM 89449
Ph: 702-588-2027

PETsMART
10000 North 31st Ave., Ste. C100
Phoenix, AZ 85051

Precise Pet Products
P.O. Box 630009
Nacogdoches, TX 75963
Ph: 602-944-7070

Pro Balanced
Gold Kist, Inc.
P.O. Box 2210
Atlanta, GA 30301
Ph: 770-393-5204

Pro Plan
Ralston Purina Company
P.O. Box 1606
St. Louis, MO 63188
Ph: 800-778-7462

Ralston Purina Company
P.O. Box 1606
St. Louis, MO 63188
Ph: 800-778-7462

Regal Pet Foods
305 West Chesapeake Avenue
Towson, MD 21204
Ph: 800-638-7006

Science Diet
Hill's Pet Nutrition, Inc.
P.O. Box 148
Topeka, KS 66601-0148
Ph: 800-445-5777

Sensible Choice
Pet Products Plus, Inc.
1600 Heritage Landing #112
St. Charles, MO 63303
Ph: 800-592-6687

Solid Gold Holistic Animal/Equine
Nutrition Center
1483 North Cuyamaca
El Cajon, CA 92020
Ph: 800-DOG-HUND

Spot's Stew
3438 East Lake Road #14
PMB 612
Palm Harbor, FL 34685
Ph: 800-426-4256
www.halopets.com/index.htm

Top Nutrition
Grama Pet, Inc.
9804 SW 138th Ave.
Miami, FL 33186
Ph: 305-383-2717

Wal-Mart
Ph: 800-WALMART

Walter Kendall
Breeder's Choice Pet Foods
16321 East Arrow Highway
Irwindale, CA 91706
1-800-255-4286

Waltham Formula
Kal Kan Pet Care
P.O. Box 58853
Vernon, CA 90058-0853
Ph: 800-525-5273

Wayne
Pet Products Plus, Inc.
1600 Heritage Landing #112
St. Charles, MO 63303
Ph: 800-592-6687

Winner's Choice
Grama Pet, Inc.
9804 SW 138th Ave.
Miami, FL 33186
Ph: 305-383-2717

Wysong Corporation
1880 North Eastman
Midland, MI 48640
Ph: 517-631-0009

ANIMAL-FRIENDLY ORGANIZATIONS

WEBSITE TO REPORT LOST OR FOUND PETS
awolpet.com

ANIMAL-ASSISTED AND PET THERAPY

Canine Companions
for Independence
P.O. Box 446
Santa Rosa, CA 95402-0446
Ph: 800-572-2275
www.caninecompanions.org

Delta Society
289 Perimeer Road East
Renton, WA 98055
Ph: 800-869-6898
www.deltasociety.org

Green Mountain Humane Society
P.O. Box 1426
White River Junction, VT 05001
Ph: 802-296-7297

Helen Woodward Animal Center
6461 El Apajo Road
P.O. Box 64
Rancho Santa Fe, CA 92067
Ph: 858-756-4117
www.animalcenter.org

Pet-A-Pet Club, Inc.
P.O. Box 40201
Redford, MI 48239
Ph: 313-535-0410

ANIMAL BLOOD BANK

HemoPet
Ph: 949-252-8455.
Pet Lifeline is a greyhound
adoption program run by
Animal Blood Bank

NUTRITION ACTIVIST

Ann N. Martin
newsage@teleport.com (email)
For information on the pet
food industry and resources
for consumer action

ADOPTION

www.aspca.org
Adoption, free and low-cost
behavior clinics, and other advice

petfinder.com
Has photos and descriptions
of animals available throughout
the U.S.

Pet Rescue
P.O. Box 393
Larchmont, NY
Ph: 914-834-8094

POISON CONTROL

National Animal Poison
Control Center
Ph: 888-4ANIHELP
Open 24 hours, 7 days a week,
staffed by veterinary toxicologists.
Call if you think your animal
may have ingested something
poisonous.

Index